Sixth Edition

STRATEGIES FOR THEORY CONSTRUCTION IN NURSING

Lorraine Olszewski Walker, RN, EdD, MPH, FAAN
The University of Texas at Austin

Kay Coalson Avant, RN, PhD, FAAN
The University of Texas Health Science Center at San Antonio

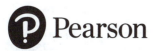

330 Hudson Street, NY, NY 10013

Vice President, Health Science and TED:
Julie Levin Alexander
Director of Portfolio Management:
Katrin Beacom
Editor in Chief: Ashley Dodge
Portfolio Manager: Pamela Fuller
Portfolio Management Assistant:
Erin Sullivan
Development Editor: Barbara Price
Associate Sponsoring Editor:
Zoya Zaman
Product Marketing Manager:
Christopher Barry
Field Marketing Manager:
Brittany Hammond
Vice President, Digital Studio and Content
Production: Paul DeLuca

Director, Digital Studio and Content
Production: Brian Hyland
Managing Producer: Jennifer Sargunar
Content Producer (Team Lead):
Faraz Sharique Ali
Content Producer: Neha Sharma
Senior Manager, Global Rights and
Permissions: Tanvi Bhatia
Operations Specialist:
Maura Zaldivar-Garcia
Cover Design: Cenveo Publisher Services
Cover Photo: Immersion Imagery/Shutterstock
Full-Service Management and
Composition: iEnergizer Aptara®, Ltd.
Printer/Binder: LSC Communications
Cover Printer: LSC Communications
Text Font: 10/12 pt, Times LT Pro

Copyright © 2019, 2011, 2005 by Pearson Education, Inc. All Rights Reserved.
Manufactured in the United States of America. This publication is protected by copyright, and permission should be obtained from the publisher prior to any prohibited reproduction, storage in a retrieval system, or transmission in any form or by any means, electronic, mechanical, photocopying, recording, or otherwise. For information regarding permissions, request forms, and the appropriate contacts within the Pearson Education Global Rights and Permissions department, please visit www.pearsoned.com/permissions/.

Acknowledgments of third-party content appear on the appropriate page within the text.

Unless otherwise indicated herein, any third-party trademarks, logos, or icons that may appear in this work are the property of their respective owners, and any references to third-party trademarks, logos, icons, or other trade dress are for demonstrative or descriptive purposes only. Such references are not intended to imply any sponsorship, endorsement, authorization, or promotion of Pearson's products by the owners of such marks, or any relationship between the owner and Pearson Education, Inc., authors, licensees, or distributors.

Library of Congress Cataloging-in-Publication Data
Names: Walker, Lorraine Olszewski, author. I Avant, Kay Coalson, author.
Title: Strategies for theory construction in nursing / Lorraine Olszewski
    Walker, RN, EdD, MPH, FAAN, The University of Texas at Austin, Kay Coalson
    Avant, RN, PhD, FAAN, The University of Texas Health Science Center at San Antonio.
Description: Sixth edition. I Boston : Pearson, Prentice Hall, [2019] I
    Includes bibliographical references and index.
Identifiers: LCCN 2017058144 I ISBN 9780134754079 I ISBN 0134754077
Subjects: LCSH: Nursing—Philosophy. I Nursing models.
Classification: LCC RT84.5 .W34 2019 I DDC 610.7301—dc23 LC record available at
    https://lccn.loc.gov/2017058144

1 18

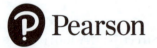

ISBN 13: 978-0-13-475407-9
ISBN 10:   0-13-475407-7

CONTENTS

PREFACE

The aim of this book remains the same as at its inception: to provide readers with a resource on theory development written from a nursing point of view. In particular, we have tried to consider the needs of the students beginning their study of theory development. Stepping into the complex philosophical and metatheoretical works on this topic can be confusing to those who have had no prior exposure to the subject matter. In addition, those works have become vastly more complex and numerous since the first edition of this book. Interest in theory development for nursing also now reaches around the globe. There is also an impatience among nurses to see the relevance of theory to practice. Students in nursing programs are also increasingly diverse in their educational backgrounds, and programs mirror that diversity by designing new educational pathways into nursing and advanced study in nursing.

In recognition of these many changing factors, we have updated chapter materials so that readers may see advances in both the context of theory development in Chapters 1, 2, and 13 and the strategies for concept, statement, and theory development (Chapters 3 to 12).

Chapter 1 provides a historical context to theory development in nursing, as well as new trends affecting theory in nursing, and global perspectives on nursing theory development and material on population- and domain-focused theories. A brief glossary and several reflective activities are provided in this chapter as well. Chapter 2 considers nursing knowledge and theory in its dynamic relationship to practice. After illustrating how theory of a phenomenon may guide nursing assessment and intervention, we cover a range of topics related to knowledge development in nursing, including evidence-based practice, practice-based evidence, and informatics and its linkages to practice and nursing theory. After considering the strategies for concept, statement, and theory development that follow, Chapter 13 covers validation and testing of concepts, statements, and theories. A new section on the central concerns in nursing knowledge has been added to this chapter as nursing advances in its 7th decade of modern knowledge development—launched in *Nursing Research* in 1952.

As in past editions, Chapter 3 provides the framework for selection of theory construction strategies. Following this, Part 2 covers the derivation strategies related to concepts, statements, and theories in Chapters 4, 5, and 6, respectively. Similarly, Part 3 presents the synthesis strategies and Part 4 presents the analysis strategies related to concepts, statements, and theories. Although some readers will still wish to focus on an isolated strategy, such as concept analysis, in general it is our view that use of a given strategy is strengthened by familiarity with its application from concept to statement to theory. We have provided updated listings and examples of use of the various strategies where these are available. Still, lesser-used strategies require use of classic examples.

NEW TO THIS EDITION

- Questions to Consider appear at the chapter opening to help link the chapter content to students' needs and interests.

- A new framework for differentiating theory derivation, theory adaptation, and theory substruction aids students in learning about new theoretical developments for each strategy.
- New discussion in Chapter 3 on the role of concepts in the advancement of nursing as a practice discipline expands the students' understanding of concept development in nursing, especially in the face of confusion about this topic in the literature stemming from philosophers of (basic) science.
- New examples of theoretical works related to derivation, synthesis, and analysis strategies aid students in learning about new theoretical developments for each strategy.

We collectively thank colleagues, former students, and our families who have contributed in numerous ways to this and to prior editions. Of course, Maggie Hank and Charles Bollinger, senior nursing editor for Appleton-Century-Crofts, made all this possible. As always and wherever you are, thanks, Charlie. We miss you.

Finally, for this edition we give special thanks to Pearson Education staff who made this edition possible: Barbara Price, Ashley Dodge, Pamela Fuller, and Zoya Zaman for supporting this sixth edition. We are also especially grateful to U.S. and international external reviewers who took the time to give advice and challenge us to make this edition even better than our vision for it.

Antonia Arnaert, RN, MPH, MPA, PhD
McGill University
Ingram School of Nursing
Montréal, Quebec, Canada

Ann M. Bowling, PhD, RN, CPNP-PC, CNE
Associate Professor
College of Nursing
Wright State University
Dayton, Ohio

Cynthia Brown, DNS, RN, AHN-BC, CNE
Associate Professor
Tanner Health System School of Nursing
University of West Georgia
Carrollton, Georgia

Latefa Dardas, PhD, PMHN
The University of Jordan
School of Nursing
Amman, Jordan

Dr. Margaret G. Landers, PhD, MSc, FFNRCSI, BNS, RNT, RGN, RM
University College Cork
School of Nursing and Midwifery
Brookfield Health Science Complex
Cork City, Ireland

Merav Ben Natan, PhD, RN
Hillel Yaffe Medical Center
Pat Matthews School of Nursing
Hadera, Israel
Tel Aviv University
Department of Nursing
Hadera, Israel

Norma Ponzoni, N, MScN, MEd, PhD(c)
McGill University
Ingram School of Nursing
Montréal, Quebec, Canada

Brandon N. Respress, PhD, RN, MPH, MSN
Assistant Professor-Clinical Track
University of Texas
Arlington, Texas

Bertha Cecilia Salazar-González, PhD, MHED, BNS
Universidad Autónoma de Nuevo León
School of Nursing
Monterrey, Nuevo León (N.L.), México

Ethel Santiago, EdD, RN, CCRN
Assistant Professor
Tanner Health System School of Nursing
University of West Georgia
Carrollton, Georgia

Catherine Witt, PhD, NNP-BC
Associate Professor, Coordinator NNP Program
Loretto Heights School of Nursing
Regis University
Denver, Colorado

L.W.
Austin, Texas

K.A.
Waco, Texas

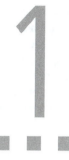

Overview of Theory and Theory Development

In Part 1, the three chapters contain a background to the history, issues, and language of theory development in nursing; its links to practice; and an overview of strategies for theory development. Using a historical lens, Chapter 1 provides an overview of major aspects of the field of nursing theory. Four levels of nursing theory development (metatheory, grand theory, middle-range theory, and practice theory) are proposed. Theoretical contributions and issues at each level are summarized. Population- and domain-focused theories and models are examined. Global efforts related to theory development in nursing are briefly reviewed. Additional reviews and summaries of substantive theories (or conceptual models) that have been important landmarks in nursing thought may be found in Fawcett (1993, 1995), Fawcett and DeSanto-Madeya (2013), Riehl and Roy (1980), and Fitzpatrick and Whall (2005) among others.

The focus of Chapter 2 is the use of knowledge and theory in nursing to inform nursing practice. We begin this chapter by showing in a simplified form how theory of a phenomenon may be used at various points to guide nursing assessment and nursing intervention. From this, we build to a fuller view of knowledge development in nursing as a tool in evidence-based practice and practice-based evidence. Advances in informatics as they relate to nursing practice are introduced. Finally, nursing practice research and theory development are considered.

In Chapter 3, the basic vocabulary used in this book is presented and defined. The elements of theorizing (concepts, statements, and theories) are examined in terms of their definitions and relationships to each other and ultimately nursing science. The basic approaches to theory construction (derivation, synthesis, and analysis) are also introduced in Chapter 3. In combining the three approaches of theorizing with the three elements, nine distinct strategies for theory development result: concept derivation, statement derivation, theory derivation, concept synthesis, statement synthesis, theory synthesis, concept analysis, statement analysis, and theory analysis. These form the substance of Parts 2, 3, and 4 of this book.

By carefully reading Chapter 3, readers should be able to make a preliminary decision about the strategy or strategies of theory development that are most relevant to their needs and interests. Although readers may be interested in only a specific development strategy, they are strongly encouraged to read the related strategies chapters. For example, a fuller understanding of theory analysis is achieved by carefully reading the chapter on statement analysis. Depending on their purposes, others may wish to read all the chapters on a given element, such as all the chapters on concept strategies. Last, some readers may simply prefer to read the parts that provide the larger context for theory development, such as Parts 1 and 5.

REFERENCES

Fawcett J. *Analysis and Evaluation of Nursing Theories*. Philadelphia, PA: Davis; 1993.

Fawcett J. *Analysis and Evaluation of Conceptual Models of Nursing*. 3rd ed. Philadelphia, PA: Davis; 1995.

Fawcett J, DeSanto-Madeya S. *Contemporary Nursing Knowledge: Analysis and Evaluation of Nursing Models and Theories*. 3rd ed. Philadelphia, PA: Davis; 2013.

Fitzpatrick JJ, Whall AL. *Conceptual Models of Nursing: Analysis and Application*. 4th ed. Upper Saddle River, NJ: Pearson Prentice Hall; 2005.

Riehl JP, Roy CR, eds. *Conceptual Models for Nursing Practice*. 2nd ed. New York, NY: Appleton-Century-Crofts; 1980.

1

■ ■ ■

Theory in Nursing: Where Have We Been? Where Are We Going?

Questions to consider before you get started reading this chapter:

▶ Have you struggled to express what is the essence of nursing's contribution to health care in an interdisciplinary context?

▶ Have you wondered why theory has been emphasized so much in nursing?

▶ Have you wondered whether theory has helped or hindered the development of the nursing profession and nursing education?

▶ Have you wondered how nursing theory enhances practice and research?

Introductory Note: These questions have been turned over in the minds of many graduate nursing students. For some, the question forms a challenge for more than superfluous jargon that will be used rarely outside the classroom. For others, the question is a thoughtful query about new and richer ways of viewing clinical experiences that are deeply familiar. For still others, the question conveys an undertone of anxiety about subject matter that looms as daunting and out of reach. In truth, most queries about why the need to study theory development in nursing are an amalgam of all three vantages. We attempt in this background chapter to briefly sketch the evolution of nursing theory development. We hope that by reading this chapter and the one that follows (Chapter 2, "Using Knowledge Development and Theory to Inform Practice") readers will be able to formulate their own thoughts and conclusions about the "why" of studying nursing theory.

THEORY DEVELOPMENT IN NURSING: A BEGINNER'S GUIDE

Nursing is a practice discipline. Nurses engage in providing complex health care to people at every level of health and illness, at every life stage, and in diverse settings. From acute care hospital units, to public health clinics, to classrooms in schools of nursing, to nursing research laboratories, nurses deal with knowledge to improve the health and well-being of individuals, families, and communities. How does theory development relate to the complex dimensions of nursing as a practice discipline? Does theory shape practice, or is practice the shaper of nursing theory? Is there such a thing as unique nursing theory? How should nursing theory influence the research process? Are there different kinds of theory? Such questions continue to be asked in nursing.

A simple view of theory development is that it provides a way to identify and express key ideas about the essence of practice. Through theory development that essence may be explored. That exploration may be focused on specific practice settings or populations. For example, the essence of practice may be studied by focusing on specific events that occur in specific contexts: body image perceptions of adolescents with eating disorders, treating persons in rural settings who struggle with drug addiction, health promotion behaviors of persons living with HIV, or services for low-income older adults struggling with maintaining cognitive function. Conversely, descriptions may focus on big picture explanations of person, health, environment, and nursing—the "metaparadigm concepts" that some have argued anchor nursing as a practice discipline (Fawcett, 1984, 1996; Fawcett & DeSanto-Madeya, 2013). Such abstract theory development may address the overall person–environment relationship as it relates to nursing and health. Regardless of how delimited or broad in scope, theory development is aimed at helping the nurse to understand practice in a more complete and insightful way. If it does not, the theory may be poorly articulated, wrong, or have limited relevance to nursing. Subsequent chapters in this book provide detailed guidance on the "how" of theory development, but beginning students should not lose sight of the "why."

Appreciating theory, however, may require some reflection on the part of nurses who have worked in busy practice environments. Often the daily demands of practice preclude asking questions about whether the current way is still the best way. However, the health care space is changing. This has resulted in the need for new and increased nursing knowledge (evidence) to lead in that space. Leadership requires knowledge for practice that is grounded in advances made through research and theory development. Dynamic trends, however, may sway how such knowledge and theory is developed. Examples of trends challenging the boundaries and methods of nursing knowledge development include (Henly et al., 2015; Wyman & Henly, 2015):

- emergence of big data,
- genomics/proteomics,
- new methodologies for developing patient-oriented outcomes,
- advances in quantitative methods,
- translational and team research,
- informatics, and
- health economics.

These emphases encourage nurses' questions about what they are about and invite innovation in the way that research, practice, and theory are viewed in nursing.

At the same time, we are reminded that core disciplinary knowledge of nursing is a critically needed component of the education and practice of nurses (Grace, Willis,

Roy, & Jones, 2016; Thorne, 2014; Villarruel & Fairman, 2015). Questions about the substance and definition of core nursing knowledge underscore the "why" that motivates theory and knowledge development. Without this core, nursing's unique and important contribution to health care of individuals, families, and communities is put at risk. We revisit this concern at the end of Chapter 13.

A HISTORICAL GLIMPSE AT THEORY IN NURSING AS A PROFESSION

From Task-Oriented Occupation to Profession

First, during the mid-twentieth century and the years that followed, nursing leaders in the United States saw theory development as a means of firmly establishing nursing as a profession, and not just a task-oriented occupation with little autonomy. Thus, theory development was inherent in the long-standing interest in defining nursing's body of knowledge. In a landmark paper early in that century, Flexner defined the characteristics of a profession. Included among Flexner's characteristics were the ideas that professions involve "intellectual operations" and "derive their raw material from science and learning" (quoted in Roberts, 1961, p. 101). Subsequent evaluations of nursing as a profession (Bixler & Bixler, 1945, 1959) specifically examined the extent to which nursing utilized and enlarged a "body of knowledge" for its practice. Indeed, Bixler and Bixler (1945, p. 730) used the term "nursing science" for this knowledge.

Interest in the body of knowledge stemmed in part from the credibility that such a body of knowledge gave to nursing as an aspiring profession. As Donaldson and Crowley forcefully stated, "the very survival of the profession may be at risk unless the discipline is defined" (1978, p. 114). However, Dickson (1993) argued subsequently that "following the male professional model" also had unintended consequences for nurses. Among these was "reluctance in the workplace to assert and trust nurses' feminine values and views of caring" (p. 80). Nonetheless, developing nursing's distinct knowledge base through theory development, research, and reflective practice was foundational to move nursing from an occupation subservient to medicine to present-day partnership among the health professions.

Second, interest in theory development was motivated by the direction and guidance that theory gave to practice. Simply stated, theory may help nurses grow and enrich their understanding of what practice is and what it can be. This intrinsic value of theory development was reflected in Bixler and Bixler's (1945) first criterion for a profession:

> A profession utilizes in its practice a well-defined and well-organized body of specialized knowledge which is on the intellectual level of . . . higher learning. (p. 730)

As the integration of professional knowledge, theory provides a more complete picture for practice than factual knowledge alone. Thus, a commitment to practice based on sound, reliable knowledge is intrinsic to the idea of a profession and practice discipline.

Theories that serve as broad conceptual frameworks for practice may also articulate the goals of a profession and its core values. Such frameworks (sometimes called *grand theories*) have aided in differentiating nursing as a distinct profession with its own goals from a mere extension of the medical profession. Consequently, many of the early grand theories (see section "Grand Nursing Theories") flowed from attempts to articulate a view of what nursing could be that extended beyond tasks and procedures.

Finally, theories that are well developed not only organize existing knowledge but also aid in making new and important innovations to advance practice. For example, Lydia Hall's theoretical work led to many of the nursing practice innovations associated with the Loeb Center for Nursing in New York (Hale & George, 1980).

Progress in Delineating Nursing's Body of Knowledge

Systematic reviews of the status of theory development in nursing have demonstrated that nursing has made substantial progress in delineating its theoretical base. Fawcett (1983), for example, cited four hallmarks of success in nursing theory development: "a metaparadigm for nursing, conceptual models for nursing, unique nursing theories, and nursing theories shared with other disciplines" (pp. 3–4). In systematically reviewing nursing research articles from 1952 to 1980, Brown, Tanner, and Padrick (1984) noted a trend for authors "to lay explicit claim to a conceptual perspective" (pp. 28–29). Indeed, over half the studies they reviewed were judged to contain explicit "conceptual perspectives" (p. 28).

Similarly, in a review of nursing research from 1977 to 1986, Moody et al. (1988) found that approximately half of the articles they analyzed contained a "theoretical perspective." Of those, however, non-nursing theories predominated. Several sources also have analyzed advances in nursing theory development. In 1988, Walker and Avant proposed four conceptual foci of nursing research phenomena: (1) health behavior and health status, (2) stress and coping, (3) developmental and health-related transitions, and (4) person–environment interactions. Subsequently, Walker (1992) identified and summarized theoretical orientations guiding parent–infant nursing science. In turn, Fawcett (1993) analyzed and evaluated nursing theories that dealt with matters, such as deliberative nursing process and human caring. More recently, nursing knowledge that is theory related has been pulled together in Fawcett's comprehensive volumes (Fawcett, 2005; Fawcett & DeSanto-Madeya, 2013).

Despite the theoretical accomplishments noted above that remain important to the progress of nursing as a practice discipline, much new and continuing work needs to be done. Nurses throughout the world face many questions about nursing and its place in the twenty-first century. Health care access and financing, need for an adequate workforce of nurses, growth of informatics and technology, and changing health care priorities confront us. An example of theory developed by nurses that is responsive to the changing health care landscape is LaCoursiere's (2001) theory of online social support and Covell's (2008) theory of nursing intellectual capital.

Nurses also confront populations of increasingly diverse clients: victims of violence and terrorism, an underclass of poor families struggling to sustain themselves, and a burgeoning population of older adults, to mention only a few. These clients come from many different ethnic backgrounds, speak many different languages, and bring new and unexpected health care needs. (See section "Population- and Domain-Focused Theories and Models" later in this chapter.) As members of the largest health profession, nurses have the potential to play leading roles in health care. It is important that they also be clear about nurses' contributions to knowledge development. Thus, although much has been achieved in nursing's theoretical development, the challenge to develop relevant and useful theories to meet the knowledge needs of nurses in the twenty-first century remains with us.

In the next sections, we first trace the evolution in nursing theory development primarily in the United States, looking at levels of theory development, and then emerging population- and domain-focused theories and models. After this we consider nursing theory development from a global (previously called *international*) perspective. (Readers interested in the history of nursing knowledge development may wish to also read Gortner's [2000] article.)

EVOLUTION OF THEORY DEVELOPMENT: METATHEORY TO PRACTICE THEORY

Overview

During the latter half of the twentieth century, the desire to develop nursing's theory base launched four levels of theory development literature. Much of this early work was launched in the United States. (*Note*: Work related to theory development in nursing globally is addressed later in this chapter.) The first of these, metatheory, focused on philosophical and methodological questions related to the development of a theory base for nursing. The second, grand nursing theories, consisted of conceptual frameworks defining broad perspectives for practice and ways of looking at nursing phenomena based on these perspectives. Third, a less abstract level of theory, middle-range theory, emerged to fill the gaps between grand nursing theories and nursing practice. Fourth, a practice-oriented level of theory, practice theory, was also advocated. In this fourth level of theory, prescriptions, or, more broadly, modalities for practice, were to be delineated. We next sketch progress made on each of these four fronts. We conclude the summary of the levels of theory development in nursing by proposing a model that depicts how levels of theory development articulate with each other. A few terms that may not be intuitively understood by readers are presented in Box 1–1. Others are explained in the text as they are presented.

Metatheory

Early Debates About Theory and Science in Nursing

Metatheory focuses on broad issues related to theory in nursing and does not generally produce any grand, middle-range, or practice theories. Issues debated at the level of metatheory include but are not limited to (1) analyzing the purpose and kind of theory

BOX 1–1   A Short Glossary

Note: Many of the terms defined below are understood and interpreted quite differently by various writers. Because language evolves, meanings can rarely be legislated. The definitions presented below should be viewed only as a guide. Other authors may pose definitions that differ substantially from these. In this book, terms are generally defined or described as they arise in text.

Discipline—"A defined field of knowledge marked by a community of scholars who are experts in the subject matter and methods of a field, a body of knowledge which may include one or more paradigms guiding scholarly work, and standards which guide the conduct of scholarly inquiry in a field" (Walker, 1992, p. 5).

Paradigm—"A family of related theories which share similar concepts and structural features rooted in a relatively shared set of starting theoretical assumptions (e.g., that the conscious mind exists; that humans are in constant interaction with their environment) as well as similar criteria of evidence" (Walker, 1992, p. 5). Other meanings include a broad philosophical approach to research and science, such as feminist paradigm or postmodern paradigm (e.g., Weaver & Olson, 2006), or a conceptual model (e.g., Fawcett, 1995).

Metaparadigm—"Global concepts [and relationships among them] that identify the phenomena of interest to a discipline" (Fawcett, 1995, p. 5). In nursing, the metaparadigm may include the core concepts of person, health, environment, and nursing as well as other considerations related to the discipline (Fawcett, 1996). The metaparadigm is generally seen as transcending paradigms.

Theory—an internally consistent group of relational statements that presents a systematic view about a phenomenon and that is useful for description, explanation, prediction, and prescription or control.

Metatheory—literally, theory about theory; not a theory in itself, but concerns related to the nature and assumptions of nursing theory.

---

needed in nursing, (2) proposing and critiquing sources and methods of theory development in nursing, and (3) proposing the criteria most suited for evaluating theory in nursing. Threaded throughout the metatheoretical literature are examinations of the meaning of nursing as a "practice discipline," that is, nursing as both science and profession. An inspection of Table 1–1 shows that metatheory has received extensive attention in nursing. Although some metatheory is accompanied by companion efforts at the grand, middle-range, or practice levels, it has been largely a separate enterprise from these other levels of theory development. Because metatheory represents many points of view about theory in nursing, it has not been consolidated into one unanimously accepted set of beliefs.

Some of the major issues debated in early nursing metatheory were the type of theory suited to nursing, how it should be developed, and the relationship of nursing theory to basic science theories (e.g., Dickoff et al., 1968a, 1968b; Wooldridge et al., 1968). Much of the early understanding of theory development in nursing drew on views of established sciences such as sociology.

TABLE 1–1   Listing of Selected Metatheoretical Papers in Nursing

Metatheoretical Papers	Sources
Towards Development of Nursing Practice Theory	Wald and Leonard (1964)
The Process of Theory Development in Nursing	McKay (1965)
Symposium: Research—How Will Nursing Define It?	"Research—How Will Nursing Define It?" (1967)
Behavioral Science, Social Practice, and the Nursing Profession	Wooldridge, Skipper, and Leonard (1968)
Conference: The Nature of Science and Nursing	"The Nature of Science and Nursing" (1968)
Theory in a Practice Discipline	Dickoff, James, and Wiedenbach (1968a, 1968b)
Symposium: Theory Development in Nursing	"Theory Development in Nursing" (1968)
Proceedings of the First Nursing Theory Conference	Norris (1969)
Conference: The Nature of Science in Nursing	"The Nature of Science in Nursing" (1969)
Proceedings of the Second Nursing Theory Conference	Norris (1970)
Proceedings of the Third Nursing Theory Conference	Norris (1971)
Nursing as a Discipline	Walker (1971a)
Three-part series based on: Toward a Clearer Understanding of the Concept of Nursing Theory	Walker (1971b, 1972); Ellis (1971); Wooldridge (1971); Folta (1971); Dickoff and James (1971)
Symposium: Approaches to the Study of Nursing Questions and the Development of Nursing Science	"Approaches to the Study of Nursing Questions and the Development of Nursing Science" (1972)
Practice Oriented Theory	"Practice Oriented Theory" (1978)
Critique: Practice Theory	Beckstrand (1978a, 1978b)
Theory Development: What, Why, How?	National League for Nursing (1978)
Fundamental Patterns of Knowing in Nursing	Carper (1978)
The Discipline of Nursing	Donaldson and Crawley (1978)
Nursing Theory and the Ghost of the Received View	Webster, Jacox, and Baldwin (1981)
The Nature of Theoretical Thinking in Nursing	Kim (1983)
Toward a New View of Science	Tinkle and Beaton (1983)
An Analysis of Changing Trends in Philosophies of Science in Nursing Theory Development and Testing	Silva and Rothbart (1984)
In Defense of Empiricism	Norbeck (1987)
Voices and Paradigms: Perspectives on Critical and Feminist Theory in Nursing	Campbell and Bunting (1991)

TABLE 1–1   Continued

Metatheoretical Papers	Sources
The Focus of the Discipline of Nursing	Newman, Sime, and Corcoran-Perry (1991)
(Mis)conceptions and Reconceptions About Traditional Science	Schumacher and Gortner (1992)
Nursing Knowledge and Human Science: Ontological and Epistemological Considerations	Mitchell and Cody (1992)
Postmodernism and Knowledge Development in Nursing	Watson (1995)
A Treatise on Nursing Knowledge Development for the 21st Century: Beyond Postmodernism	Reed (1995)
A Case for the "Middle Ground": Exploring the Tensions of Postmodern Thought in Nursing	Stajduhar, Balneaves, and Thorne (2001)
Nursing Research and the Human Sciences	Malinski (2002)
A New Foundation for Methodological Triangulation	Risjord, Dunbar, and Moloney (2002)
Understanding Paradigms Used for Nursing Research	Weaver and Olson (2006)
What Constitutes Core Disciplinary Knowledge	Thorne (2014)
Profession at the Crossroads: A Dialog Concerning the Preparation of Nursing Scholars and Leaders	Grace, Willis, Roy, and Jones (2016)

Critique and Expansion of Views of Science and Theory

Following this early period, recognition of changes in the philosophy of science itself subsequently influenced nursing metatheory. In a critical analysis of the philosophy of science embraced by nursing, Webster et al. (1981) called for "exorcising the ghost of the Received View from nursing" (p. 26). They argued that nurses had uncritically accepted a number of doctrines about the nature of science that were prominent in the 1930s. Based on assumptions of logical positivism, the received view doctrines included beliefs such as "theories are either true or false," "science has nothing to say about values," and "there is a single scientific method" (pp. 29–30). Jacox and Webster (1986) noted the emergence of alternate philosophies of science, including historicism. They suggested that expanding the philosophical positions adopted in nursing enriched both nursing theories and research.

In a related criticism, Silva and Rothbart (1984) distinguished between two major schools of philosophy of science, logical empiricism and historicism. They asserted that these two schools differed in several fundamental ways, including the underlying conception of science. Logical empiricists, they asserted, emphasize understanding science as a product; historicists understand science from the standpoint of process (pp. 3–5). Similarly, they proposed that logical empiricists and historicists differ in their ideas about the goals of philosophy of science and the components of science. Finally, Silva and Rothbart claimed that logical empiricists assess scientific progress in terms of acceptance or rejection of theories, whereas historicists emphasize the number of scientific problems solved. While noting a stable commitment among nurses to logical empiricism, they acknowledged an emerging diversity in conceptual frameworks and research methods congruent with historicist perspectives.

As nurses reconsidered the metatheoretical assumptions of the discipline, their interest in alternate methodologies for nursing theory and research was spawned (e.g., Chinn, 1985; Gorenberg, 1983). Research methodologists increasingly acknowledged distinct quantitative (Atwood, 1984) and qualitative (Benoliel, 1984) approaches. There are many ways to differentiate these two approaches. One of the most apparent differences is the use of statistical tests in drawing inferences within quantitative approaches and the use of text analysis to portray experiences of participants in qualitative approaches. Another way is by reference to the underlying philosophical foundations of the two approaches, such as an empiricist versus phenomenological or other philosophical stance (Monti & Tingen, 1999; Weaver & Olson, 2006). Some authors proposed integrating both methods within research studies (Goodwin & Goodwin, 1984). The philosophical ferment about the nature and method of science not only was a major focus of nursing metatheory but also enlarged the approaches advocated for nursing research.

Furthermore, challenges to traditional science by researchers espousing qualitative methods led to clarification of traditional science as understood in nursing. For example, Schumacher and Gortner (1992) corrected common misinterpretations in nursing about traditional science, such as warrants for knowledge claims and universality of laws. Readers who wish more detailed information about philosophy of science and nursing metatheory will find classic reviews in Stevenson and Woods (1986), Suppe and Jacox (1985), and Newman (1992).

Two additional philosophical perspectives introduced into debates about nursing science, theory, and ethics are critical theory and feminism (e.g., Allen, 1985; Campbell & Bunting, 1991; Holter, 1988; Liaschenko, 1993). Both approaches share a common goal of addressing power imbalances inherent in existing social structures that shape the conduct and goals of science as well as human communication.

Critical theory, as applied to nursing (Allen, 1985; Holter, 1988), builds on the philosophical writings of theorists such as Habermas (1971). According to Campbell and Bunting (1991), "In keeping with its Marxist roots, the critical theory epistemology from its inception dictated that knowledge should be used for emancipatory political aims" (p. 4). Critical theory moves beyond existing empirical and interpretive sciences. Through analysis, critical theory reveals ideological positions inherent but unrecognized in existing social structures and scientific methods. For example, qualitative research approaches that stress personal meaning have shortcomings from the perspective of critical theory. "For the critical theorist, personal meanings are shaped by societal structures and communication processes and are therefore all too often ideologic, historically bound, and distorted" (p. 5).

Similarly, *feminist* approaches aim at realigning social and scientific enterprises in ways that free women from the domination of prevailing, entrenched male structures. As a philosophical approach, feminism is focused at exposing ideology and social conventions that favor men as a group and constrain women as a group. According to Campbell and Bunting (1991), feminist approaches emphasize "unity and relatedness," "contextual orientation," "the subjective," and the "centrality of gender and idealism" (pp. 6–7). Thus, Allen (1985) points out the need to recognize that "one's [scientific] framework is not arbitrary or free of value interests" (p. 64). Finally, Im and Meleis (2001) have explicated six facets of gender-sensitive theories, such as voice and perspective.

Indeed, feminism is part of a broader *postmodern* philosophical movement challenging modern philosophy and science, including the modern metatheory of nursing. Postmodernism is defined more by rejecting tenets of modern philosophy than by "any agreement on substantive doctrines or philosophical questions" (Audi, 1995). Because postmodernism undercuts most knowledge derived from traditional scientific methods and rejects "grand narratives," some nursing scholars have called for cautious and thoughtful application of postmodern positions in nursing (Reed, 1995; Stajduhar et al., 2001). For a historical review of postmodernism and the issues and opportunities it poses for education, practice, and research, see Whall and Hicks (2002) and Kermode and Brown (1996).

Efforts to Find a Middle Way

Still, a number of factors continue to drive efforts to find new ways to bridge perceived methodological and philosophical barriers to integrative approaches to nursing science and theory:

- the growing complexity and discontinuity of health care,
- concerns about continuing health disparities,
- a funding emphasis on biobehavioral research, and
- inputs from many health-related disciplines into the body of health research.

Examples of such efforts include Risjord, Dunbar, and Moloney's idea of a "blending" metaphor for "integration of qualitative and quantitative research into a holistic, dynamic model for nursing inquiry" (2002, p. 275). Johnston (2005), another example, proposed "communicative understanding" to promote respect and receptivity in conversations between researchers using qualitative and quantitative methods. Others have turned to neopragmatism or other alternative philosophical approaches to overcome barriers to communication and knowledge integration rooted in existing methodological and philosophical stances (Isaacs, Ploeg, & Tompkins, 2009; Warms & Schroeder, 1999; Weaver & Olson, 2006). Such efforts acknowledge the pluralistic nature of nursing theory and research but recognize that the ultimate goal is to provide an integrative basis for the care that nurses provide. (For further readings in the philosophy of science, see the list of "Additional Readings" at the end of this chapter.) Box 1–2 presents an exercise on philosophical foundations of nursing knowledge development.

BOX 1–2   Philosophical Foundations/Paradigms of Nursing Knowledge Development: One or Multiple?

Many authors have struggled to resolve this question. It lies at the heart of a number of issues related to development of nursing scholarship and theory development. To guide you in forming your view on this issue, consider your area of practice or research interest.

> **Reflection:** How would you describe it? Is it one spanning biological and psychosocial aspects of nursing? Are community factors also important? Is understanding of the patient or client as person central to this area? Read one or both of the following articles to help you form your view. (*Note*: Many authors use the term *paradigm* to refer to what we have called *philosophical foundations*.) Consider how your area of practice or research would be influenced according to whether your approach was based on only one or multiple philosophical views/paradigms.

> **Your View:** If you think that one philosophical view (such an empiricism or post-positivism) is needed in your area, which view is it? If you think that multiple philosophical views are needed in your area, which ones are these? Write out your rationale.

Suggested readings:

Monti EJ, Tingen MS. Multiple paradigms of nursing science. *J Adv Nurs*. 1999;21(4):64–80.
Weaver K, Olson JK. Understanding paradigms used for nursing research. *J Adv Nurs*. 2006;53:459–469.

Grand Nursing Theories

Grand theories are abstract and give a broad perspective to the goals and structure of nursing practice. Not all grand theories are at the same level of abstraction or have exactly the same scope. On the whole, however, they have as their goal explicating a worldview useful in understanding key concepts and principles within a nursing perspective, yet they are not limited enough to be classified as middle-range theories. In a similar vein, Fawcett (1989) used the term "conceptual models" for those "global ideas about the individuals, groups, situations, and events of interest to a discipline" (p. 2).

Grand theories have made an important contribution in conceptually sorting out nursing from the practice of medicine by demonstrating the presence of distinct nursing perspectives. Although there may be some disagreement on what works constitute grand theories, Table 1–2 shows a representative listing of writings that figured in the historical development of nursing theory during the twentieth century. A number of these theories also have associated websites. Because websites may change, we encourage readers who may wish to locate such sites to simply type the words *nursing theory* into the search box of their Internet browser.

TABLE 1–2   Representative Grand Nursing Theories

Author(s)	Date	Publication
Peplau	1952	*Interpersonal Relations in Nursing*
Orlando	1961	*The Dynamic Nurse–Patient Relationship*
Wiedenbach	1964	*Clinical Nursing: A Helping Art*
Henderson	1966	*The Nature of Nursing*
Levine	1967	*The Four Conservation Principles of Nursing*
Ujhely	1968	*Determinants of the Nurse–Patient Relationship*
Rogers	1970	*An Introduction to the Theoretical Basis of Nursing*
King	1971	*Toward a Theory of Nursing*
Orem	1971	*Nursing: Concepts of Practice*
Travelbee	1971	*Interpersonal Aspects of Nursing*
Neuman	1974	The Betty Neuman Health-Care Systems Model
Roy	1976	*Introduction to Nursing: An Adaptation Model*
Newman	1979	Toward a Theory of Health
Johnson	1980	The Behavioral System Model for Nursing
Parse	1981	*Man-Living-Health*
Erickson, Tomlin, and Swain	1983	*Modeling and Role Modeling*
Leininger	1985	Transcultural Care Diversity and Universality
Watson	1985	*Nursing: Human Science and Human Care*
Roper, Logan, and Tierney	1985	*The Elements of Nursing*
Newman	1986	*Health as Expanding Consciousness*
Boykin and Schoenhofer	1993	*Nursing as Caring*

Most grand theories were developed from the early 1960s through the 1980s. Peplau's (1952) exposition of nursing and its educative function with patients was an early example of grand nursing theory. Grand theories in the 1960s, such as Orlando's *The Dynamic Nurse–Patient Relationship* (1961) and Wiedenbach's *Clinical Nursing: A Helping Art* (1964), focused on defining concepts centered in the nurse–patient relationship. For example, Wiedenbach emphasized the patient's "need-for-help" as distinct from nurse-defined patient needs. Orlando differentiated deliberative and automatic nursing actions. These two theorists' work helped nurses clarify and respond to patients' needs and behaviors with the benefit of a theoretical perspective.

Subsequent grand theories shifted from a focus on the nurse–patient relationship to more expansive concepts. For example, Rogers (1970) stressed a holistic perspective on the life process of man. A multilevel systems model developed by King (1971) included the major concepts of perception, interpersonal relations, social systems, and health. Johnson (1980) constructed a model of the client as a behavioral system composed of seven subsystems. Johnson's thinking was further reflected in Auger's (1976) behavioral systems model, which includes eight subsystems: the affiliative, dependency, ingestive, achievement, aggressive, eliminative, sexual, and restorative.

Whereas nurses might deal with medical and physiological data in the Johnson and Auger grand theories, the approach to these is distinctively a behavioral one.

Later grand theories attempted to capture the phenomenological aspects of nursing. For example, Watson adopted a "phenomenological-existential" orientation in her theory of human care (1985, p. *x*). Others, such as Leininger's (1985) transcultural care theory, paved the way for nursing's response to more culturally diverse client groups. Development of grand theories also expanded to outside the United States, for example, the Roper–Logan–Tierney theory in the United Kingdom (Roper et al., 1985). (Readers interested in brief biographies of nurse theorists and their nursing theories, including ones developed outside the United States, may find Johnson and Webber's [2015] chapter on nursing theory and nursing theorists of interest, as well as Parker and Smith's [2010] edited volume.)

Although the grand nursing theories provide global perspectives for nursing practice, education, and research, many have limitations. By virtue of their generality and abstractness, many grand nursing theories are untestable in their present form (see Chapter 13 on theory testing). They offer general perspectives for practice or curriculum organization in nursing, but by their very nature and purpose, most would require major revision and expansion before testing would be possible. In revising and refining grand nursing theories, (1) vague terminology would need to be clarified and (2) interrelationships between concepts in the theories would need to be delineated with sufficient precision so that predictions can be made. Several theorists published revisions of their works in an effort to clarify and further elaborate them (e.g., see King, 1981; Orem, 1995; Roy & Andrews, 1991, 1999; Roy & Roberts, 1981).

Nevertheless, many grand theories pose formidable problems for those wishing to test them. These problems relate to still another problem in grand theories: absent or weak linkages between terminology in the theories and their observational indicators. This is the point on which Suppe and Jacox (1985) critique the tests of the grand theory of Rogers: Such tests are contingent on "auxiliary claims that provide most of the testable content" (p. 249). Fawcett and Downs (1986) are even more forceful as they assert, "a conceptual model [and/or grand theory] cannot be tested directly. Rather, the propositions of a conceptual model are tested indirectly through the empirical testing of theories that are derived or linked with the model. If the findings of theory-testing research support the theory, then it is likely that the conceptual model is credible" (p. 89).

Thus, it would appear that a layer of theory is needed between grand theories and their empirical dimensions. This layer is congruent with the idea of middle-range theory as proposed here. McQuiston and Campbell (1997), for example, have illustrated the process (substruction) whereby an intermediate layer of theory was applied to Orem's (1995) theory to enhance its testability. For detailed analysis and evaluation of the status (including theory testing) of grand theories such as those of Johnson, King, Levine, Neuman, Orem, Rogers, and Roy, see Fawcett (1989, 1995, 2005) and Fawcett and DeSanto-Madeya (2013). An extensive review of research guided by the Roy model may be found in the work of the Boston Based Adaptation Research in Nursing Society (1999). Reviews of research based on Orem's model may be found in Taylor, Geden, Isaramalai, and Wongvatunyu (2000) and Biggs (2008).

Although some nurses have focused their work on the problems of testing grand theories, others have directed their attention to areas of commonality among grand theories

(Flaskerud & Halloran, 1980). Fawcett concluded, "A review of the literature on theory development in nursing reveals a consensus about the central concepts of the discipline— person, environment, health, and nursing" (1984, p. 84). As the broadest area of consensus within the nursing discipline, these concepts constitute its metaparadigm (Fawcett, 1989). In a related vein, Meleis (1985) identified the following as "domain concepts": nursing client, transitions, interaction, nursing process, environment, nursing therapeutics, and health (p. 184). Fuller elaboration of some of the metaparadigm concepts was provided by Smith's (1981) analysis of health's four models and Kleffel's (1991) exploration of the environmental domain. Others, such as Newman et al. (1991), however, have put forth alternative versions of the nursing defining foci, with the concepts of health and caring. Reed (2000), however, critiqued "caring" as overly focused on nurses' practice and proposed "embodiment" as "a core concept in understanding" patients' experiences of health and illness (p. 131). New and revised proposals for the core concepts defining nursing include concepts such as "humanization" and "choice" (Willis, Grace, & Roy, 2008) and "mutual process" and "consciousness" (Newman, Smith, Pharris, & Jones, 2008).

Finally, a series of changes in the late twentieth century conspired to put grand theories somewhat out of vogue. Perhaps because of difficulties in theory testing (see above), several authors have suggested that a gradual, and perhaps undeserved, devaluation of grand theories occurred in nursing (Barnett, 2002; DeKeyser & Medoff-Cooper, 2001; Silva, 1999; Tierney, 1998). On another front, the liberalization of nursing program accreditation criteria pertaining to conceptual frameworks may have contributed to de-emphasizing the role of grand theories in nursing education. Finally, growth of postmodern thinking in certain quarters of nursing has led to the discounting of grand theory as a suitable level of discourse for nursing. Nevertheless, some nurses have argued that grand theories, despite their limitations, continue to have merit in the development of the nursing discipline (Barnett, 2002; Reed, 1995; Silva, 1999), and arguments continue in favor of or in opposition to the role of nursing grand theories in nursing scholarly development (Parse, 2008). (See Box 1–3 for a reflection on the disparagement of nurse theorists.)

BOX 1–3   The Disparagement of Twentieth-Century Nurse Theorists

In stopping to chat several years ago with a historically important nursing theorist at a meeting I (LOW) was attending, she conveyed the following to me, "Nursing theory has become a dirty word. I'm often confronted by nurses who say to me: 'Oh, you're the one!'" She continued her account of personal verbal abuses she had experienced from nurses because of her theoretical work.

> **Reflection:** Why is this happening? Is there something amiss about the way nurse theorists' work is being used in nursing education? Are nurses sensitive to the difference between challenging a set of ideas versus the writer of the ideas? What are the past and present contributions and limitations of nurse theorists' works to the development of the nursing discipline?

> **Reading and Discussion:** Read the following article and then consider the scenario and reflection above:

Nelson S, Gordon S. The rhetoric of rupture: Nursing as a practice with a history? *Nurs Outlook.* 2004:52;255–261.

Middle-Range Theories

In view of difficulties inherent in testing grand theories, a more workable level of theory development was proposed (Jacox, 1974; See, 1981; Liehr & Smith, 1999) and utilized in nursing: middle-range theories. Theories of this level contain a limited number of concepts and are limited in scope as well. Because of these characteristics, middle-range theories are testable, yet sufficiently general to still be scientifically interesting. Thus, middle-range theories not only share some of the conceptual economy of grand theories but also provide the specificity needed for usefulness in research and practice. Consequently, middle-range theories have gained increasing appeal in nursing (Lenz, 1998; Peterson & Bredow, 2017; Smith & Liehr, 2014). Although middle-range theories from other disciplines are used in nursing science and research (Fawcett, 1999, 2006; Lenz, 1998), nursing-based middle-range theories are increasingly evident.

An early example of middle-range theory developed in nursing is Mishel's (1988) uncertainty theory developed to explain "how patients cognitively process illness-related stimuli and construct meaning in these events" (p. 225). Uncertainty influences patients' appraisal, coping, and adaptation. Uncertainty itself is influenced by stimuli frame and structure providers. Under certain conditions of continual uncertainty, Mishel (1990) proposes that factors such as social resources aid people to view uncertainty as a "natural" condition. In such a view, "instability and fluctuation are natural and increase the person's range of possibilities" (p. 261).

Two examples of more recently developed middle-range theories in nursing include Covell's (2008) organizational model of nursing intellectual capital (NIC) and Butterfield, Postma, and ERRNIE research team's (2009) TERRA (translational environmental research in rural areas) framework. In Covell's (2008) model of nursing intellectual capital, nursing human capital and nursing structural capital are two interrelated concepts that are at the core of the theory. Nursing human capital is defined as "the knowledge, skills and experience of nurses," whereas nursing structural capital is defined as "nursing knowledge converted into information that exists within practice guidelines" (Covell, 2008, p. 97). Nursing human capital is influenced by nurse staffing and employer support of nurse development. In turn, nursing human capital influences both patient outcomes and organizational outcomes; nursing structural capital also contributes to patient outcomes. In contrast, Butterfield et al. (2009) focused their TERRA framework on environmental health, which is rooted in concerns about environmental and social justice. This framework places environmental risk reduction interventions within the larger context of environmental health inequities, which in turn are influenced by macrodeterminants. For other examples of middle-range theories developed in nursing, see Table 1–3. (*Note*: Readers who are interested in reading further about middle-range theories are referred to "Additional Readings" at the end of the chapter, including the works of Peterson and Bredow [2017] and Smith and Liehr [2014].)

In addition to middle-range theories, two related yet narrower scope theories are microtheory (Higgins & Moore, 2000) and situation-specific theory (Im, 2005; Im & Meleis, 1999a). These were introduced into nursing to bring theoretical understanding of delimited clinical situations. Davis and Simms (1992), for example, proposed that microtheory was suitable for procedures involving intravenous therapy and injection administration. Im and Meleis (1999a) illustrated the use of situation-specific theory

TABLE 1–3   Examples of Middle-Range Theories Developed In Nursing

Theory	Source
Interaction model of client health behavior	Cox (1982)
Theory of smoking relapse	Wewers and Lenz (1987)
Uncertainty theory	Mishel (1988, 1990)
Theory of caring	Swanson (1991)
Theory of mastery	Younger (1991)
Symptom management model	University of California, San Francisco School of Nursing Symptom Management Faculty Group (1994)
Theory of culture brokering	Jezewski (1995)
Theory of unpleasant symptoms	Lenz, Suppe, Gift, Pugh, and Milligan (1995); Lenz, Pugh, Milligan, Gift, and Suppe (1997)
Health promotion model (revised)	Pender (1996)
Theory of nurse-expressed empathy and patient outcomes	Olson and Hanchett (1997)
Theory of chronotherapeutic intervention for pain	Auvil-Novak (1997)
Theory of chronic sorrow	Eakes, Burke, and Hainsworth (1998)
Self-regulation theory	Johnson (1999)
Theory of transitions	Meleis, Sawyer, Im, Messias, and Schumacher (2000)
Theory of comfort	Kolcaba (2001)
Theory of adapting to diabetes mellitus	Whittemore and Roy (2002)
Theory of caregiver stress	Tsai (2003)
Theory of adaptation to chronic pain	Dunn (2004)
Theory of health promotion for preterm infants	Mefford (2004)
Theory of patient advocacy	Bu and Jezewski (2007)
Theory of nursing intellectual capital	Covell (2008)
Individual and family self-management theory	Ryan and Sawin (2009)
Theory of music and its effects on physical activity and health	Murrock and Higgins (2009)
TERRA (translational environmental research in rural areas) framework	Butterfield et al. (2009)
Theory of spiritual well-being in illness	O'Brien (2014)
Theory of parental end-of-life decision making (after child's bone-marrow transplant)	Rishel (2014)
Transcendent pluralism (nonviolent social transformation)	Perry (2015)

in depicting the experiences of menopause among Korean immigrant women (Im & Meleis, 1999b). As these examples show, the focus and range of abstraction of middle-range theories and related theories are likely to widen as emerging health needs and advances in science and technology are coupled with increasing diversity of clients served by nurses.

Practice Theory

One outgrowth of nursing metatheory has been the idea of a distinct type of theory for nursing as a practice discipline (Dickoff et al., 1968a; Jacox, 1974; Wald & Leonard, 1964; Walker, 1971a, 1971b; Wooldridge et al., 1968). Wald and Leonard (1964) were early proponents of nursing practice theory, a form of theory that was causal in nature and included variables that could be modified by nurses. The essence of practice theory was a desired goal and prescriptions for action to achieve the goal. Jacox (1974), in proposing her idea of practice theory, provided the following succinct description:

> It is theory that says given this nursing goal (producing some desired change or effect in the patient's condition), these are the actions the nurse must take to meet the goal (produce the change). For example, a nursing goal may be to prevent a postoperative patient from becoming hypona-tremic. Nursing practice theory states that, to prevent hyponatremia, a particular set of actions must be taken. (p. 10)

Dickoff et al. (1968a) advocated a model of "practice-oriented theory" in which four phases of theorizing were to lead to the theory base for nursing practice. These phases included factor-isolating, factor-relating, situation-relating, and situation-producing or prescriptive theory. These four phases roughly paralleled the acts of description, explanation, prediction, and control. Situation-producing or prescriptive theory comprised three components: goal content (desired situations), prescriptions, and a survey list. An example of the prescription component offered by Dickoff et al. (1968a) was "Registered nurses, let the patient take his own medication as soon as he is able" (p. 424). The survey list was an intricately developed, yet vague component related to activity. Nonetheless, the Dickoff et al. (1968a, 1968b) proposal for practice theory did not provide clear and specific procedures to use in actually constructing a practice theory.

After the ideas of practice theory, situation-producing theory, or prescriptive the-ory were proposed, they did not lead immediately to development of any actual theories of this type. Some reasons for the slow growth of these types of theories may be that the early expositions used examples that sounded very procedural and consequently inspired little excitement. Another reason may be that formulating theory for practice requires a well-developed body of nursing science on effective nursing interventions.

Subsequently, progress did occur in the knowledge base for nursing practices. For example, in the Conduct and Utilization of Research in Nursing project (Haller, Reynolds, & Horsley, 1979), research-based knowledge was transferred into "proto-cols for nursing practice" (p. 45). Among the practice protocols studied were (1) sensa-tion information: distress, (2) intravenous cannula change regimen, (3) prevention of decubiti by means of small shifts of body weight, and (4) deliberate nursing: pain

TABLE 1–4   Examples of Practice Theories Developed In Nursing

Theory	Source
Theory of balance between analgesia and side effects	Good and Moore (1996)
Theory of the peaceful end of life	Ruland and Moore (1998)
Theory of acute pain management in infants and children	Huth and Moore (1998)

reduction. Similarly, clinical guideline statements such as those proposed by the Panel for the Prediction and Prevention of Pressure Ulcers in Adults (1992) provided a further example of statements developed to guide care of persons. Further, several books devoted to nursing interventions have expanded the foundations of nursing practices (Bulechek & McCloskey, 1985; McCloskey & Bulechek, 2000; Snyder, 1992), including a taxonomy of nursing interventions (Iowa Intervention Project, 1992). That latter taxonomy continues to be updated (Bulechek, Butcher, Dochterman, & Wagner, 2012).

Of particular interest are efforts to blend middle-range theory with prescriptive theory (Good & Moore, 1996). These hybrid efforts elevate the resulting practice theory above simple dictates or imperatives for practice. Although the relational statements of these theories are stated in predictive versus prescriptive (ought or should) language, they come the closest yet to developing theory that is useful in actual practice. Examples of this emerging version of practice theory are shown in Table 1–4. Box 1–4 presents an exercise for readers.

BOX 1–4   Middle-Range Theory and Practice Theory

Middle-range theories are usually seen as more useful than grand theories because they may serve as the basis for developing nursing practice theories. Consider the description of practice theory as comprising these two components:

1. a nursing goal and
2. a nursing care action to meet the goal (Jacox, 1974).

Activity: Examine a middle-range theory cited in Table 1–3 that is related to your area of practice or research interest. Look for concepts in the middle-range theory that could guide development of a practice theory. Does this middle-range theory have the necessary potential nursing goals and actions to formulate a practice theory statement? Do you need to first modify the middle-range theory before you would be able to formulate the needed goal and action?

Try to develop a practice theory statement from the middle-range theory using this suggested format: to ____[*insert a nursing goal based on the middle-range theory*]__, these actions should be taken: ____[*insert one or more specific nursing actions based on the middle-range theory*]__.

Reflection: How easy or difficult was it to develop the practice theory statement? Were the practice theory goal and actions you were able to extract from the middle-range theory specific enough that these could be considered a guide for practice? If you were unsuccessful in extracting any practice theory statements, what were some of the shortcomings of the middle-range theory that you used?

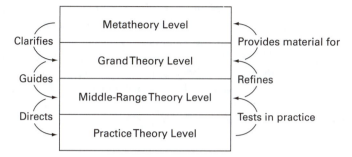

FIGURE 1–1 Linkages among levels of theory development.

Linkages Among Levels of Theory Development

After reading the preceding sections, it should be clear that one cannot reasonably ask at what level nursing theory development should occur: Work has been and is being done at each level. A more fitting question is, how are the levels of theory development related to each other? In Figure 1–1, we propose a model of the linkages between and among the four levels of theory development. Metatheory, through analysis of issues about nursing theory, clarifies the methodology and roles of each level of theory development in a practice discipline. In turn, each level of theory provides material for further analysis and clarification at the level of metatheory. Grand nursing theories by their global perspectives serve as guides and heuristics for the phenomena of special concern at the middle-range level of theory. For example, the Roy adaptation model (Roy, 1976; Roy & Andrews, 1991, 1999; Roy & Roberts, 1981), a grand theory, served as the basis for several middle-range theories: a theory of adapting to diabetes mellitus (Whittemore & Roy, 2002), a theory of caregiver stress (Tsai, 2003), and a theory of adaptation to chronic pain (Dunn, 2004). The Levine (1967) model served as the foundation for a middle-range theory of health promotion for preterm infants developed by Mefford (2004). In yet another example, O'Brien (2014) used the theoretical work of Travelbee (1971) as a point of departure in developing a middle-range theory of spiritual well-being in illness. Furthermore, middle-range theories, as they are tested in reality, become reference points for further refining grand nursing theories to which they may be connected (see an example of this connection in Gill and Atwood [1981]). Middle-range theories also direct the prescriptions of practice theories aimed at concrete goal attainments. Finally, practice theory, which is constructed from scientifically based propositions about reality, tests (if only indirectly) the empirical validity of those propositions as practices are incorporated in patient care. Those propositions most relevant to practice theory are likely to come from middle-range theories because their language is more easily tied to concrete situations. Despite the variety of linkages between the levels of theory development, none of them directly represent actual methods or strategies for theory construction.

POPULATION- AND DOMAIN-FOCUSED THEORIES AND MODELS

Overview

In the preceding section, theories were viewed in relation to levels of abstraction, but usually these were not delimited to a specific population. Within nursing, there has been an increasing interest in population-focused theories and models, often centered on a defining population characteristic such as age, ethnicity and race, or gender. Because of the limits of what is possible within a single chapter, we have focused here primarily on population-focused theories and models related to racial/ethnic populations. Subsequent to this, we briefly focus on emerging domain-focused (or phenomenon-specific) theories and models. In contrast, rather than emphasizing specific populations, domain-focused theories and models emphasize the central phenomena and problems that make up the world of practice in caring for persons, families, and communities, for example, symptom management.

Population-Focused Theories and Models

Because of the cultural, racial, and ethnic diversity of the United States, our consideration of population-focused knowledge and theory development will be directed primarily at certain theoretical advances in the U.S. context, but may be applicable to similarly diverse countries. Our literature review was based on a combination of computerized and hand searches. The minimal number of sources found through computerized searches may indicate a limitation of descriptors attached to nursing theory-related articles pertaining to ethnic populations. Omission of a work in our review may simply reflect the limits of our search methods and is not a statement of a work's importance.

A key concern expressed within literature focused on ethnic minority populations was potential mismatch between the views and values inherent in extant nursing theories and those held by ethnic minority populations. Orem's (1991) theory was an example of a grand theory analyzed for such potential incongruence. For example, Roberson and Kelley (1996) proposed that Orem's theory reflects Western values such as self-reliance and self-direction that may be incongruent in cultural groups that value interdependence and harmony. They further propose that the biomedical orientation in Orem's theory may be incongruent with traditional health practices. In a review of several international and U.S.-based studies, Roberson and Kelley concluded that the theory insufficiently delineated how culture affects health, thereby limiting "the theory's usefulness for guiding culturally competent nursing care" (p. 27). In an analysis of an inductive study couched in Orem's (1991) theory, Villarruel and Denyes (1997) reported that self-care agency and dependent-care agency (separate terms in Orem's theory) were difficult to differentiate in their study of Mexican Americans. They noted that caring for others was highly valued in this cultural group.

Because of concern about the misfit of theories developed from a dominant culture perspective when applied to ethnic minority groups, efforts have been undertaken to develop frameworks, concepts, and perspectives that are congruent with specific cultural groups. At the concept level, Dancy et al. (2001) explored the concept of empowerment within two urban housing projects. After reviewing the literature on empowerment, they documented the impact of the urban housing project environments on the outreach team members' observations, feelings, and thoughts. Using content analysis, they explored the negative impact of the housing project environment on their own feelings of empowerment. Im and Meleis (1999b) applied the idea of situation-specific theory to investigate the phenomenon of menopause among Korean immigrants to the United States. Their findings derived from this specific group of women were then used to modify a more general model of transition experiences.

Loxe and Struthers (2001) used focus group data to design a nursing conceptual framework for Native American culture. Examples of key concepts in the conceptual framework were the following: caring, traditions, respect, and holism. In a related work, Jensen-Wunder (2002) developed a nursing practice model from her experiences with a Lakota community. Starting from a commitment to human becoming (Parse, 1995), Jensen-Wunder developed the model, Indian Health Initiatives, using symbols and beliefs derived from Lakota culture. To increase understanding of how to promote health among Chinese immigrants in the United States, Zeng, Sun, Gray, Li, and Liu (2014) developed a conceptual model for this population. Their model development was based on a synthesis of the literature.

Critical scholarship and ways of knowing also have been applied to articulation of frameworks and methodologies for study of cultural groups and cultural-gender groups. Turton (1997), for example, developed the health worldview-orienting framework for ethnographic research on health promotion among the Ojibwe community. Boutain (1999) proposed combining critical social theory and African American studies methods as a more powerful way for nurses to study the health and social context of African Americans. Two other nurses described womanism (Taylor, 1998) and womanist ways of knowing (Banks-Wallace, 2000) as forms of gender-centered thought of value to nursing scholarship focused on the context and health of African American women.

Although race and ethnicity define many of the population-focused theories and models, the scope of such theories and models embraces a variety of populations that may be viewed through the lens of race, ethnicity, socioeconomic status, gender, disability, immigrant status, and sexual minority status. Using the term "vulnerable populations," Flaskerud and Winslow (1998) propose a model of health research in which *relative risk, resource availability*, and *health status* are key concepts that mutually influence each other and are in turn affected by research, practice, and ethical and policy analysis. A related model proposed by Rew, Hoke, Horner, and Walker (2009) focuses on health disparities research. In this second model, *research collaborations* influence *health disparities communities, community-based interventions*, and *health disparities outcomes*. In this model, health disparities communities are viewed as having assets, risk factors, and barriers to services.

In conclusion, important beginning contributions are being made in developing population-focused theories and models in the United States. On a more cautionary note, though, Kikuchi (2005) has warned of culture-specific theories that are founded on moral relativism. This concern is exemplified when such theories are at odds with issues of human rights, such as in the treatment of women and children.

Domain-Focused Theories and Models

Domain-focused theories and models make distinctive contributions to practice by their emphasis on the phenomena and problems encountered in the nursing care of persons, families, and communities. Domain-focused theories or models are likely to reside at the middle-range level. It is, however, their content focus that is of particular concern because that content addresses central problems of practice. Domain-focused theories and models have high potential for advancing practice if they are clearly artic-ulated, supported by research findings (qualitative, quantitative, or both), and translat-able to practice situations. Although there are several contained in Table 1–3, we focus on one domain-focused theory, the symptom management model (SMM) developed by the University of California, San Francisco School of Nursing Symptom Management Faculty Group (1994; Dodd et al., 2001; Humphreys et al., 2014). Because of its emerg-ing application across a variety of symptom-related practice problems delineated by Dodd et al. (2001), it is of particular relevance to practice situations.

As defined in the context of the SMM, a symptom is "a subjective experience reflecting changes in the biopsychosocial functioning, sensations, or cognition of an individual" (Dodd et al., 2001, p. 669). Although a number of terms are contained in the model, at its core are three central and interrelated concepts: *symptom experience*, *symptom management strategies*, and *symptom outcomes*. Each of these is influenced by factors stemming from the *person*, *environment*, and *health and illness*. Of particu-lar interest is the generative nature of the SMM reflected in its application to a number of clinical problems, such as fatigue in care of persons with HIV/AIDS (Voss, Dodd, Portillo, & Holzemer, 2006) and symptom management of diabetes among African Americans (Skelly, Leeman, Carlson, Soward, & Burns, 2008).

In focusing on domain-focused theories here, we are not introducing a new level of theory or a new type of theory. Rather we use this terminology to point to theories and models that have high potential to inform the problems encountered in person-centered nursing practice. Further growth of domain-focused theories and models provides a foundation for nursing assessments, nursing interventions, and nursing outcomes of care. In so doing, domain-focused theories may give rise to the elusive practice theories envisioned in the 1960s.

GLOBAL NURSING THEORY DEVELOPMENT ISSUES AND EFFORTS

Overview

The growth of global nursing knowledge development has been exponential. Besides the presence of numerous journals in national languages, a survey conducted in 2000 by McConnell identified 82 English-language nursing journals published outside the United States and originating from 13 countries. In addition, several leading U.S. nursing journals (*Nursing Science Quarterly* and the *Journal of Nursing Scholarship*) contain sections devoted to global nursing scholarship. These are overt signs of the burgeoning scientific and theoretical growth of global efforts to advance nursing as a scholarly discipline.

Still, reviewing the global literature on nursing theory is difficult because theo-retical thinking often grows through personal interactions that are not always fully reflected in published literature. Searches of literature databases may uncover articles of interest in non-English-language journals, but costs of translation may make those sources beyond easy reach. Bearing in mind these challenges, we focused on global theory development and theoretical thinking in articles published in English. Our coverage, thus, is only a partial consideration of global efforts of nursing theory development. Furthermore, because of the breadth of global theory development literature, our review is necessarily selective and illustrative.

Issues and Global Contributions

As interest in nursing theory development spread globally, the nursing community struggled with a number of issues and concerns: the value and contribution of theory (Allison, McLaughlin, & Walker, 1991; Biley & Biley, 2001; Draper, 1990; Poggenpoel, 1996; Searle, 1988); concern about the uncritical adoption of U.S.-origin nursing theories, values, and knowledge schemes (Draper, 1990; Ketefian & Redman, 1997; Lawler, 1991; Salas, 2005); questioning the need for unique nursing knowledge (Nolan, Lundh, & Tishelman, 1998); disparagement or questioning of grand theories (Daly & Jackson, 1999; Nolan et al., 1998); advocating contextual or delimited scope theories (Daly & Jackson, 1999; Draper, 1990; Nolan et al., 1998); and questioning the effectiveness of imposing theories using a top-down strategy (Kenney, 1993). For example, Nolan et al. (1998) argued that grand nursing theories fail to meet the needs of practice because they are too far removed from reality to be useful to practitioners. (Box 1–5 presents an exercise for readers on whether there can be an international theory of nursing.)

Articulation of these issues by the preceding authors indicated that theoretical work based on the American experience may need to be modified to fit other countries, or may be incompatible with cultural and other considerations for application in some countries (Salas, 2005). Despite this, others have recognized the opportunity for more widespread benefit and enhanced progress by certain cross-national and global knowledge-building efforts. Thus, knowledge that can cross borders prevents the age-old problem of reinventing the wheel. Nursing diagnosis and related nomenclature was one such area of international collaboration (Casey, 2002; Ehnfors, 2002; Goosen, 2002; Ketefian & Redman,

---

BOX 1–5 "Why There Cannot Be an International Theory of Nursing"

In an article with the above title, Mandelbaum (1991) challenged the idea that nursing theories can be applicable globally. Among her reasons for that belief was that "each region must define the concepts [person, environment, health, and nursing] in the way most readily understood and applicable to the needs of indigenous people" (p. 53).

Read one or both of the following articles for critical views about nursing theory.

Salas AS. Toward a north–south dialogue: Revisiting nursing theory (from the south). *Adv Nurs Sci.* 2005;28(1):17–24.

Gustafson DL. Transcultural nursing theory from a critical cultural perspective. *Adv Nurs Sci.* 2005;28(1):2–16.

> **Reflection:** Based on your readings and your experience, is Mandelbaum's view still applicable today with increased globalization of trade, travel, and electronic communication, such as on the Internet? Are there commonalities, for example, about nursing, health, and illness that transcend cultural beliefs of specific groups? Or, to the contrary, do cultural differences in the way that health and illness are understood make it impossible for theories related to nursing to be applicable globally?

1997). However, the expansion of nursing diagnoses and related systems of classification was not without their detractors (Lawler, 1991; Nolan et al., 1998).

Examples of the range of countries in which nurses have written about the conceptual, metatheoretical, historical, or educational issues and achievements related to developing and applying nursing theory include the following: Sweden (Lutzen & da Silva, 1995; Willman & Stoltz, 2002); United Kingdom (Smith, 1987); Canada (Major, Pepin, & Légault, 2001; Rodgers, 2000); Australia (Daly & Jackson, 1999); Finland (Leino-Kilpi & Suominen, 1998); Japan (Hisama, 2001); Iceland (Jonsdottir, 2001); India (Sirra, 1986); South Africa (Searle, 1988); Slovenia (Starc, 2009); Turkey (Ustun & Gigliotti, 2009), and Iran (Hoseini, Alhani, Khosro-Panah, & Behjatpour, 2013).

Additional examples of metatheoretical and philosophical topics that have been addressed in the global literature related to nursing theory and knowledge development are displayed in Table 1–5. In an early contribution that was unique in the Australian nursing literature, Emden and Young (1987) reported on a Delphi study conducted with nursing experts on issues related to theory development. Expert opinion was sought on seven issues, such as whether nursing theory development was "critical to the advancement of professional nursing" and "nursing should develop its

TABLE 1–5   Examples of Foundational Global Discourse Related to Nursing Theory and Knowledge Development

Author Country or Countries	Author(s)	Topic or Focus
Australia	Emden and Young (1987)	Integrative review of "trends and issues" in nursing theory development; Delphi study
Sweden and Norway	Lundh, Söder, and Waerness (1988)	Critique of nursing process and nursing theories
United Kingdom	Draper (1990)	Contributions of nursing theory and impediments to its development in the United Kingdom
Australia	Holden (1991)	Critical examination of dualism, idealism, and materialism as theories of mind applied in nursing
United Kingdom	Reed and Robbins (1991)	Proposed and illustrated inductive theory "testing"
Australia	Bruni (1991)	Discourse analysis of literature related to nursing as a profession and knowledge development
Sweden	Dahlberg (1994)	Exposition of holistic perspective and gender-related barriers to application in practice
Sweden	Lutzen and da Silva (1995)	Linguistic issues, nursing methodology, concept of care, trends
Australia	Holmes (1996)	Summary of postmodern critiques of traditional science; alternative philosophical stances for nursing summarized

TABLE 1–5 Continued

Author Country or Countries	Author(s)	Topic or Focus
Australia	Kermode and Brown (1996)	Critically examine postmodernism and its potential weaknesses for advancing nursing
United Kingdom	Timpson (1996)	Theory-practice relationship in nursing
Canada	Baker (1997)	Critical analysis of cultural relativism, including its use in nursing theories
United Kingdom and Sweden	Nolan et al. (1998)	Critique grand nursing theory, critique unique nursing knowledge, advocate middle-range theory
Korea	Shin (2001)	Taoism, Buddhism, and Confucianism as related to nursing theory in Korea
United Kingdom	Allmark (2003)	Reconsideration of Popper's philosophy of science in nursing
Chile/Canada	Salas (2005)	Critical review of use of U.S. nursing theories in the Latin American context
Canada	Weaver and Olson (2006)	Paradigms used for nursing research
Canada	Kirkham and Browne (2006)	Social justice in nursing discourse
Canada	Pesut and Johnson (2008)	Philosophical inquiry in relation to other nursing methodologies
New Zealand and Iceland	Litchfield and Jonsdottir (2008)	Participatory paradigm proposed as the basis for nursing as a practice discipline
Norway and Sweden	Fagerstrom and Bergbom (2010)	Application of Hegelian dialectics to nursing

own unique research traditions" (p. 27). Detailed presentation of the expert opinions on issue statements represents one of the few studies of this kind and may be of interest to readers in a number of countries outside Australia. More recently, scholars have made important contributions to philosophical issues related to nursing theory development. Examples include the writings of Falk-Rafael (2005) and Kirkham and Browne (2006) on social justice in nursing discourse and the consideration of neopragmatism (Isaacs et al., 2009) in nursing. Box 1–6 presents a reflective exercise related to social justice and theory in nursing for interested readers.

Theoretical Developments

Another branch of global nursing literature on theory development has focused on theorizing about nursing and nursing care. The foundations for such works lay in the pioneering writing of Florence Nightingale in her 1859 volume, *Notes on Nursing*. Recent examples of conceptual or theoretical works are presented in Table 1–6. Related efforts

BOX 1–6   Is Social Justice a Consideration in Developing Nursing Theory?

Social justice is an ethical concept that is gaining increasing attention among nurses globally (e.g., Kirkham & Browne, 2006). What is social justice and how might it pertain to nursing theory development and nursing practice? If you want to first learn more about the meaning of social justice, place the words *social justice definition health* or *social justice definition nursing* into the search box of your Internet browser and examine the sources you find.

Read one or more of the following articles about social justice and consider what relevance this concept has to theory development in nursing.

Clingerman E, Fowles E. Foundations for social justice-based actions in maternal/infant nursing. *J Obstet Gynecol Neonatal Nurs.* 2010;39:320–327.

Kirkham SR, Browne AJ. Toward a critical theoretical interpretation of social justice discourses in nursing. *Adv Nurs Sci.* 2006;29:324–339.

Schim SM, Benkert R, Bell SE, Walker DS, Danford CA. Social justice: Added metaparadigm concept for urban health nursing. *Public Health Nurs.* 2007;24:73–80.

Reflection: Based on your reading, how do you see social justice influencing theory development in nursing? How do you see social justice-based theories influencing nursing practice? Does that influence differ based on whether you consider nursing in your country or nursing globally?

TABLE 1–6   Examples of Global Theorizing About Nursing and Nursing Care

Author(s)	Nature of work
Roper et al. (1985)	Roper–Logan–Tierney nursing model
Minshull, Ross, and Turner (1986)	Human needs nursing model
Sarvimäki (1988)	Theory of nursing care
Andersen (1991)	Nursing activity model
Chao (1992)	Concept of caring
Eriksson (2002)	Exposition of caring science
Wong, Pang, Wang, and Zhang (2003)	Chinese definition of nursing
Yoshioka-Maeda et al. (2006)	Japanese purpose-focused public health nursing model
Scheel, Pedersen, and Rosenkrands (2008)	Interactional nursing theory
Halldorsdottir (2008)	Theory of the nurse–patient relationship
Starc (2009)	Human capital conversion model
Boggatz and Dassen (2011)	Model of seeking nursing care among older adults
Hoseini, Alhani, Khosro-Panah, and Behjatpour (2013)	Concept of nursing from Islam sources
Forsberg, Lennerling, Fridh, Karlsson, and Nilsson (2015)	Perceived threat of graft rejection risk
Zandi, Vanaki, Shiva, Mohammadi, and Bagheri-Lankarani (2016)	Caring model for women becoming mothers by surrogacy

have focused on critiquing and applying nursing theories. For example, Tierney (1998) examined the contributions and criticisms of the Roper–Logan–Tierney (1985) nursing model. Whall, Shin, and Colling (1999) examined a derivative of Nightingale's thought for suitability to care of cognitively impaired elders in Korea, whereas Clift and Barrett (1998) tested a power framework in three German-speaking countries, and da Nobrega and Coler (1994) used nursing theory as a basis of nursing diagnoses in Brazil. Other global theoretical works focus on specific patient populations, including nurses' practice models for patients with dermatological conditions (Kirkevold, 1993), decision making in adult and gerontology care settings (Lauri et al., 2001), analysis of a pediatric care model (Lee, 1998), and development or application of theory to the care of psychiatric patients (Mavundla, Poggenpoel, & Gmeiner, 2001; Poggenpoel, 1996).

Theories of U.S. origin have also been the subject of global application, as well as critique. The following are a few examples: de Villiers and van der Wal (1995) applied Leininger's (1991) model to curriculum development in South Africa, whereas Bruni (1988) critiqued earlier elements of the theory. Similarly, Morales-Mann and Jiang (1993) critically examined Orem's (1991) theory in light of fit with Chinese culture, whereas Lauder (2001) critiqued the theory in relation to self-neglect. In a related vein, Baker (1997) critically examined the issue of cultural relativism in nursing theory and practice. Examples of still other U.S.-origin nursing theories in global usage include Parse's (1999) theory utilized in Switzerland (Maillard-Struby, 2009) and in a multinational study (Baumann, 2002); application and testing of King's (1981) theory within three countries (Frey, Rooke, Sieloff, Messmer, & Kameoka, 1995); and dissemination of the Roy model to countries in Latin America and Asia (Roy, Whetsell, & Frederickson, 2009).

In conclusion, despite being limited to English-language sources, the global literature related to nursing theory that we reviewed was rich and diverse. The range of theoretical works includes metatheoretical and critical work and covers a variety of needs and contexts. There is no evidence of one predominating theory in the literature that we reviewed. Indeed, there was much skepticism about imposing theories from outside a country (Salas, 2005). (Also see "Additional Readings" at the end of this chapter related to global nursing theory development.)

Summary

In this chapter, we have presented a summary of historical circumstances that spawned theory development in nursing. Next, we provided a compressed history of the many achievements made in developing the theoretical bases for nursing practice and research. In so doing, we have tried to capture the wide-ranging nature of theory development in nursing, including:

- metatheory to practice theory,
- population- and domain-focused theory, and
- global contributions to theory development in nursing.

Still, as noted throughout this chapter, the concerns and phenomena needed in nursing practice and research continue to grow and change. In the next chapter, we look in more detail at the role of nursing theory and knowledge development in relation to nursing practice. In subsequent chapters, we present strategies to aid in further development of theory in nursing. In the final chapter, we turn to concept, statement, and theory testing, and conclude with a focus on the scope of and central concerns in nursing knowledge.

References

Allen DG. Nursing research and social control. *Image*. 1985;17:58–64.

Allison SE, McLaughlin K, Walker D. Nursing theory: A tool to put nursing back into nursing administration. *Nurs Adm Q*. 1991;15(3):72–78.

Allmark P. Popper and nursing theory. *Nurs Philos*. 2003;4:4–16.

Andersen BM. Mapping the terrain of the discipline. In: Gray G, Pratt R, eds. *Towards a Discipline of Nursing*. Melbourne, Australia: Churchill Livingstone; 1991.

Approaches to the study of nursing questions and the development of nursing science. Symposium. *Nurs Res*. 1972;21:484–517.

Atwood JR. Advancing nursing science: Quantitative approaches. *West J Nurs Res*. 1984;6(3):9–15.

Audi R. *The Cambridge Dictionary of Philosophy*. Cambridge, England: Cambridge University Press; 1995.

Auger JR. *Behavioral Systems and Nursing*. Englewood Cliffs, NJ: Prentice Hall; 1976.

Auvil-Novak SE. A middle-range theory of chronotherapeutic intervention for postsurgical pain. *Nurs Res*. 1997;46:66–71.

Baker C. Cultural relativism and cultural diversity: Implications for nursing practice. *Adv Nurs Sci*. 1997;20(1):3–11.

Banks-Wallace J. Womanist ways of knowing: Theoretical considerations for research with African American women. *Adv Nurs Sci*. 2000;22(3):33–45.

Barnett EAM. What is nursing science? *Nurs Sci Q*. 2002;15:51–60.

Baumann SL. Toward a global perspective of the human sciences. *Nurs Sci Q*. 2002;15:81–84.

Beckstrand J. The need for a practice theory as indicated by the knowledge used in the conduct of practice. *Res Nurs Health*. 1978a;1:175–179.

Beckstrand J. The notion of a practice theory and the relationship of scientific and ethical knowledge to practice. *Res Nurs Health*. 1978b;1:131–136.

Benoliel JQ. Advancing nursing science: Qualitative approaches. *West J Nurs Res*. 1984;6(3):1–8.

Biggs A. Orem's self-care deficit nursing theory: Update on the state of the art and science. *Nurs Sci Q*. 2008;21:200–206.

Biley A, Biley FC. Nursing models and theories: More than just passing fads. *Theoria J Nurs Theory*. 2001;10(2):5–10.

Bixler G, Bixler RW. The professional status of nursing. *Am J Nurs*. 1945;45:730–735.

Bixler G, Bixler RW. The professional status of nursing. *Am J Nurs*. 1959;59:1142–1147.

Boggatz T, Dassen T. Why older persons seek nursing care: Towards a conceptual model. *Nurs Inq*. 2011;18(3):216–225.

Boston Based Adaptation Research in Nursing Society. *Roy Adaptation Model-Based Research: 25 Years of Contributions to Nursing Science*. Indianapolis, IN: Center Nursing Press; 1999.

Boutain DM. Critical nursing scholarship: Exploring critical social theory with African American studies. *Adv Nurs Sci*. 1999;21(4):37–47.

Boykin A, Schoenhofer S. *Nursing as Caring: A Model for Transforming Practice*. New York, NY: National League for Nursing Press; 1993.

Brown JS, Tanner CA, Padrick KP. Nursing's search for scientific knowledge. *Nurs Res.* 1984;33:26–32.

Bruni N. A critical analysis of transcultural theory. *Aust J Adv Nurs.* 1988;5(3):26–32.

Bruni N. Nursing knowledge: Processes of production. In: Gray G, Pratt R, eds. *Towards a Discipline of Nursing.* Melbourne, Australia: Churchill Livingstone; 1991.

Bu X, Jezewski MA. Developing a mid-range theory of patient advocacy through concept analysis. *J Adv Nurs.* 2007;57:101–110.

Bulechek GM, Butcher HK, Dochterman JM, Wagner C. *Nursing Interventions Classification (NIC).* 6th ed. St. Louis, MO: Mosby Elsevier, 2012.

Bulechek GM, McCloskey JC, eds. *Nursing Interventions: Treatments for Nursing Diagnoses.* Philadelphia, PA: Saunders; 1985.

Butterfield P, Postma J, ERRNIE research team. The TERRA framework: Conceptualizing rural environmental health inequities through an environmental justice lens. *Adv Nurs Sci.* 2009;32(2):107–117.

Campbell JC, Bunting S. Voices and paradigms: Perspectives on critical and feminist theory in nursing. *Adv Nurs Sci.* 1991;13(3):1–15.

Carper BA. Fundamental patterns of knowing in nursing. *Adv Nurs Sci.* 1978;1(1):13–23.

Casey A. Standardization and nursing terminology. In: Oud N, ed. *ACENDIO 2002: Proceedings of the Special Conference of the Association of Common European Nursing Diagnoses, Interventions and Outcomes in Vienna.* Bern, Switzerland: Verlag Hans Huber; 2002.

Chao Y. A unique concept of nursing care. *Int Nurs Rev.* 1992;39(6):181–184.

Chinn PL. Debunking myths in nursing theory and research. *Image.* 1985;17:45–49.

Clift J, Barrett E. Testing nursing theory cross-culturally. *Int Nurs Rev.* 1998;45(4):123–126, 128.

Covell CL. The middle-range theory of nursing intellectual capital. *J Adv Nurs.* 2008;63:94–103.

Cox CL. An interaction model of client health behavior: Theoretical prescription for nursing. *Adv Nurs Sci.* 1982;5:41–56.

Dahlberg K. The collision between caring theory and caring practice as a collision between feminine and masculine cognitive style. *J Holist Nurs.* 1994;12:391–401.

Daly J, Jackson D. On the use of nursing theory in nurse education, nursing practice, and nursing research in Australia. *Nurs Sci Q.* 1999;12:342–345.

Dancy BL, McCreary L, Daye M, Wright J, Simpson S, Williams C. Empowerment: A view of two low-income African-American communities. *J Natl Black Nurses Assoc.* 2001;12:49–52.

da Nobrega MML, Coler MS. The utilization of Horta's Basic Human Needs Theory in the identification and classification of nursing diagnoses in Brazil. In: Carroll-Johnson RM, Paquette M, eds. *Classification of Nursing Diagnoses: Proceedings of the Tenth Conference.* Philadelphia, PA: Lippincott; 1994.

Davis B, Simms CL. Are we providing safe care? *Can Nurse.* 1992;88(1):45–47.

DeKeyser FG, Medoff-Cooper B. A non-theorist perspective on nursing theory: Issues of the 1990s. *Sch Inq Nurs Pract.* 2001;15:329–341.

de Villiers L, van der Wal D. Putting Leininger's nursing theory "culture care diversity and universality" into operation in the curriculum—Part 1. *Curationis.* 1995;18(4):56–60.

Dickoff J, James P. Commentary on Walker's "Toward a clearer understanding of the concept of nursing theory": Clarity to what end? *Nurs Res.* 1971;20:499–502.

Dickoff J, James P, Wiedenbach E. Theory in a practice discipline, part I. *Nurs Res.* 1968a;17:415–435.

Dickoff J, James P, Wiedenbach E. Theory in a practice discipline, part II. *Nurs Res.* 1968b;17:545–554.

Dickson GL. The unintended consequences of a male professional ideology for the development of nursing education. *Adv Nurs Sci.* 1993;15(3):67–83.

Dodd M, Janson S, Facione N, Faucett J, Froelicher ES, Humphreys J, et al. Advancing the science of symptom management. *J Adv Nurs.* 2001;33:668–676.

Donaldson SK, Crowley DM. The discipline of nursing. *Nurs Outlook.* 1978;26:113–120.

Draper P. The development of theory in British nursing: Current position and future prospects. *J Adv Nurs.* 1990;15(1):12–15.

Dunn KS. Toward a middle-range theory of adaptation to chronic pain. *Nurs Sci Q.* 2004;17:78–84.

Eakes G, Burke ML, Hainsworth MA. Middle-range theory of chronic sorrow. *Image.* 1998; 30:179–184.

Ehnfors M. The development of the VIPS-model in Nordic countries. In: Oud N, ed. *ACENDIO 2002: Proceedings of the Special Conference of the Association of Common European Nursing Diagnoses, Interventions and Outcomes in Vienna.* Bern, Switzerland: Verlag Hans Huber; 2002.

Ellis R. Commentary on Walker's "Toward a clearer understanding of the concept of nursing theory": Reaction to Walker's article. *Nurs Res.* 1971;20:493–494.

Emden C, Young W. Theory development in nursing: Australian nurses advance global debate. *Aust J Adv Nurs.* 1987;4(3):22–40.

Erickson HC, Tomlin EM, Swain MAP. *Modeling and Role Modeling: A Theory and Paradigm of Nursing.* Englewood Cliffs, NJ: Prentice Hall; 1983.

Eriksson K. Caring science in a new key. *Nurs Sci Q.* 2002;15:61–65.

Fagerstrom L. Bergbom I. The use of Hegelian dialectics in nursing science. *Nurs Sci Q.* 2010;23:79–84.

Falk-Rafael A. Speaking truth to power: Nursing's legacy and moral imperative. *Adv Nurs Sci.* 2005;28:212–223.

Fawcett J. Hallmarks of success in nursing theory development. In: Chinn PL, ed. *Advances in Nursing Theory Development.* Rockville, MD: Aspen; 1983.

Fawcett J. The metaparadigm of nursing: Present status and future refinements. *Image.* 1984;16:84–87.

Fawcett J. *Analysis and Evaluation of Conceptual Models of Nursing.* 2nd ed. Philadelphia, PA: Davis; 1989.

Fawcett J. *Analysis and Evaluation of Nursing Theories.* Philadelphia, PA: Davis; 1993.

Fawcett J. *Analysis and Evaluation of Conceptual Models of Nursing.* 3rd ed. Philadelphia, PA: Davis; 1995.

Fawcett J. On the requirements for a metaparadigm: An invitation to dialogue. *Nurs Sci Q.* 1996;9:94–97.

Fawcett J. The state of nursing science: Hallmarks of the 20th and 21st centuries. *Nurs Sci Q.* 1999;12:311–318.

Fawcett J. *Contemporary Nursing Knowledge: Analysis and Evaluation of Nursing Models and Theories.* 2nd ed. Philadelphia, PA: Davis; 2005.

Fawcett J. Commentary: Finding patterns of knowing in the work of Florence Nightingale. *Nurs Outlook.* 2006;54:275–277.

Fawcett J, DeSanto-Madeya S. *Contemporary Nursing Knowledge: Analysis and Evaluation of Nursing Models and Theories.* 3rd ed. Philadelphia, PA: Davis; 2013.

Fawcett J, Downs F. *The Relationship of Theory and Research.* Norwalk, CT: Appleton-Century-Crofts; 1986.

Flaskerud JH, Halloran EJ. Areas of agreement in nursing theory development. *Adv Nurs Sci.* 1980;3(1):1–7.

Flaskerud JH, Winslow BJ. Conceptualizing vulnerable populations health-related research. *Nurs Res.* 1998;47:69–78.

Folta JR. Commentary on Walker's "Toward a clearer understanding of the concept of nursing theory": Obfuscation or clarification: A reaction to Walker's concept of nursing theory. *Nurs Res.* 1971;20:496–499.

Forsberg A, Lennerling A, Fridh I, Karlsson V, Nilsson M. Understanding the perceived threat of the risk of graft rejections: A middle-range theory. *Glob Qual Nurs Res*. 2015:1–9.

Frey MA, Rooke L, Sieloff C, Messmer PR, Kameoka T. King's framework and theory in Japan, Sweden, and in the United States. *Image*. 1995;27:127–130.

Gill BP, Atwood JR. Reciprocy and helicy used to relate mEGF and wound healing. *Nurs Res*. 1981;30:68–72.

Good M, Moore SM. Clinical practice guidelines as a new source of middle-range theory: Focus on acute pain. *Nurs Outlook*. 1996;44:74–79.

Goodwin LD, Goodwin WL. Qualitative vs. quantitative research or qualitative and quantitative research? *Nurs Res*. 1984;33:378–380.

Goosen W. The international nursing minimum data set (J-NMDS): Why do we need it? In: Oud N, ed. *ACENDIO 2002: Proceedings of the Special Conference of the Association of Common European Nursing Diagnoses, Interventions and Outcomes in Vienna*. Bern, Switzerland: Verlag Hans Huber; 2002.

Gorenberg B. The research tradition of nursing: An emerging issue. *Nurs Res*. 1983;32:347–349.

Gortner SR. Knowledge development in nursing: Our historical roots and future opportunities. *Nurs Outlook*. 2000;48:60–67.

Grace PJ, Willis DG, Roy C, Jones DA. Profession at the crossroads: A dialog concerning the preparation of nursing scholars and leaders. *Nurs Outlook*. 2016;64:61–70.

Habermas J. *Knowledge and Human Interests*. Shapiro J, trans. Boston, MA: Beacon Press; 1971.

Hale K, George JB, Lydia Hall. In: George JB, ed. *Nursing Theories: The Base for Professional Nursing Practice*. Englewood Cliffs, NJ: Prentice Hall; 1980.

Halldorsdottir S. The dynamics of the nurse–patient relationship: Introduction of a synthesized theory from the patient's perspective. *Scand J Caring Sci*. 2008;22:643–652.

Haller KB, Reynolds MA, Horsley JA. Developing research-based innovation protocols: Process, criteria, and issues. *Res Nurs Health*. 1979;2:45–51.

Henderson V. *The Nature of Nursing*. New York, NY: Macmillan; 1966.

Henly SJ, McCarthy DO, Wyman JF, Heitkemper MM, Redeker NS, Titler MG, et al. Emerging areas of science: Recommendations for nursing science education from the Council for the Advancement of Nursing Science idea festival. *Nurs Outlook*. 2015;63(4):398–407.

Higgins PA, Moore SM. Levels of theoretical thinking in nursing. *Nurs Outlook*. 2000;48:179–183.

Hisama KK. The acceptance of nursing theory in Japan: A cultural perspective. *Nurs Sci Q*. 2001;14:255–259.

Holden RJ. In defence of Cartesian dualism and the hermeneutic horizon. *J Adv Nurs*. 1991;16:1375–1381.

Holmes CA. Resistance to positivist science in nursing: An assessment of the Australian literature. *Int J Nurs Pract*. 1996;2(4):172–181.

Holter IM. Critical theory. *Sch Inq Nurs Pract*. 1988;2:223–232.

Hoseini ASS, Alhani F, Khosro-Panah A-H, Behjatpour A-K. A concept analysis of nursing based on Islamic sources: Seeking remedy. *Int J Nurs Knowl*. 2013;24(3):142–149.

Humphreys J, Janson S, Donesky D, Dracup K, Lee KA, Puntillo K, et al. Theory of symptom management. In: Smith MJ, Liehr PR, eds. *Middle Range Theory for Nursing*. New York, NY: Springer; 2014.

Huth MM, Moore SM. Prescriptive theory of acute pain management in infants and children. *J Soc Pediatr Nurses*. 1998;3:23–32.

Im E. Development of situation-specific theories: An integrative approach. *Adv Nurs Sci*. 2005;28(2):137–151.

Im E, Meleis AI. Situation-specific theories: Philosophical roots, properties, and approach. *Adv Nurs Sci*. 1999a;22(2):11–24.

Im E, Meleis AI. A situation-specific theory of Korean immigrant women's menopausal transition. *Image*. 1999b;31:333–338.

Im E, Meleis AI. An international imperative for gender-sensitive theories in women's health. *J Nurs Scholarsh*. 2001;33:309–314.

Iowa Intervention Project, McCloskey JC, Bulechek GM, eds. *Nursing Interventions Classification (NIC)*. St. Louis, MO: Mosby; 1992.

Isaacs S, Ploeg J, Tompkins C. How can Rorty help nursing science in the development of a philosophic 'foundation'? *Nurs Philos*. 2009;10:81–90.

Jacox A. Theory construction in nursing: An overview. *Nurs Res*. 1974;23:4–13.

Jacox AK, Webster G. Competing theories of science. In: Nicoll LH, ed. *Perspectives on Nursing Theory*. Boston, MA: Little, Brown; 1986.

Jensen-Wunder L. Indian health initiatives: A nursing practice model. *Nurs Sci Q*. 2002;15:32–35.

Jezewski MA. Evolution of a grounded theory: Conflict resolution through culture brokering. *Adv Nurs Sci*. 1995;17(3):14–30.

Johnson BM, Webber PB. *An Introduction to Theory and Reasoning in Nursing*. 4th ed. Philadelphia, PA: Lippincott Williams Wilkins; 2015.

Johnson DE. The behavioral system model for nursing. In: Riehl JP, Roy C, eds. *Conceptual Models for Nursing Practice*. 2nd ed. New York, NY: Appleton-Century-Crofts; 1980.

Johnson JE. Self-regulation theory and coping with physical illness. *Res Nurs Health*. 1999;22:435–448.

Johnston N. Beyond the methods debate: Toward embodied ways of knowing. In: Ironside PM, ed. *Beyond Method: Philosophical Conversations in Health Care Research and Scholarship*. Madison, WI: The University of Wisconsin Press; 2005, pp. 259–296.

Jonsdottir H. Nursing theories and their relation to knowledge development in Iceland. *Nurs Sci Q*. 2001;14:165–168.

Kenney T. Nursing models fail in practice. *Br J Nurs*. 1993;2(2):133–136.

Kermode S, Brown C. The postmodernist hoax and effects on nursing. *Int J Nurs Stud*. 1996;33:375–384.

Ketefian S, Redman RW. Nursing science in the global community. *Image*. 1997;29:11–15.

Kikuchi JF. Cultural theories of nursing responsive to human needs and values. *J Nurs Scholarsh*. 2005;37:302–307.

Kim HS. *The Nature of Theoretical Thinking in Nursing*. Norwalk, CT: Appleton-Century-Crofts; 1983.

King I. *Toward a Theory of Nursing*. New York, NY: Wiley; 1971.

King I. *A Theory for Nursing: Systems, Concepts, Process*. New York, NY: Wiley; 1981.

Kirkevold M. Toward a practice theory of caring for patients with chronic skin disease. *Sch Inq Nurs Pract*. 1993;7:37–57.

Kirkham SR, Browne AJ. Toward a critical theoretical interpretation of social justice discourses in nursing. *Adv Nurs Sci*. 2006;29:324–339.

Kleffel D. Rethinking the environment as a domain of nursing knowledge. *Adv Nurs Sci*. 1991;14(1):40–51.

Kolcaba K. Evolution of the mid range theory of comfort for outcomes research. *Nurs Outlook*. 2001;49:86–92.

LaCoursiere SP. A theory of online social support. *Adv Nurs Sci*. 2001;24(1):60–77.

Lauder W. The utility of self-care theory as a theoretical basis for self-neglect. *J Adv Nurs*. 2001;34:545–551.

Lauri S, Salanterä S, Chalmers C, Ekman S, Kim HS, Käppeli S, et al. An exploratory study of clinical decision-making in five countries. *J Nurs Scholarsh*. 2001;33:83–90.

Lawler J. In search of an Australian identity. In: Gray G, Pratt R, eds. *Towards a Discipline of Nursing*. Melbourne, Australia: Churchill Livingstone; 1991.

Lee P. An analysis and evaluation of Casey's conceptual framework. *Int J Nurs Stud.* 1998;35(4):204–209.

Leininger MM. Transcultural care diversity and universality. *Nurs Health Care.* 1985;6:209–212.

Leininger MM. *Culture Care Diversity and Universality: A Theory of Nursing.* New York; NY: National League for Nursing; 1991.

Leino-Kilpi H, Suominen T. Nursing research in Finland from 1958 to 1995. *Image.* 1998;30:363–367.

Lenz ER. Role of middle range theory for nursing research and practice. Part I. Nursing research. *Nurs Leadersh Forum.* 1998;3(1):24–33.

Lenz ER, Pugh LC, Milligan RA, Gift A, Suppe F. The middle-range theory of unpleasant symptoms: An update. *Adv Nurs Sci.* 1997;19(3):14–27.

Lenz ER, Suppe F, Gift AG, Pugh LC, Milligan RA. Collaborative development of middle-range nursing theories: Toward a theory of unpleasant symptoms. *Adv Nurs Sci.* 1995;17(3):1–13.

Levine M. The four conservation principles of nursing. *Nurs Forum.* 1967;6(1):45–59.

Liaschenko J. Feminist ethics and cultural ethos. *Adv Nurs Sci.* 1993;15(4):71–81.

Liehr P, Smith MJ. Middle range theory: Spinning research and practice to create knowledge for the new millennium. *Adv Nurs Sci.* 1999;21(4):81–91.

Litchfield MC, Jonsdottir H. A practice discipline that's here and now. *Adv Nurs Sci.* 2008;31(1):79–91.

Loxe J, Struthers R. A conceptual framework of nursing in Native American culture. *J Nurs Scholarsh.* 2001;33:279–283.

Lundh U, Söder M, Waerness K. Nursing theories: A critical view. *Image.* 1988;20:36–40.

Lutzen K, da Silva AB. Delineating the domain of nursing science in Sweden—Some relevant issues. *Värd i Norden.* 1995;15(1):4–7.

Maillard-Struby FV. Transforming while affirming those we serve: Parse's theory in Switzerland. *Nurs Sci Q.* 2009;22:212–213.

Major FA, Pepin JI, Légault AJ. Nursing knowledge in a mostly French-speaking Canadian province: From past to present. *Nurs Sci Q.* 2001;14:355–359.

Malinski VM. Nursing research and the human sciences. *Nurs Sci Q.* 2002;15:14–20.

Mandelbaum J. Why there cannot be an international theory of nursing. *Int Nurs Rev.* 1991;38:53–55, 48.

Mavundla TR, Poggenpoel M, Gmeiner A. A model of facilitative communication for the support of general hospital nurses nursing mentally ill people: Part I: Background, problem statement and research methodology. *Curationis.* 2001;24(1):7–14.

McCloskey JC, Bulechek GM. *Nursing Intervention Classification (NIC).* 3rd ed. St. Louis, MO: Mosby; 2000.

McKay RP. *The Process of Theory Development in Nursing.* Dissertation. New York, NY: Columbia University; 1965.

McQuiston CM, Campbell JC. Theoretical substruction: A guide for theory testing research. *Nurs Sci Q.* 1997;10:117–123.

Mefford LC. A theory of health promotion for preterm infants based on Levine's conservation model of nursing. *Nurs Sci Q.* 2004;17:260–266.

Meleis AI. *Theoretical Nursing.* Philadelphia, PA: Lippincott; 1985.

Meleis AI, Sawyer LM, Im E, Messias DKH, Schumacher K. Experiencing transitions: An emerging middle-range theory. *Adv Nurs Sci.* 2000;23(1):12–28.

Minshull J, Ross K, Turner J. The Human Needs Model of nursing. *J Adv Nurs.* 1986;11:643–649.

Mishel MH. Uncertainty in illness. *Image.* 1988;20:225–231.

Mishel MH. Reconceptualization of the uncertainty in illness theory. *Image.* 1990;22:256–261.

Mitchell GJ, Cody WK. Nursing knowledge and human science: Ontological and epistemological considerations. *Nurs Sci Q.* 1992;5:54–61.

Monti EJ, Tingen MS. Multiple paradigms of nursing science. *J Adv Nurs.* 1999;21(4):64–80.

Moody LE, Wilson ME, Smyth K, Schwartz R, Tittle M, Van Cott ML. Analysis of a decade of nursing practice research: 1977–1986. *Nurs Res.* 1988;37:374–379.

Morales-Mann ET, Jiang SL. Applicability of Orem's conceptual framework: A cross-cultural point of view. *J Adv Nurs.* 1993;18:737–741.

Murrock CJ, Higgins PA. The theory of music, mood, and movement to improve health outcomes. *J Adv Nurs.* 2009;65:2249–2257.

National League for Nursing. *Theory Development: What, Why, How?* New York, NY: National League for Nursing; 1978.

The nature of science and nursing. *Nurs Res.* 1968;17:484–512.

The nature of science in nursing. *Nurs Res.* 1969;18:388–411.

Neuman B. The Betty Neuman health-care systems model: A total person approach to patient problems. In: Riehl JP, Roy C, eds. *Conceptual Models for Nursing Practice.* New York, NY: Appleton-Century-Crofts; 1974.

Newman MA. Toward a theory of health. In: *Theory Development in Nursing.* Philadelphia, PA: Davis; 1979.

Newman MA. *Health as Expanding Consciousness.* St. Louis, MO: Mosby; 1986.

Newman MA. Prevailing paradigms in nursing. *Nurs Outlook.* 1992;40:10–13, 32.

Newman MA, Sime AM, Corcoran-Perry SA. The focus of the discipline of nursing. *Adv Nurs Sci.* 1991;14(1):1–6.

Newman MA, Smith MC, Pharris MD, Jones D. The focus of the discipline revisited. *Adv Nurs Sci.* 2008;31(1):E16–E27.

Nightingale F. *Notes on Nursing: What It Is and What It Is Not.* London: Harrison; 1859. Reprinted 1946. Philadelphia, PA: Lippincott.

Nolan M, Lundh U, Tishelman C. Nursing's knowledge base: Does it have to be unique? *Br J Nurs.* 1998;7(5):270, 272–276.

Norbeck JS. In defense of empiricism. *Image.* 1987;19:28–30.

Norris CM, ed. *Proceedings of the First Nursing Theory Conference.* Kansas City, MO: University of Kansas Medical Center, Department of Nursing; 1969.

Norris CM, ed. *Proceedings of the Second Nursing Theory Conference.* Kansas City, MO: University of Kansas Medical Center, Department of Nursing; 1970.

Norris CM, ed. *Proceedings of the Third Nursing Theory Conference.* Kansas City, MO: University of Kansas Medical Center, Department of Nursing; 1971.

O'Brien ME. *Spirituality in Nursing: Standing on Holy Ground.* 5th ed. Burlington, MA: Jones & Bartlett; 2014.

Olson J, Hanchett E. Nurse-expressed empathy, patient outcomes, and development of a middle-range theory. *Image.* 1997;29:71–76.

Orem D. *Nursing: Concepts of Practice.* New York, NY: McGraw-Hill; 1971.

Orem D. *Nursing: Concepts of Practice.* 4th ed. St. Louis, MO: Mosby; 1991.

Orem D. *Nursing: Concepts of Practice.* 5th ed. St. Louis, MO: Mosby; 1995.

Orlando IJ. *The Dynamic Nurse–Patient Relationship.* New York, NY: Putnam; 1961.

Panel for the Prediction and Prevention of Pressure Ulcers in Adults. *Pressure Ulcers in Adults: Prediction and Prevention.* Clinical Practice Guideline, No. 3. Rockville, MD: Agency for Health Care Policy and Research, PHS, USDHHS; May 1992. AHCPR publication 92-0047.

Parker ME, Smith MC. *Nursing Theories & Nursing Practice.* 3rd ed. Philadelphia, PA: Davis; 2010.

Parse RR. *Man-Living-Health: A Theory of Nursing.* New York, NY: Wiley; 1981.

Parse RR, ed. *Illuminations: The Human Becoming Theory in Practice and Research.* New York, NY: National League for Nursing; 1995.

Parse RR. *Hope: An International Human Becoming Perspective.* Sudbury, MA: Jones & Bartlett; 1999.

Parse RR. Nursing knowledge development: Who's to say how? (Editorial). *Nurs Sci Q.* 2008;21:101.

Pender NJ. *Health Promotion in Nursing Practice.* 3rd ed. Stamford, CT: Appleton & Lange; 1996.

Peplau HE. *Interpersonal Relations in Nursing.* New York, NY: Putnam; 1952.

Perry DJ. Transcendent pluralism: A middle-range theory of nonviolent social transformation through human and ecological dignity. *Adv Nurs Sci.* 2015;38(4):317–329.

Pesut B, Johnson J. Reinstating the 'queen': Understanding philosophical inquiry in nursing. *J Adv Nurs.* 2008;61:115–121.

Peterson SJ, Bredow TS. *Middle Range Theories: Application to Nursing Research.* 4th ed. Philadelphia, PA: Wolters Kluwer; 2017.

Poggenpoel M. Psychiatric nursing research based on nursing for the whole person theory. *Curationis.* 1996;19(3):60–62.

Practice oriented theory, part I. *Adv Nurs Sci.* 1978;1(1):1–95.

Reed J, Robbins I. Models of nursing: Their relevance to the care of elderly people. *J Adv Nurs.* 1991;16:1350–1357.

Reed PG. A treatise on nursing knowledge development for the 21st century: Beyond postmodernism. *Adv Nurs Sci.* 1995;17(3):70–84.

Reed PG. Nursing reformation: Historical reflections and philosophic foundations. *Nurs Sci Q.* 2000;13:129–133.

Research—How will nursing define it? *Nurs Res.* 1967;16:108–129.

Rew L, Hoke MM, Horner SD, Walker L. Development of a dynamic model to guide health disparities research. *Nurs Outlook.* 2009;57:132–142.

Rishel CJ. An emerging theory on parental end-of-life decision making as a stepping stone to new research. *Appl Nurs Res.* 2014;27:261–264.

Risjord MW, Dunbar SB, Moloney MR. A new foundation for methodological triangulation. *J Nurs Scholarsh.* 2002;34:269–275.

Roberson MR, Kelley JH. Using Orem's theory in transcultural settings: A critique. *Nurs Forum.* 1996;31(3):22–28.

Roberts MA. *American Nursing: History and Interpretation.* New York, NY: Macmillan; 1961:101.

Rodgers SJ. The role of nursing theory in standards of practice: A Canadian perspective. *Nurs Sci Q.* 2000;13:260–262.

Rogers ME. *An Introduction to the Theoretical Basis of Nursing.* Philadelphia, PA: Davis; 1970.

Roper N, Logan WW, Tierney AJ. *The Elements of Nursing.* 2nd ed. Edinburgh, Scotland: Churchill Livingstone; 1985.

Roy C. *Introduction to Nursing: An Adaptation Model.* Englewood Cliffs, NJ: Prentice Hall; 1976.

Roy C, Andrews HA. *The Roy Adaptation Model: The Definitive Statement.* Norwalk, CT: Appleton & Lange; 1991.

Roy C, Andrews HA. *The Roy Adaptation Model.* 2nd ed. Norwalk, CT: Appleton & Lange; 1999.

Roy C, Roberts SL. *Theory Construction in Nursing: An Adaptation Model.* Englewood Cliffs, NJ: Prentice Hall; 1981.

Roy C, Whetsell MV, Frederickson K. The Roy adaptation model and research: Global perspective. *Nurs Sci Q.* 2009;22:209–211.

Ruland CM, Moore SM. Theory construction based on standards of care: A proposed theory of the peaceful end of life. *Nurs Outlook.* 1998;46:169–175.

Ryan P, Sawin KJ. The individual and family self-management theory: Background and perspectives on context, process, and outcomes. *Nurs Outlook.* 2009;57:217–225.

Salas AS. Toward a north–south dialogue: Revisiting nursing theory (from the south). *Adv Nurs Sci.* 2005;28(1):17–24.

Sarvimäki A. Nursing care as a moral, practical, communicative and creative activity. *J Adv Nurs.* 1988;13:462–467.

Scheel ME, Pedersen BD, Rosenkrands V. Interactional nursing—A practice-theory in the dynamic field between the natural, human and social sciences. *Scand J Caring Sci.* 2008;22:629–636.

Schumacher KL, Gortner SR. (Mis)conceptions and reconceptions about traditional science. *Adv Nurs Sci.* 1992;14(4):1–11.

Searle C. Nursing theories: What is our commitment? *Nurs RSA Verpleging.* 1988;3(2):15–17, 19, 21.

See EM. Theories of middling-range generality in the development of nursing theory. Paper presented at the meeting of the Nursing Theory Think Tank, Denver, 1981.

Shin KR. Developing perspectives on Korean nursing theory: The influences of Taoism. *Nurs Sci Q.* 2001;14:346–353.

Silva MC. The state of nursing science: Reconceptualizing for the 21st century. *Nurs Sci Q.* 1999;12:221–226.

Silva MC, Rothbart D. An analysis of changing trends in philosophies of science in nursing theory development and testing. *Adv Nurs Sci.* 1984;6(2):1–13.

Sirra E. An approach to systematic nursing. *Nurs J India.* 1986;77(1):3–5, 28.

Skelly AH, Leeman J, Carlson J, Soward ACM, Burns D. Conceptual model of symptom-focused care for African Americans. *J Nurs Scholarsh.* 2008;40:261–267.

Smith JA. The idea of health: A philosophic inquiry. *Adv Nurs Sci.* 1981;3(3):43–50.

Smith L. Application of nursing models to a curriculum: Some considerations. *Nurse Educ Today.* 1987;7(3):109–115.

Smith MJ, Liehr PR, eds. *Middle Range Theory for Nursing.* 3rd ed. New York: Springer; 2014.

Snyder M. *Independent Nursing Interventions.* 2nd ed. New York, NY: Delmar; 1992.

Stajduhar KI, Balneaves L, Thorne SE. A case for the "middle ground": Exploring the tensions of postmodern thought in nursing. *Nurs Philos.* 2001;2:72–82.

Starc A. Nursing professionalism in Slovenia: Knowledge, power, and ethics. *Nurs Sci Q.* 2009;22:371–374.

Stevenson JS, Woods NF. Nursing science and contemporary science: Emerging paradigms. In: Sorensen GE, ed. *Setting the Agenda for the Year 2000.* Kansas City, MO: American Academy of Nursing; 1986.

Suppe F, Jacox AK. Philosophy of science and the development of nursing theory. In: Werley HH, Fitzpatrick JJ, eds. *Annual Review of Nursing Research.* 1985;3:241–267.

Swanson KM. Empirical development of a middle range theory of caring. *Nurs Res.* 1991;40:161–166.

Taylor JY. Womanism: A methodologic framework for African American women. *Adv Nurs Sci.* 1998;21(1):53–64.

Taylor SG, Geden E, Isaramalai S, Wongvatunyu S. Orem's self-care deficit nursing theory: Its philosophic foundation and the state of the science. *Nurs Sci Q.* 2000;13:104–110.

Theory development in nursing. *Nurs Res.* 1968;17:196–227.

Thorne S. (2014). What constitutes core disciplinary knowledge? *Nurs Inq.* 2014;21(1):1–2.

Tierney AJ. Nursing models: Extant or extinct? *J Adv Nurs.* 1998;28:377–385.

Timpson J. Nursing theory: Everything the artist spits is art? *J Adv Nurs.* 1996;23:1030–1036.

Tinkle MB, Beaton JL. Toward a new view of science. *Adv Nurs Sci.* 1983;5(3):27–36.

Travelbee J. *Interpersonal Aspects of Nursing.* Philadelphia, PA: Davis; 1971.

Tsai P. A middle-range theory of caregiver stress. *Nurs Sci Q.* 2003;16:137–145.

Turton CLR. Ways of knowing about health: An Aboriginal perspective. *Adv Nurs Sci.* 1997;19(3):28–36.

Ujhely G. *Determinants of the Nurse–Patient Relationship.* New York, NY: Springer; 1968.

University of California, San Francisco School of Nursing Symptom Management Faculty Group. A model for symptom management. *Image.* 1994;26:272–276.

Ustun B, Gigliotti E. Nursing research in Turkey. *Nurs Sci Q.* 2009;22:206–208.

Villarruel AM, Denyes MJ. Testing Orem's theory with Mexican Americans. *Image.* 1997;29:283–288.

Villarruel AM, Fairman JA. The Council for the Advancement of Nursing Science, Idea Festival Advisory Committee: Good ideas that need to go further. *Nurs Outlook.* 2015;63(4):436–438.

Voss JG, Dodd M, Portillo C, Holzemer W. Theories of fatigue: Application to HIV/AIDS. *J Assoc Nurses AIDS Care.* 2006;17:37–50.

Wald FS, Leonard RC. Towards development of nursing practice theory. *Nurs Res.* 1964;13:309–313.

Walker LO. *Nursing as a Discipline.* Dissertation. Bloomington, IN: Indiana University; 1971a.

Walker LO. Toward a clearer understanding of the concept of nursing theory. *Nurs Res.* 1971b;20:428–435.

Walker LO. Rejoinder to commentary: Toward a clearer understanding of the concept of nursing theory. *Nurs Res.* 1972;21:59–62.

Walker LO. *Parent–Infant Nursing Science: Paradigms, Phenomena, Methods.* Philadelphia, PA: Davis; 1992.

Walker LO, Avant KC. *Strategies for Theory Construction in Nursing.* 2nd ed. Norwalk, CT: Appleton & Lange, 1988.

Warms CA, Schroeder CA. Bridging the gulf between science and action: The "new fuzzies" of neopragmatism. *Adv Nurs Sci.* 1999;22(2):1–10.

Watson J. *Nursing: Human Science and Human Care.* Norwalk, CT: Appleton-Century-Crofts; 1985.

Watson J. Postmodernism and knowledge development in nursing. *Nurs Sci Q.* 1995;8:60–64.

Weaver K, Olson JK. Understanding paradigms used for nursing research. *J Adv Nurs.* 2006;53:459–469.

Webster G, Jacox A, Baldwin B. Nursing theory and the ghost of the received view. In: McCloskey JC, Grace HK, eds. *Current Issues in Nursing.* Boston, MA: Blackwell; 1981.

Wewers ME, Lenz E. Relapse among ex-smokers: An example of theory derivation. *Adv Nurs Sci.* 1987;9(2):44–53.

Whall AL, Hicks FD. The unrecognized paradigm shift in nursing: Implications, problems, and opportunities. *Nurs Outlook.* 2002;50:72–76.

Whall AL, Shin YH, Colling KB. A Nightingale-based model of dementia care and its relevance for Korean nursing. *Nurs Sci Q.* 1999;12:319–323.

Whittemore R, Roy C. Adapting to diabetes mellitus: A theory synthesis. *Nurs Sci Q.* 2002;15:311–317.

Wiedenbach E. *Clinical Nursing: A Helping Art.* New York, NY: Springer; 1964.

Willis DG, Grace PJ, Roy C. A central unifying focus for the discipline: Facilitating humanization, meaning, choice, quality of life, and healing in living and dying. *Adv Nurs Sci.* 2008;31(1):E28–E40.

Willman A, Stoltz P. Yes, no, or perhaps: Reflections on Swedish human science nursing research development. *Nurs Sci Q.* 2002;15:66–70.

Wong TK, Pang SM, Wang CS, Zhang CJ. A Chinese definition of nursing. *Nurs Inq.* 2003;10;79–80.

Wooldridge PJ. Commentary on Walker's "Toward a clearer understanding of the concept of nursing theory": Meta-theories of nursing: A commentary on Walker's article. *Nurs Res.* 1971;20:494–495.

Wooldridge P, Skipper JK, Leonard RC. *Behavioral Science, Social Practice, and the Nursing Profession.* Cleveland, OH: Case Western Reserve; 1968.

Wyman JF, Henly SJ. PhD programs in nursing in the United States: Visibility of American Association of Colleges of Nursing core curriculum elements and emerging areas of science. *Nurs Outlook*. 2015;63(4):390–397.

Yoshioka-Maeda K, Taguchi A, Murashima S, Asahara K, Anzai Y, Arimoto A, et al. Function and practice of public health nursing in Japan: A trial to develop the Japanese purpose-focused public health nursing model. *J Nurs Manag*. 2006;14:483–489.

Younger JB. A theory of mastery. *Adv Nurs Sci*. 1991;14(1):76–89.

Zandi M, Vanaki Z, Shiva M, Mohammadi E, Bagheri-Lankarani N. Security giving in surrogacy motherhood process as a caring model for commissioning mothers: A theory synthesis. *Jpn J Nurs Sci*. 2016;13(3):331–344.

Zeng B, Sun W, Gray RA, Li C, Liu T. Towards a conceptual model of diabetes self-management among Chinese immigrants in the United States. *Int J Environ Res Public Health*. 2014;11(7):6727–6742.

Additional Readings

Readers who wish to do additional reading in the philosophy, philosophy of science, and philosophy of nursing science will find resources below: many are classics, of interest. Introductory readings are signified by an asterisk (*).

Aronson JL. *A Realist Philosophy of Science*. London, England: Macmillan; 1984.

Cole S. *Making Science: Between Nature and Society*. Cambridge, MA: Harvard University; 1992.

Curd M, Cover JA, eds. *Philosophy of Science: The Central Issues*. New York, NY: W.W. Norton; 1998.

Dahnke MD, Dreher HM, eds. *Philosophy of Science for Nursing Practice: Concepts and Applications*. 2nd ed. New York, NY: Springer; 2016.

Feyerabend P. *Against Method: Outline of an Anarchistic Theory of Knowledge*. London, England: Verso; 1975.

Fiske DW, Shweder RA, eds. *Metatheory in Social Science*. Chicago, IL: University of Chicago Press; 1986.

Giere RN. *Explaining Science: A Cognitive Approach*. Chicago, IL: University of Chicago Press; 1988.

Glymour C. *Theory and Evidence*. Princeton, NJ: Princeton University Press; 1980.

Godfrey-Smith P. *Theory and Reality: An Introduction to the Philosophy of Science*. Chicago, IL: University of Chicago Press; 2003.

Harre R. *Varieties of Realism: A Rationale for the Natural Sciences*. New York, NY: Basil Blackwell; 1986.

*Klee R. *Introduction to the Philosophy of Science: Cutting Nature at Its Seams*. Oxford, England: Oxford University Press; 1997.

Klemke ED, Hollinger R, Rudge DW, Kline AD, eds. *Introductory Readings in the Philosophy of Science*. 3rd ed. Amherst, NY: Prometheus Books; 1998.

Kuhn TS. *The Structure of Scientific Revolutions*. 2nd ed. Chicago, IL: University of Chicago Press; 1970.

Lakatos I, Musgrave A, eds. *Criticism and the Growth of Knowledge*. London, England: Cambridge University Press; 1970.

Laudan L. *Progress and Its Problems: Toward a Theory of Scientific Growth*. Berkeley, CA: University of California Press; 1977.

*Okasha S. *Philosophy of Science: A Very Short Introduction*. Oxford, England: Oxford University Press; 2002.

*Omery A, Kasper CE, Page GG, eds. *In Search of Nursing Science*. Thousand Oaks, CA: Sage; 1995.

*Phillips DC. *Philosophy, Science, and Social Inquiry*. New York, NY: Pergamon; 1987.

Phillips DC. *The Social Scientist's Bestiary: A Guide to Fabled Threats to, and Defenses of, Naturalistic Social Science*. New York, NY: Pergamon; 1992.

Popper KR. *Conjectures and Refutations: The Growth of Scientific Knowledge*. New York, NY: Harper & Row; 1965.

Psillos S. *Scientific Realism: How Science Tracks Truth*. London, England: Routledge; 1999.

Risjord M. *Nursing Knowledge: Science, Practice, and Philosophy*. Oxford, UK: Wiley-Blackwell; 2010.

*Rodgers BL. *Developing Nursing Knowledge: Philosophical Traditions and Influences*. Philadelphia, PA: Lippincott Williams & Wilkins; 2005.

*Suppe F. Response to "positivism and qualitative nursing research." *Sch Inq Nurs Pract*. 2001;15:389–397.

Weimer WW. *Notes on the Methodology of Scientific Research*. Hillsdale, NJ: Erlbaum; 1979.

Readers who wish to do additional reading related to middle-range theory may find the following resources of interest.

Peterson SJ, Bredow TS. *Middle Range Theories: Application to Nursing Research*. 4th ed. Philadelphia, PA: Wolters Kluwer; 2017.

Smith MJ, Liehr PR, eds. *Middle Range Theory for Nursing*. 3rd ed. New York, NY: Springer; 2014.

Readers who wish to do additional readings related to development of global nursing theory may find the following resources of interest.

Adams T. The idea of revolution in the development of nursing theory. *J Adv Nurs*. 1991;16:1487–1491.

Bailey J. Reflective practice: Implementing theory. *Nurs Stand*. 1995;9(46):29–31.

Barker PJ, Reynolds W, Stevenson C. The human science basis of psychiatric nursing: Theory and practice. *J Adv Nurs*. 1997;25:660–667.

Bostrom I, Hall-Lord M, Larsson G, Wilde B. Nursing theory based changes of work organisation in an ICU: Effects on quality of care. *Intensive Crit Care Nurs*. 1992;8(1):10–16.

Brieskorn-Zinke M. The relevance of health sciences for nursing [in German]. *Pflege*. 1998;11(3):129–134.

Castledine G. Where are the British models? Nursing models. *Nurs Times*. 1985;81(43):22.

Chalmers KI. Giving and receiving: An empirically derived theory on health visiting practice. *J Adv Nurs*. 1992;17:1317–1325.

Cook SH. Mind the theory/practice gap in nursing. *J Adv Nurs*. 1991;16:1462–1469.

Eldh A. Monograph review: Critical appraisal: Nursing theories in practice, education and research. *Theoria J Nurs Theory*. 2001;10(3):17–19.

Emden C. Nursing knowledge: An intriguing journey. *Aust J Adv Nurs*. 1987–1988;5(2):33–45.

Evans AM. Philosophy of nursing: Future directions. *Aust N Z J Ment Health Nurs*. 1995;4(1):14–21.

Gray G, Pratt R. *Towards a Discipline of Nursing*. Melbourne, Australia: Churchill Livingstone; 1991.

Gray G, Pratt R. *Scholarship in the Discipline of Nursing*. Melbourne, Australia: Churchill Livingstone; 1995.

Hauge S. From focusing on illness to focusing on health in nursing [in Norwegian]. *Värd i Norden*. 1997;17(1):18–24.

Hopkins S, McSherry R. Debate: Is there a great divide between nursing theory and practice? *Nurs Times*. 2000;96(17):16.

Kyriacos U, van der Walt A. Attitudes of diploma-prepared and graduate registered nurses towards nursing models: A comparative study. *Curationis*. 1996;19(3):2–6.

Laschinger HK, Duff V. Attitudes of practicing nurses towards theory-based nursing practice. *Can J Nurs Adm.* 1991;4(1):6–10.

Mattice M. Parse's theory of nursing in practice: A manager's perspective. *Can J Nurs Adm.* 1991;4(1):11–13.

Mulholland J. Assimilating sociology: Critical reflections on the "sociology in nursing" debate. *J Adv Nurs.* 1997;25:844–852.

Muller E, Reipschlager C. The drawing up of a classification system for nursing science for the University Library in Bremen—A contribution to the development of nursing as a science [in German]. *Pflege.* 1997;10(5):292–298.

Norberg A, Wickstrom E. The perception of Swedish nurses and nurse teachers of the integration of theory with nursing practice. An explorative qualitative study. *Nurse Educ Today.* 1990;10(1):38–43.

Quiquero A, Knights D, Meo CO. Theory as a guide to practice: Staff nurses choose Parse's theory. *Can J Nurs Adm.* 1991;4(1):14–16.

Scott H. More clinical skills but not at the expense of theory. *Br J Nurs.* 1999;8:910.

Smith JP. *Models, Theories, and Concepts.* London, England: Blackwell Scientific; 1994.

Smith M, Cusack L. The Ottawa Charter—From nursing theory to practice: Insights from the area of alcohol and other drugs. *Int J Nurs Pract.* 2000;6(4):168–173.

Tornstam L. Caring for the elderly: Introducing the theory of gerotranscendence as a supplementary frame of reference for caring for the elderly. *Scand J Caring Sci.* 1996;10(3):144–150.

Wang Y, Li X. Cross-cultural nursing theory and Chinese nursing today [in Chinese]. *Chin Nurs Res.* 2000;14(6):231–232.

2

■ ■ ■

Using Knowledge Development and Theory to Inform Practice

Questions to consider before you get started reading this chapter:

▶ Are you confused about how theory relates to practice?

▶ Have you thought how knowledge is developed in a scientific and practice discipline?

▶ Have you wondered how nursing knowledge development, evidence-based practice, and informatics are related, and whether these ideas are compatible or at odds with each other?

Introductory Note: If you answered yes to any of these questions, then this is the chapter you should read before you proceed to use the rest of this book. Without a good grasp of the relationships between knowledge, theory, research, and practice, you will likely encounter difficulties understanding the strategies put forward in the following chapters.

We often encounter the question, "Why do we need theory? It isn't relevant to practice." Our answer usually begins with another question relating to a complementary field such as physiology (e.g., Starling's law) or pharmacology (e.g., drug interactions using chemical theory). Then, we point out that nurses use those sorts of theories on a daily basis and that they are certainly relevant to practice. This allows us to suggest that in the same way we need theories in nursing to describe and explain our thinking and to predict the outcomes of our nursing care. In an era of increasing focus on the need for quality and safety in patient care, nurses need to be able to demonstrate the effectiveness and efficiency of their care. Theories and the research that develops and tests them can help in this endeavor. This chapter will explore the interactions between theory, research, and practice and how together they form a matrix to improve patient care.

INTRODUCTION

The purpose of science is to develop knowledge. That knowledge is often summarized or synthesized into a theory. Theories guide both research and practice. Theories that are useful in nursing practice describe phenomena, explain how things work, predict results, or prescribe interventions or therapies (An, Hayman, Panniers, & Carty, 2007). A theory may, for instance, describe how antecedent incidents such as poor labeling (A) are related to subsequent outcomes such as medication errors (C). Or a theory may predict that one type of intervention is more efficacious or cost-effective than another intervention. In Figure 2–1, we show how theory can be used as a framework for nursing practice in what we are calling the *Theory of a Phenomenon*. The origins of the Theory of a Phenomenon may stem from one or more types of nursing scholarship, including literature synthesis derived from practice. In this simplified schematic of a theory, antecedent conditions lead to mediating events that then affect good or poor nursing outcomes. Furthermore, nurses can use the concepts (A, B, and C) and their linkages (arrows linking concepts) to extrapolate assessments and interventions at various early, mid-, or late points in the development of the phenomenon. Figure 2–1 is much like a road map to help you get your bearings and help you achieve your goal. The Theory of a Phenomenon is especially helpful when routine approaches are only partially effective or when challenges to usual practice arise.

Despite the usefulness of theory to guide our practice, often there are no theories that apply to the situation in which we find ourselves. This is partly due to the fact that nursing is still young as a science. However, the lack of needed theory does not excuse

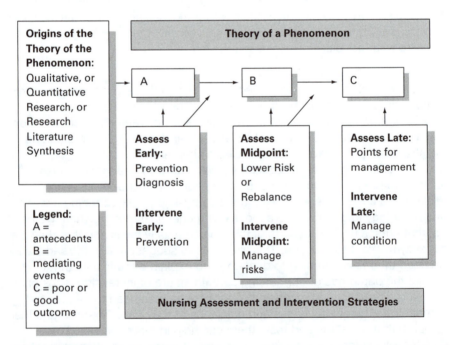

FIGURE 2–1 Simple schematic figure of theory as a framework for nursing assessment and intervention.

us from the obligation to develop the knowledge that will lead to those theories (Clark, 2000). Thus, in this chapter, we consider not only theory but also the broader context of knowledge development related to nursing practice.

Nurses are knowledge workers and have been so since the beginning of modern nursing. They systematically use knowledge from nursing and other sciences to inform their care. But nurses don't just *use* information, they *produce* it as well, and on a daily basis. Whether it is documenting in a patient record, writing clinical guidelines, or publishing research findings, nurses are expected to provide evidence of their practice. The quality of the information they produce and how that information is stored and maintained also significantly affect how it is used. Without adequate production and sharing of information and evidence, nursing care and decisions are hampered (Avant, 2008; Bakken-Henry, 1995; Calvert et al., 2013; Goosen, 2002; Keenan et al., 2002).

In an era of serious health care reform, nurses are positioned to provide many of the health care services needed in any system that emerges. However, it is critical that nurses are able to show that they are efficient and effective providers of those services. They must demonstrate that they can provide safe, quality care that is cost-effective as well.

Providing evidence of effectiveness requires interactions among the fields of evidence-based practice research, practice-based evidence research, improvement science, team science, informatics and information science, and theory development. All of these are pieces of the quality/safety puzzle. Without all of the pieces, the full picture of how nursing care affects patient outcomes cannot be made explicit. In this chapter, we will explore the issues of evidence and practice, informatics as it relates to evidence and practice, and finally discuss development of knowledge and theory in direct patient care.

EVIDENCE-BASED PRACTICE AND PRACTICE-BASED EVIDENCE

Definitions of these two fields demonstrate their interconnectedness. **Evidence-based practice (EBP)** has been defined in several ways. Sackett, Rosenberg, Gray, Haynes, and Richardson (1996) define it as "the conscientious, explicit and judicious use of current best evidence about the care of individual patients . . . integrating individual clinical expertise with the best available external clinical evidence from systematic research" (p. 71). French (2002) refers to it as "the systematic interconnecting of scientifically generated evidence with the tacit knowledge of the expert practitioner to achieve a change in a particular practice for the benefit of a well defined client/patient group" (p. 74). Roberts (1998) states, "EBP uses evidence gleaned from research to establish sound clinical practice" (p. 24). Finally, Eisenberg (1998) contends that "evidence-based clinical practice draws on the findings of research to provide information to improve patient care for each individual, while at the same time challenging researchers to address the questions for which clinicians and patients most urgently need information." EBP protocols use a system of grading evidence based most often on the medical model, although some nursing models such as the Joanna Briggs model (Pearson, Wiechula, Court, & Lockwood, 2005), the ACE Star Model of Knowledge Transformation (Stevens, 2012), and others are available as well. As it is beyond the scope of this chapter to fully discuss EBP models, you are encouraged to read about them in one of the references above or one of the several journals that relate to EBP for further clarification of the methods.

Although there is some concern about the current emphasis on EBP for nursing (French, 2002; Jennings, 2000; Jennings & Loan, 2001) because it is philosophically based on the medical evidence-based model (EBM), we believe that evidence of good practice is always important. However, the concerns are also valid ones that need to be kept in mind during any discussion of EBP in particular. For these and other reasons, hierarchies of evidence have been developed that encompass the additional practice concerns, such as harm, diagnosis, prognosis, human response, and meaning (Grace & Powers, 2009).

The concerns are expressed because the medical EBM focuses only on medical diagnoses, single interventions, and meta-analyses and uses the randomized controlled trial (RCT) as the gold standard for evidence (Kitson, 1997). Jennings and French both point out that nurses have misunderstood the term and its underlying intent and question whether nursing really wants to concentrate large portions of energy only on specific interventions and RCTs. They are not alone in this concern. Berwick (2009) has expressed a similar concern when it comes to many quality improvement initiatives, especially those that take place in highly complex systems or involve multidimensional interventions. Nurses who espouse using EBP because they think it will help them achieve better quality care across the spectrum of nursing arenas and help them demonstrate "how nursing works" may want to be very specific about what they mean when they use the term *evidence-based research* or *practice*. The potential exists for nursing science to find itself in a situation where it is severely constrained in its purposes and scope.

Doane and Varcoe (2008) postulate that the interconnections between theory, evidence, and practice may be "lost in translation" (p. 3), as nurses try to "live/translate/enact knowledge" (p. 3) in complex arenas of practice. Decisions that are evidence based are often hampered because many interventions have limited formal research evidence to support them, or there are serious barriers to the implementation of the practices (Millenson, 1997; Retsas, 2000). The situation is improving, but lack of sufficient evidence impedes the implementation of EBP (Schwartz-Barcott, Patterson, Lusardi, & Farmer, 2002; van Achterberg, Schoonhoven, & Grol, 2008). In fact, Melnyk, Fineout-Overholt, Gallagher-Ford, and Kaplan (2012) and Lavin, Harper, and Barr (2015) found that although nurses were generally positive about using EBP, they often encountered significant barriers when attempting to implement it.

Nevertheless, the EBP movement is strong and has resulted in multiple clinical practice guidelines for such issues as prevention and management of obesity in children (Fitch et al., 2013), assessment and management of pressure ulcers (Registered Nurses' Association of Ontario, 2016), prevention of catheter-associated urinary tract infections (Wald, Fink, Makic, & Oman, 2012), and more. (The guidelines can be accessed through the Agency for Healthcare Research and Quality [AHRQ] website.) In addition, the U.S. federal government has funded the Clinical Translational Science Awards (Zerhouni, 2005) and the Patient-Centered Outcomes Research Institute (Adashi & Selby, 2012) to assist in moving research to the point of care more quickly.

Zerenstein and Treweek (2009) suggest that there is often a "mismatch between the clinical context in which clinicians must make decisions and the clinical context of the randomized trials that they must use for evidence . . . " (p. 999). They propose the use of what Schwartz and Lellouch (1967) called a pragmatic attitude toward clinical trials that makes them more relevant to the actual clinicians who must use them to make decisions. Pragmatic trials focus more on whether the intervention works in normal practice situations, can be applied flexibly, and is directly applicable and relevant to participants, clinicians, and policy makers rather than stricter, more tightly controlled trials. For the purpose of this book, we prefer to use this broader understanding of evidence-based research. We believe the concept of EBP should include any of the following: any steps in the nursing process (assessment, diagnosis, goal setting, interventions, outcomes, or evaluation), decision support, quality improvements, safety monitoring, standards and guidelines, expert opinions, and workload evaluations and staffing.

Horn and Gassaway (2007) have suggested a means to overcome the problem of using only RCTs as the basis for EBP: mining large databases to gather the data needed to demonstrate quality and effectiveness. They called it **practice-based evidence (PBE)**. PBE attempts to capture in-depth, comprehensive information about patient characteristics, processes of care, and outcomes while controlling for patient differences. Increasingly sophisticated information technology provides the means to capture complex patient data and seamlessly incorporate them into electronic health records (EHRs). Large systems of patient records can provide researchers and theorists a means to search for meaningful and explanatory relationships across large data sets.

This idea of using big data (the term is used to mean large data sets as well as data analytics) has been around since the end of the last century. Internet browsers, advertisements on the Internet, and online shopping are examples of the use of big data. Large quantities of data are available on any one of these databases, making our lives both easier and more complex. Many health care organizations are storing their big data in data warehouses that may lead to the problems of volume, velocity, and variety that Laney (2001) first discussed. As more and more data (volume) of different types (variety) are put into a system, and more and more people try to access them (velocity), managing the data becomes extremely complex, requiring a fairly sophisticated information technology and usually a common categorization vocabulary such as the Systematized Nomenclature of Medicine—Clinical Terms (SNOMED International, 2017) in order to access and use the data.

Of course, databases require that information entered into them is coded so that it can be retrieved and used more than once. If the data are not coded correctly, they will not be reliable or retrievable. Coded nursing data are usually found in good standardized nursing language classifications such as NANDA-International nursing diagnoses (Herdman & Kamitsuru, 2018), the Nursing Intervention Classification (Bulecheck, Butcher, Dochterman, & Wagner, 2013), and the Nursing Outcomes Classification (Moorhead, Johnson, Maas, & Swanson, 2013) or one of the other American Nurses Association–recognized terminologies. (We will speak more of this later in this chapter.)

Thus, the theories or hypotheses generated from these large data sets may be richer and more reliable and valid than those theories or hypotheses tested in RCTs, where the population of interest and the number of variables tested must necessarily be constrained to achieve the desired control of the research design. The problem with using such large databases, of course, is that the data used are only as reliable as the data that were entered. If monitors are faulty or a practitioner enters inaccurate data, then false conclusions may be drawn from that data. This model works well as long as there are electronic warehouses of information that can be used for many purposes. So, good documentation and adequate information are critical to the process.

The issues of good documentation, adequate information to inform decisions, and best practices have been around since formal nursing began. It seems informatics and EBPs have been uniquely interrelated phenomena of concern to nurses throughout our history.

> In attempting to arrive at the truth, I have applied everywhere for information, but in scarcely an instance have I been able to obtain hospital records fit for any purpose of comparison. If they could be obtained they would enable us to decide many other questions besides the one alluded to. They would show the subscribers how their money was being spent, what good was really being done with it, or whether the money was not doing mischief rather than good; . . . And if wisely used, these improved statistics would tell more the relative value of particular operations and modes of treatment than we have means of ascertaining at present. They would enable us, besides, to ascertain the influence of the hospital . . . upon the course of operations and diseases passing through its wards; and the truth thus ascertained would enable us to save life and suffering and to improve the treatment and management of the sick. (Nightingale, 1863, pp. 175–176)

Nightingale had it right 150 years ago. There is a significant link between good evidence and the outcomes of nursing work. Nurses rely heavily on sufficient, appropriate, and timely information in the delivery of care. Without sufficient and appropriate information, decision making is hampered and quality of care is jeopardized. The quality and types of information available significantly impact the kinds and quality of decisions made (Brazelton, Knuckles, & Lyons, 2017). As Nightingale suggested, whether needed information is available and retrievable for use also impacts the quality of patient outcomes and decisions made. In fact, Ireson and Velotta (1998) suggest that seeming unwillingness to *use* evidence in practice is, in part, due to nurses being unable to retrieve evidence or needing evidence that is not available. This problem partially accounts for the long lag-time between completion of research studies and use of the findings in practice and is one of the stimuli for the increased focus on issues of translational research. Moreover, Resnick (2008) suggests that the gap between evidence and application may also be due to factors such as political agendas, funding constraints, or the cyclic nature of the amount of public attention focused on an issue.

Currently, for example, there are numerous discussions related to **improvement science**, a relatively new field within the evidence-based movement that has arisen from the Institute of Medicine (IOM) quality and safety reports (IOM, 2000, 2001) and the Quality and Safety Education for Nurses (QSEN) initiatives (Cronenwett et al., 2007). The studies arising in this field are primarily related to quality and safety improvement programs. In focus and methodology, they look surprisingly like the pragmatic trials proposed by Schwartz and Lellouch. What we found most interesting in our brief review was a call for the use of sound theory to guide the research being conducted and to compellingly predict intervention success (IOM, 2001; Shojania & Grimshaw, 2005). A good example of how this can be initiated is Brant, Beck, and Miaskowski's (2009) careful comparisons of two models and two theories commonly used to guide symptom management research. Their analysis revealed that each of the four models/theories contained gaps, did not address such issues as symptom resolution, and often lacked essential definitions for some of the concepts. However, they were clear that although new models needed to be generated that would reduce the flaws in the current models, theory-driven research was the best method for studying the phenomenon of symptom management.

So far, we have discussed the ideas of EBP and PBE. But how is this relevant to theory development? Figure 2–2 is an effort to show the interrelationships among EBP, PBE, research, and practice. The figure demonstrates that the interactions are iterative and feed into one another. Practice generates questions and problems to be solved. PBE research can answer some of the questions but may also generate hypotheses about diagnoses or interventions that could be tested in RCTs. The accumulation of evidence from these trials can be captured in EBP research, which results in the composition of sound clinical guidelines for practice. Using the guidelines in practice allows for evaluations of their quality, safety, and efficacy through PBE research.

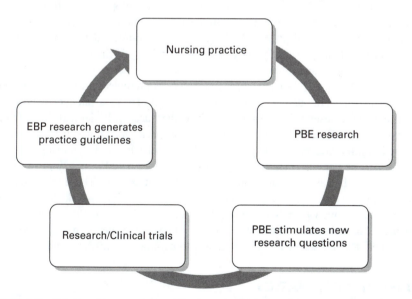

FIGURE 2–2   Relationships among practice-based evidence, evidence-based practice, research, and practice.   *Source*: Avant KC. Developing knowledge for nursing practice: Mid-range theory and nursing diagnosis. Paper presented at the 14th Annual Meeting of the Japan Society of Nursing Diagnosis. Kyoto, Japan, July 2008.

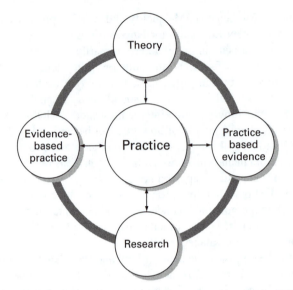

FIGURE 2–3   Relationships between practice, theory, research, and the PBE/EBP cycle.   *Source*: Avant KC. Developing knowledge for nursing practice: Mid-range theory and nursing diagnosis. Paper presented at the 14th Annual Meeting of the Japan Society of Nursing Diagnosis. Kyoto, Japan, July 2008.

In Figure 2–3, we show how EBP and PBE relate to practice, research, and theory. Practice is the central and core phenomenon. It is the basis for our existence and the focus of our work. All other aspects of knowledge development are framed around it and interact with it. Theory not only guides practice but also generates models for testing in research through PBE or EBP. Research and clinical data provide evidence for EBP or PBE that can subsequently generate practice guidelines and/or theory. The process is interactive and iterative.

Our review of EBP brings us full circle to issues presented in Chapter 1 related to the historical context of nursing knowledge development. The idea that nursing practice is evidence based represents the fulfillment of the earlier ideas of Bixler and Bixler (1945), wherein "a well-defined and well-organized body of specialized knowledge" (p. 730) was proposed as a requirement of the professional status of nursing. For nursing, however, practice must be not only evidence based but also theory based. In nursing, values and perspectives of the patient or client are central to the care process. Those values and perspectives, though often criticized as overly grand, remain the benchmarks for what gives nursing its distinctive view of care among the health professions. As Sampselle (2007) so aptly put it, "research requires a 2-way transfer of knowledge" between the scientists and the communities they serve. This is particularly true for nursing research and theory.

NURSING INFORMATICS

Returning to Nightingale's issue of evidence for use in practice and decision support leads us into the discussion of information and how we generate, store, use, and retrieve it. The advent of inexpensive and very efficient computers and information systems has pushed health care systems and health care workers into the information age with a vengeance. The amazing growth of electronic patient records has significantly changed the way patient care is documented. In addition, there has been a relative explosion of nursing research related to interventions, outcomes, effectiveness of care, cost of care, and so forth as a result of the availability of large databases for mining as we discussed above.

Nursing informatics has been defined as "a combination of computer science, information science and nursing science designed to assist in the management and processing of nursing data, information and knowledge to support the practice of nursing and the delivery of nursing care" (Graves & Corcoran, 1989, p. 227). Hannah, Ball, and Edwards (1994) define it as "the use of information technologies in relation to those functions within the purview of nursing, and that are carried out by nurses when performing their duties" (p. 3). Turley (1996) calls nursing informatics "the interaction of cognitive science, computer science, and information science resting on a base of nursing science" (p. 309). Informatics provides some of the infrastructure for managing, storing, retrieving, and working with various forms of nursing data, information, and evidence. Finally, the Scope and Practice of Nursing Informatics Standards of the ANA (2008) defines it as "a specialty that integrates nursing science, computer science, and information science to manage and communicate data, information, knowledge and wisdom in nursing practice" (p. 1).

In the fourth edition of this book, we mentioned Heller, Oros, and Durney-Crowley's (2000) 10 trends they believed would be highly significant factors in nursing in the twenty-first century. Three of the trends were mentioned as highly relevant. First was the technological explosion, which enumerated the dramatic changes in computers, information systems, and telecommunications; technological changes in patient care and diagnostics; and improvements in accessibility of clinical data. The second trend related to the cost of health care, the changes in health care systems, and the lack of insurance coverage by huge numbers of persons. The third trend, the significant advance in nursing science and research, highlighted the increasing numbers of studies that provided a scientific basis for nursing care to improve patient outcomes. Thus, 3 of the 10 trends related directly to informatics and EBP, emphasizing the importance these trends would have over the next few years. And in fact, the authors were correct. These trends have been significant and continue to be significant. In the next section, we document the increasing emphasis on the relationships between informatics, research, and theory development.

Model and Theory Development in Informatics and Evidence-Based Practice

Most of the theoretical work in this area was in the EBP domain. Very little was found in the informatics literature in nursing with the exception of Turley's (1996) model and Matney, Avant, and Stagger's (2015) theory of wisdom discussed later. This is not to say that informatics lacks a theoretical base, but it does tend to be information science based; it is not focused on nursing theory. However, both Bakken-Henry (1995) and the IOM (2001) have called explicitly for informatics theories.

Similarly, other authors called for better theoretical underpinnings for EBP and decision making and the knowledge development that drives these efforts (Elkan,

Blair, & Robinson, 2000; Fawcett, Watson, Neuman, Walker, & Fitzpatrick, 2001; Liehr & Smith, 1999; Thompson, 1999; Walker, 1999). Although each took a somewhat different approach, each suggested that integrating and expanding what nursing views as evidence would promote growth of knowledge and allow for sound middle-range theory development in nursing. Each suggested that EBP and the research that directs it should be theory based. This approach would allow for a more comprehensive view of nursing knowledge as it guides practice. Three of the articles actually proposed models or methods for theory development (Elkan et al., 2000; Fawcett et al., 2001; Thompson, 1999). This is encouraging to see. For the first several years of the movement toward EBP, there was little mention of theory as a basis for evidence, or vice versa.

In what have become classic articles, authors proposed development of middle-range theory based on the use of clinical guidelines (Gooch, 1991; Good & Moore, 1996) and standards of care (Ruland & Moore, 1998). The authors suggested that guidelines and standards are fruitful grounds for developing middle-range theory that is directly linked to practice. They argued that standards and guidelines directly link to nursing interventions and outcomes. Good and Moore even proposed a method for developing theory from guidelines and demonstrated how it can be done. The results lead to a theory synthesis (see Chapter 9) that is relevant to practice. We would like to see more work using this type of method. The guidelines are out there. All that is needed are willing minds.

Three groups of authors actually proposed models or theories related to EBP or informatics. Kolcaba (2001) presented a fascinating discussion of the development of the middle-range theory of comfort and its eventual use for outcomes research. She carefully detailed the steps taken to build and refine the theory and demonstrated how using the theory in outcomes research benefited not only the patients but also some institutional outcomes related to nurse productivity. Smith et al. (2002) used the caregiving effectiveness model to predict the outcomes of family members' caregiving on technology-dependent elders in the home. The authors found that nurses were very willing to use the verified relational statements in the model to generate nursing interventions. Mitchell, Ferketich, and Jennings (1998) and the American Academy of Nursing Expert Panel on Quality Health Care proposed a dynamic model for quality health outcomes. They suggested that the model is broad enough to allow for research on system-level interventions and outcomes at both individual and systems levels, to guide formation of relevant clinical databases, and to help researchers identify key variables for study.

The two theories proposed for informatics in the literature we reviewed were those by Turley (1996) and Matney et al. (2015). Turley proposed that nursing informatics be based within the three fields of cognitive science, computer science, and information science, but resting on a base of nursing science. He envisioned a model of three-dimensional Venn diagrams encapsulated within the science base of nursing. He proposed that research is needed at each of the intersections within the model, but all of it be focused within the context of nursing. It provides a very clear view of the field of nursing informatics. Matney, Avant, and Staggers found no clear definition for the concept of "wisdom" in the Nursing Informatics Scope and Standards (ANA,

2008) model of the relationships among data, information, knowledge, and wisdom. Using theory derivation and synthesis strategies, they proposed a model of wisdom in action that clearly shows the interactions and relationships between the four concepts. This model is now incorporated in the 2014 version of the Standards.

Although evidence may vary by type and source, as we have said earlier, one of the first criteria for evidence is that it be available and retrievable so that it can be used. Developing theories related to informatics use in practice can provide direction to programmers, software developers, and vendors. Such theories may assist in determining what nursing data are relevant to input, store, maintain, and retrieve and how to represent that data in their products. Without adequate theories of what nursing information is critical and how the data types are related to each other, developers and vendors cannot be responsive to nursing's particular needs for evidence to advance practice.

Information technology now drives much of our communications, keeps us in touch with each other and the world, and provides consumers with instant information about health care services, new drugs, and the latest in health technology. Consumers are becoming very knowledgeable about best practices related to their particular health situations. It is important that nurses keep up to date with the rapid development of such technology and use it appropriately.

NURSING PRACTICE RESEARCH AND THEORY DEVELOPMENT

Over a decade ago, Blegen and Tripp-Reimer (1997) suggested that established taxonomies of nursing languages might constitute the basis for middle-range theory development for nursing practice. They contended that linking nursing diagnosis concepts with interventions to predict expected outcomes is a reasonable way to construct theory that is relevant to and supports EBP. We will take up this idea and explore it a bit further.

Despite the sometimes draconic ways in which nursing diagnosis is taught within the nursing process, thus turning off many nurses to the whole idea of care planning, standardized nursing languages are important to the documentation of nursing care. More and more vendors of EHR software are using one or more of these nursing terminologies to populate the nursing care sections of their programs. Standardized nursing languages are the entry point for accessing nursing data from most EHRs. Without such coded information, the data are not retrievable and thus cannot be used to develop new terminology, discover new relations among concepts, determine the effects of nursing interventions, or demonstrate effectiveness of nursing care on patient outcomes. The very core of PBE research methods depends on the accessibility of large sets of data including nursing data in order to conduct the studies. Having standardized nursing concepts in these data sets allows for an amazing variety of studies to be conducted relating to many aspects of patient care, nursing management, and cost-effectiveness evaluation.

Most of the standardized languages are still in development. This is to be expected as no terminology should ever become stagnant. Some of the nursing languages (e.g., NANDA, NIC, NOC, Omaha) have significant evidence to support the inclusion of any particular term or concept, although not all. Most of the language development groups welcome input and new submissions or suggestions for additions or deletions to their terminologies. The more the languages are developed, strengthened, added to, and revised, the more we can use them to study nursing care.

In the next few paragraphs, we will show how we used a NANDA nursing diagnosis to develop a small theory. (This was part of a presentation one of us [Avant] did on middle-range theory development for the Japanese Nursing Diagnosis Association in July 2008.) Using defining characteristics, related factors, and possible outcomes, we can generate a middle-range theory of impaired home maintenance. (This diagnosis can be found in *Nursing Diagnoses: Definitions and Classifications,* 2018–2020, p. 242.) The definition of the diagnosis was "inability to independently maintain a safe growth-promoting immediate environment."

To develop the theory, we chose the defining characteristics of overtaxed family members, disorderly and unclean surroundings, unavailability of cooking and cleaning equipment, and presence of vermin. Next, we chose the related factors of impaired functioning, insufficient family organization, and inadequate support systems. Then we modified or collapsed some of the defining characteristics and related factors to form new concepts. Unavailability of cooking and cleaning equipment was modified to *insufficient or inadequate equipment.* Presence of vermin and disorderly and unclean surroundings were collapsed to *unhygienic environment.* Impaired functioning was modified to include *physical or mental functioning.*

Next, we examined the new concepts for relationships and hierarchies. We determined that there were a set of antecedent conditions and a set of intermediate conditions that led to the undesirable outcome of impaired home maintenance. The antecedent conditions were

- impaired mental or physical functioning,
- inadequate support systems,
- insufficient family organization, and
- inadequate or insufficient equipment.

The intermediate conditions were

- overtaxed family members and
- unhygienic environment.

The final theoretical model is presented in Figure 2–4. Though this model is used primarily for illustrative purposes, it demonstrates how using a standardized language facilitates theory development.

We believe that using standardized languages is an efficient means to clearly link the elements of practice, research, evidence, and theory into a meaningful program for knowledge development in practice. However, there are other models that are equally efficient for generating theory for practice. Figure 2–1, which we presented at the beginning of this chapter, provides another example or approach to theory development in practice, using the nursing process or clinical reasoning model as a guide. In fact, this entire book is dedicated to showing you how to do just that. In this chapter, we are merely giving examples of what is to come.

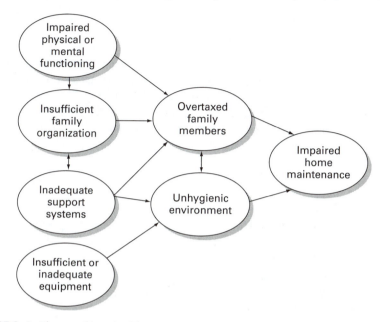

FIGURE 2–4   Theory of impaired home maintenance.

In Figure 2–1, if you start on the left side of the model, you can see that the origins of any theory to guide practice may be research or literature on the phenomenon of interest. Synthesizing the literature and reviewing research findings will ground you in what is already known. If there is not any research or literature on the phenomenon but it is a problem you see in practice, then you must take a step back from theory development and choose one of the concept or statement development strategies you will find later in this book. Moving across the top of the model, you will see that antecedents lead to mediating events that in turn lead to either good outcomes or poor ones. This level of the model might be your guide in determining methods for studying the phenomenon of interest. (In fact, if you look at Figure 2–4, you can see that it looks very similar to the top level of Figure 2–1.) The bottom level of the model relates to assessment and intervention strategies. As you can see, assessing early relates to early diagnosis of any problems or life situations that might be troubling, while early intervention leads to prevention. If the assessment occurs at a later time such as the midpoint of the process, perhaps after diagnosis has occurred and prevention is no longer feasible, then the object is to rebalance the system or lower the risk of further problems. Thus, interventions at this point are directed at managing risks. If the assessment occurs late in the process, the object becomes to determine management points in care and to subsequently manage the condition appropriately over time with a view to maintaining function and quality of life.

There are yet other models for linking evidence, research, and practice to develop knowledge. The ones we show here are but examples to whet your appetite. In the forthcoming chapters, we will help you learn more about other strategies for developing theory.

Summary

We have been very impressed with the amount of theoretical work done to date relating to nursing theory and knowledge development. We hope that such strides in development will continue over the course of the next several years. With the large numbers of young researchers entering the ranks, we look forward to exciting new theory development across the globe. We continue to urge novice researchers and theorists to "think outside the box," be fearless in trying new ideas, and, most of all, enjoy the process.

Practice Exercise

Access the three websites listed below. All three are nursing focused. Compare the similarities and differences. Which one is more comprehensive? Which one gives you the greatest understanding of what EBP is? Do any of them discuss the idea of PBE?

- The Joanna Briggs Institute (http://joannabriggs.org/)
- The ACE STAR EBP website (http://www.acestar.uthscsa.edu)
- http://libguides.ohsu.edu/ebptoolkit

References

Adashi EY, Selby JV. PCORI: What is it: How does it work? The Director explains. *Medscape One-on-One: News and Perspectives.* May 18, 2012.

An JY, Hayman LL, Panniers T, Carty B. Theory development in nursing and healthcare informatics: A model explaining and predicting information and communication technology acceptance by healthcare consumers. *Adv Nurs Sci.* 2007;30(3):E37–E49.

ANA. *Nursing Informatics: Scope and Standards of Practice.* Silver Springs, MD: American Nurses Association; 2008, 2014.

Avant KC. Developing knowledge for nursing practice: Mid-range theory and nursing diagnosis. Paper presented at the 14th Annual Meeting of the Japan Society of Nursing Diagnosis, Kyoto, Japan, July 2008.

Bakken-Henry S. Informatics: Essential infrastructure for quality assessment and improvement in nursing. *J Am Med Inform Assoc.* 1995;(2):169–182.

Berwick DM. The science of improvement. *JAMA.* 2009;299(10):1182–1184.

Bixler G, Bixler RW. The professional status of nursing. *Am J Nurs.* 1945;45:730–735.

Blegen MA, Tripp-Reimer T. Implications of nursing taxonomies for middle-range theory development. *Adv Nurs Sci.* 1997;19(3):37–49.

Brant JM, Beck S, Miaskowski C. Building dynamic models and theories to advance the science of symptom management research. *J Adv Nurs.* 2009;66(1):228–240.

Brazelton, NC, Knuckles MC, Lyons AM. Clinical documentation improvement and nursing informatics. *Comput Inform Nurs.* 2017;35(6);271–277.

Bulecheck G, Butcher J, Dochterman J, Wagner C, eds. *Nursing Interventions Classification (NIC).* 6th ed. St. Louis, MO: Elsevier; 2013.

Calvert M, Blazeby J, Altman DG, Revicki DA, Moher D, Brundage MD. Reporting of patient-reported outcomes in randomized trials: The Consort Pro extension. *JAMA.* 2013;309(8):814–822.

Clark J. Old wine in new bottles: Delivering nursing in the 21st century. *J Nurs Scholarsh.* 2000;32(1):11–15.

Cronenwett L, Sherwood G, Barnsteiner J, Disch J, Johnson J, Mitchell P, et al. Quality and safety education for nurses. *Nurs Outlook.* 2007;55(3):122–131.

Doane GH, Varcoe C. Knowledge translation in everyday nursing: From evidence-based to inquiry-based practice. *Adv Nurs Sci.* 2008;31(4):283–295.

Eisenberg JM. The effectiveness of clinical care: Is there any evidence? Plenary paper presented at ANA Council for Nursing Research Pre-conference on Research Utilization, San Diego, CA, June 1998.

Elkan R, Blair M, Robinson JJA. Evidence-based practice and health visiting: The need for theoretical underpinnings for evaluation. *J Adv Nurs.* 2000;31(6):1316–1323.

Fawcett J, Watson J, Neuman B, Walker PH, Fitzpatrick JJ. On nursing theories and evidence. *J Nurs Scholarsh.* 2001;33(2):115–119.

Fitch A, Fox C, Bauerly K, Gross A, Heim C, Judge-Dietz J, et al. *Prevention and Management of Obesity for Children and Adolescents.* Bloomington, MN: Institute for Clinical Systems Improvement; 2013.

French P. What is the evidence on evidence-based nursing? An epistemological concern. *J Adv Nurs.* 2002;37(3):250–257.

Gooch S. Management: Speaking out on violence. *Nurs Stand.* 1991;5(15):52–53.

Good M, Moore SM. Clinical practice guidelines as a new source of middle-range theory: Focus on acute pain. *Nurs Outlook.* 1996;44(2):74–79.

Goosen W. The International Nursing Minimum Data Set (J-NMDS): Why do we need it? In: Oud N, ed. *ACENDIO2002: Proceedings of the Special Conference of the Association of Common European Nursing Diagnoses, Interventions and Outcomes in Vienna.* Bern, Switzerland: Verlag Hans Huber; 2002.

Grace JT, Powers BA. Claiming our core: Appraising qualitative evidence for nursing questions about human response and meaning. *Nurs Outlook.* 2009;57:27–34.

Graves J, Corcoran S. The study of nursing informatics. *Image.* 1989;21(4):227–231.

Hannah K, Ball M, Edwards M. *Introduction to Nursing Informatics.* New York, NY: Springer-Verlag; 1994.

Heller BR, Oros MT, Durney-Crowley J. The future of nursing education: 10 trends to watch. *Nurs Health Care Perspect.* 2000;21(1):9–13.

Herdman H, Kamitsuru S, eds. *Nursing Diagnoses: Definitions and Classifications, 2018–2020.* 11th ed. New York, NY: Thieme; 2018.

Horn S, Gassaway J. Practice-based evidence study design for comparative effectiveness research. *Med Care.* 2007;45(10):S50–S57.

Institute of Medicine. *Building a Safer Health System.* Washington, DC: National Academy Press; 2000.

Institute of Medicine, Committee on Quality Health Care in America. *Crossing the Quality Chasm: A New Health System in the 21st Century.* Washington, DC: National Academy Press; 2001.

Ireson CL, Velotta CL. Accessibility to knowledge for research-based practice. In: Moorhead S, Delaney C, eds. *Information Systems Innovations for Nursing: New Visions and Ventures.* Thousand Oaks, CA: Sage Publications; 1998, pp. 94–105.

Jennings BM. Evidence-based practice: The road best traveled? *Res Nurs Health.* 2000;23:343–345.

Jennings BM, Loan LA. Misconceptions among nurses about evidence-based practice. *J Nurs Scholarsh.* 2001;33(2):121–127.

Keenan GM, Stocker JR, Geo-Thomas AT, Soparkar NR, Barkauskas VH, Lee JL. The HANDS project: Studying and refining the automated collection of cross-setting clinical data. *Comput Inform Nurs.* 2002;20(3):89–100.

Kitson A. Using evidence to demonstrate the value of nursing. *Nurs Stand.* 1997;11(28):34–39.

Kolcaba K. Evolution of the midrange theory of comfort for outcomes research. *Nurs Outlook.* 2001;49(2):86–92.

Laney D. 3D data management: Controlling data volume, velocity, and variety. *Application Delivery Strategies.* Feb.6, 2001: File 949.

Lavin MA, Harper E, Barr N. Health information technology, patient safety, and professional nursing care documentation in acute care settings. *Online J Issues Nurs.* 2015;20(2):6.

Liehr P, Smith MJ. Middle-range theory: Spinning research and practice to create knowledge for the new millennium. *Adv Nurs Sci.* 1999;21(4):81–91.

Matney S, Avant K, Staggers N. Toward an understanding of wisdom in nursing. *Online J Issues Nurs.* 2015;21(1):9.

Melnyk BM, Fineout-Overholt E, Gallagher-Ford L, Kaplan L. The state of evidence-based practice in US nurses: Critical implications for nurse leaders and educators. *JONA.* 2012;42(9):410–417.

Millenson MI. *Demanding Medical Evidence: Doctors and Accountability in the Information Age.* Chicago, IL: University of Chicago Press; 1997.

Mitchell PH, Ferketich S, Jennings BM. Quality health outcomes model. Report of the American Academy of Nursing Expert Panel. *J Nurs Scholarsh.* 1998;30(1):43–46.

Moorhead S, Johnson M, Maas M, Swanson E, eds. *Nursing Outcomes Classification.* 5th ed. St. Louis, MO: Mosby; 2013.

Nightingale F. *Notes on Hospitals.* London, England: Longman, Green, Longman, Roberts and Green; 1863, pp. 175–176.

Pearson A, Wiechula R, Court A, Lockwood C. The JBI model of evidence-based healthcare. *Int J Evid Based Healthcare.* 2005;3(8):207–215. Registered Nurses' Association of Ontario. *Assessment and Management of Pressure Injuries for the Interprofessional Team.* 3rd ed. Toronto, Ontario: Author; 2016.

Resnick MD. *Res Ipsa Loquitur:* "The thing speaks for itself" so why isn't evidence enough for enactment? *Fam Community Health Suppl 1.* 2008;31(16):S5–S14.

Retsas A. Barriers to using nursing research evidence in nursing practice. *J Adv Nurs.* 2000;3(3):599–606.

Roberts K. Evidence-based practice: An idea whose time has come. *Collegian.* 1998;5(3):24–27.

Ruland CM, Moore SM. Theory construction based on standards of care: A proposed theory of the peaceful end of life. *Nurs Outlook.* 1998;46(4):169–175.

Sackett DL, Rosenberg WMC, Gray JAM, Haynes RB, Richardson WS. Evidence-based medicine: What it is and what it isn't. *Br Med J.* 1996;312(7023):71–72.

Sampselle CM. Nickel-and-dimed in America: Underserved, understudied, and underestimated. *Fam Community Health Suppl 1.* 2007;50(15):S4–S14.

Schwartz O, Lellouch J. Explanatory and pragmatic attitudes in therapeutical trials. *J Chronic Dis.* 1967;20:637–648.

Schwartz-Barcott D, Patterson BJ, Lusardi P, Farmer BC. From practice to theory: Tightening the link via three fieldwork strategies. *J Adv Nurs.* 2002;39(3):281–289.

Shojania KG, Grimshaw JM. Evidence-based quality improvement: The state of the science. *Health Affairs.* 2005;24(1):138–150.

Smith CE, Pace K, Kochinda C, Kleinbeck SVM, Koehler J, Popkess-Vawter S. Caregiving effectiveness model evolution to a midrange theory of home care: A process for critique and replication. *Adv Nurs Sci.* 2002;25(1):50–64.

SNOMED International. SNOMED Clinical Terms. 2017.

Stevens KR. *Star Model of EBP: Knowledge Transformation.* San Antonio, TX: Academic Center for Evidence-Based Practice, The University of Texas Health Science Center at San

Antonio; 2012. Thompson C. A conceptual treadmill: The need for "middle ground" in clinical decision making theory in nursing. *J Adv Nurs.* 1999;30(5):1222–1229.

Turley JP. Toward a model for nursing informatics. *Image.* 1996;28(4):309–313.

van Achterberg T, Schoonhoven L, Grol R. Nursing implementation science: How evidence-based nursing requires evidence-based implementation. *J Nurs Scholarsh.* 2008;40(4):302–310.

Wald HL, Fink RM, Makic MB, Oman KS. Catheter-associated urinary tract infection prevention. In: Boltz M, Capezuti E, Fulmer T, Zwicker D, eds. *Evidence-Based Geriatric Nursing Protocols for Best Practice.* 4th ed. New York, NY: Springer Publishing Company; 2012, pp. 388–408.

Walker LO. Is integrative science necessary to improve nursing practice? *West J Nurs Res.* 1999;21(1):94–102.

Zerenstein M, Treweek S. What kind of randomized trials do we need? (Commentary). *Can Med Assoc J.* 2009;180(10):998–999.

Zerhouni EA. Translational and clinical science—Time for a new vision. *N Engl J Med.* 2005;353:1621–1623.

Additional Readings

Adams T. The idea of revolution in the development of nursing theory. *J Adv Nurs.* 1991;16:1487–1491.

Alpay L, Russell A. Information technology training in primary care: The nurses' voice. *Comput Inform Nurs.* 2002;20(4):136–142.

Bailey J. Reflective practice: Implementing theory. *Nurs Stand.* 1995;9(46):29–31.

Bakken-Henry S, Holzemer WL, Tallberg M, Grobe S, eds. *Informatics: The Infrastructure for Quality Assessment & Improvement in Nursing.* San Francisco, CA: UC Nursing Press; 1994.

Barker PJ, Reynolds W, Stevenson C. The human science basis of psychiatric nursing: Theory and practice. *J Adv Nurs.* 1997;25:660–667.

Bjornsdottir K. Language, research and nursing practice. *J Adv Nurs.* 2001;33(2):159–166.

Bliss-Holtz J. Using Orem's theory to generate nursing diagnoses for electronic documentation. *Nurs Sci Q.* 1996;9(3):121–125.

Bostrom I, Hall-Lord M, Larsson G, Wilde B. Nursing theory based changes of work organisation in an ICU: Effects on quality of care. *Intensive Crit Care Nurs.* 1992;8(1):10–16.

Bowles KH, Naylor MD. Nursing intervention classification systems. *Image.* 1996;28(4):303–308.

Brieskorn-Zinke M. The relevance of health sciences for nursing [in German]. *Pflege.* 1998;11(3):129–134.

Broome ME. Outcomes research: Practice counts! *J Soc Pediatr Nurses.* 1999;4(2):83–84.

Chalmers KI. Giving and receiving: An empirically derived theory on health visiting practice. *J Adv Nurs.* 1992;17:1317–1325.

Cook SH. Mind the theory/practice gap in nursing. *J Adv Nurs.* 1991;16:1462–1469.

Eldh A. Monograph review: Critical appraisal: Nursing theories in practice, education and research. *Theoria J Nurs Theory.* 2001;10(3):17–19.

Emden C. Nursing knowledge: An intriguing journey. *Aust J Adv Nurs.* 1987–1988;5(2):33–45.

Evans AM. Philosophy of nursing: Future directions. *Aust N Z J Ment Health Nurs.* 1995;4(1):14–21.

Gould D. Teaching theories and models of nursing: Implications for a common foundation programme for nurses. *Recent Adv Nurs.* 1989;(24):93–105.

Gray G, Pratt R. *Scholarship in the Discipline of Nursing.* Melbourne, Australia: Churchill Livingstone; 1995.

Gray G, Pratt R. *Towards a Discipline of Nursing.* Melbourne, Australia: Churchill Livingstone; 1991.

Greenwood J. Reflective practice: A critique of the work of Argyris and Schon. *J Adv Nurs.* 1993;18:1183–1187.

Grobe SJ. The infrastructure for quality assessment and quality improvement. In: Bakken-Henry S, Holzemer WL, Tallberg M, Grobe S, eds. *Informatics: The Infrastructure for Quality Assessment & Improvement in Nursing.* San Francisco, CA: UC Nursing Press; 1994.

Grobe SJ, Pluyter-Wenting ESP, eds. *Nursing Informatics: An International Overview for Nursing in a Technological Era.* Amsterdam, The Netherlands: Elsevier; 1994.

Hauge S. From focusing on illness to focusing on health in nursing [in Norwegian]. *Värd i Norden.* 1997;17(1):18–24.

Hopkins S, McSherry R. Debate: Is there a great divide between nursing theory and practice? *Nurs Times.* 2000;96(17):16.

Kyriacos U, van der Walt A. Attitudes of diploma-prepared and graduate registered nurses towards nursing models: A comparative study. *Curationis.* 1996;19(3):2–6.

Laschinger HK, Duff V. Attitudes of practicing nurses towards theory-based nursing practice. *Can J Nurs Adm.* 1991;4(1):6–10.

Lewis T. Leaping the chasm between nursing theory and practice. *J Adv Nurs.* 1988;13:345–351.

Matney S, Avant K, Staggers N. Toward an understanding of wisdom in nursing. *Online J Issues Nurs.* 2015;21(1):9.

Mulholland J. Assimilating sociology: Critical reflections on the "sociology in nursing" debate. *J Adv Nurs.* 1997;25:844–852.

Muller E, Reipschlager C. The drawing up of a classification system for nursing science for the University Library in Bremen—A contribution to the development of nursing as a science [in German]. *Pflege.* 1997;10(5):292–298.

Norberg A, Wickstrom E. The perception of Swedish nurses and nurse teachers of the integration of theory with nursing practice. An explorative qualitative study. *Nurse Educ Today.* 1990;10(1):38–43.

Oud N, ed. *ACENDIO 2002: Proceedings of the Special Conference of the Association of Common European Nursing Diagnoses, Interventions and Outcomes in Vienna.* Bern, Switzerland: Verlag Hans Huber; 2002.

Prowse MA, Lyne PA. Clinical effectiveness in the post-anaesthesia care unit: How nursing knowledge contributes to achieving intended patient outcomes. *J Adv Nurs.* 2000;31(5):1115–1124.

Quiquero A, Knights D, Meo CO. Theory as a guide to practice: Staff nurses choose Parse's theory. *Can J Nurs Adm.* 1991;4(1):14–16.

Scott H. More clinical skills but not at the expense of theory. *Br J Nurs.* 1999;8:910.

Smith JP. *Models, Theories, and Concepts.* London, England: Blackwell Scientific; 1994.

Smith M, Cusack L. The Ottawa Charter—From nursing theory to practice: Insights from the area of alcohol and other drugs. *Int J Nurs Pract.* 2000;6(4):168–173.

Tornstam L. Caring for the elderly: Introducing the theory of gerotranscendence as a supplementary frame of reference for caring for the elderly. *Scand J Caring Sci.* 1996;10(3):144–150.

Wang Y, Li X. Cross-cultural nursing theory and Chinese nursing today [in Chinese]. *Chin Nurs Res.* 2000;14(6):231–232.

Warren J, Hoskins L. *NANDA's Nursing Diagnosis Taxonomy: A Nursing Database.* ANA Steering Committee on Databases to Support Clinical Nursing Practice. Washington, DC: ANA Publishing; 1995.

Zielstorff RD, Hudgings CI, Grobe SJ. The National Commission on Nursing Implementation Project Task Force on Nursing Information Systems. *Next-Generation Nursing Information Systems.* Washington, DC: ANA Publishing; 1993.

3

■ ■ ■

Approaches to Theory Development

Questions to consider before you get started reading this chapter:

▶ Are you seeking some guidance on how to pull together some observations you have made about a recurring pattern you have seen in practice?

▶ Are you a graduate student who needs to develop a literature-based "framework" for a thesis or dissertation?

▶ Are you looking for a way to clarify what you see as confusion about the way terms describing a nursing problem are used in the literature or in practice?

Introductory Note: The questions above are some of the reasons nurses and others in the health field have looked for guidance or methods for developing and refining concepts, statements, and theories. Experienced researchers and theorists probably are not even aware of how they put theory together. But for novices, learning some systematic ways of examining ideas and putting relationships together allows them to practice until they find ways that work for them. Although hard thinking, careful observation, and clear definitions are the best tools of the potential theory builder, they are not always enough for the beginner. Structure is helpful when you are a novice or when you are trying a new way to examine a phenomenon. This chapter gives a brief overview of both the elements of theory and the approaches to theory construction. It includes a consideration of concepts, their role in theories, and recent criticisms of focusing on concepts in theory development. This chapter also focuses on statement formation and its role in knowledge development and theory building. In addition to focusing on these elements, the chapter also introduces the strategies of derivation, synthesis, and analysis.

INTRODUCTION

The historical review of theory development in nursing in Chapter 1 shows the key role it has played in the evolution of nursing as a scholarly discipline. In nursing practice and some areas of nursing research, however, all too often there is an absence of theory, or the theory in use fails to incorporate a nursing perspective. For example, most behavioral change theories used by nurses do not include concepts pertaining to interactions between clients and nurses or health care providers. Yet counseling done by nurses and other health care professionals may be a key aspect of behavioral changes to promote health or manage disease. In recognition of this omission, Cox (1982) developed a model of health behavior that incorporated interactions between clients and health professionals. This is one example of why theory development by nurses has been and continues to be needed to enrich practice and research. More recently, nurses have developed theories to gain understanding of emerging challenges in practice. For example, Zandi, Vanaki, Shiva, Mohammadi, and Bagheri-Lankarani (2016) developed a theoretical model for caring for women becoming mothers by surrogacy.

Clear and explicit methods of theory construction can facilitate development of concepts, statements, and theories in a nursing context. In this chapter, our basic framework for strategies of theory development is laid out. In subsequent chapters, specific strategies for constructing theory, such as concept synthesis, are described, for the most part, from the vantage point of middle-range theory. The strategies are presented with emphasis on theory construction. Readers interested in theory evaluation are referred to the works of Hardy (1978), Fawcett (2005), and Parse (2005).

We do not propose to present a set of ironclad rules for theory construction in this book. What we propose is rather a comprehensive set of strategies that can augment the intuitive processes that theorists already use in forming concepts, statements, and theories. We see strategies as guidelines for activities. As guidelines, strategies give theorists their bearings but do not remove the burden of creative work from the theorist.

Both proponents and opponents of organized approaches to theory construction exist. We, of course, believe that using explicit approaches to theory construction can facilitate development of theory. Others would argue otherwise. Opponents see theory development as a non-rule-governed activity. Successful theorizing is, for them, based on the creativity of the theorist. We agree that creativity is a key ingredient in successful theorizing. In this line, Hempel (1966, p. 15) argued that there are no rules for mechanically deriving hypotheses or theories from data. We also agree with this assertion.

Even good methods, however, cannot salvage a poor idea. In turn, slavishly following a method that is unsuitable can ruin the best of ideas. Users of this book should try to strike a realistic balance between their intuitive processes and the strategies contained herein. As guidelines, the strategies function as points of reference on a creative journey. They are markers along the way to keep the traveler reasonably on course.

To discuss theory building in a meaningful way, we must have some basic understanding among ourselves about the meanings of certain terms that will be used throughout the following chapters. This chapter is devoted to explaining these basic terms and demonstrating, in a general way, how they are related to each other. It is very important to be sure that agreement on meanings of terms is established at the beginning of our discussion. Three basic elements of theory building and three basic approaches for working with these elements will occupy our attention in this chapter.

The three elements are concepts, statements, and theories. The three approaches are derivation, synthesis, and analysis. We will demonstrate the relationship of the elements to the approaches in the "Strategy Selection" section of this chapter.

ELEMENTS OF THEORY BUILDING

Concepts

The very basis of any theory depends on the identification and explication of the concepts to be considered in it. Yet many attempts to describe, explain, or predict phenomena start without a clear understanding of what is to be described, explained, or predicted. Thus, sound concept development is a critical task in any effort to develop theory. As noted by Hardy (1974), concepts are the basic building blocks of theory, and we will comment on critiques of this idea at the end of this section. A **concept** is a mental image of a phenomenon, an idea, or a construct in the mind about a thing or an action. It is not the thing or action, only the image of it (Kaplan, 1964). Concept formation begins in infancy, for concepts help us categorize or organize our environmental stimuli. Concepts help us identify how our experiences are similar or equivalent by categorizing all the things that are alike about them. Concept formation is thus a very efficient way of learning.

Concepts have different levels of abstractness (Reynolds, 1971). **Primitive concepts** are those that have a common shared meaning among all individuals in a culture. For instance, a primitive concept like the color blue cannot be defined other than by giving examples of blue and not blue. **Concrete concepts** are those that can be defined by primitive concepts, are limited by time and space, and are observable. **Abstract concepts** are also capable of being defined by primitive or concrete concepts, but they are independent of time and space (Reynolds, 1971). The concept of temperature, for instance, is abstract, whereas the concept of "temperature today in Kansas City" is concrete because it is dependent on a specific place and time.

Language is the means by which we express a concept. The language names (terms or words) we use to express concepts are useful in communicating our ideas to other people. These names or terms are *not* the concepts themselves but are only our way of communicating the concepts. Thus, the names or terms may be found to be adequate or inadequate at times when we are attempting to get someone to understand our ideas or are trying to define something completely new. If the name or term we are using to attempt to define our concept is inadequate, we may need to refine or change the name, but the concept itself remains the same.

Some authors and researchers use the terms *concept* and *variable* interchangeably. When concepts are defined operationally, that is, the definitions contain within them the means of measuring the concepts, they can be considered variables for the purposes of research. Nevertheless, in the context of discussions about theory development, ideas and their names remain concepts.

Concepts allow us to classify our experiences in a meaningful way both to ourselves and to others. Classifying experiences is a very useful and efficient ability. The ability to express a relationship between two or more concepts is even more useful and efficient.

Despite usefulness of clear concepts in communication, the idea that concepts are the basic building blocks of theory has been criticized. According to Bergdahl and Berterö (2016), "concepts are not the building blocks of theory" (p. 2559). In making this assertion, they frame much of their argument based on philosophical analyses pertaining to advanced natural sciences, not practice disciplines like nursing. Because nursing is a discipline with knowledge and theoretical development aimed at under-standing and enhancing the multiple dimensions of the nursing care process, we argue that it is important to consider concepts in this larger view, and not simply from one of the natural sciences. This larger view is reflected in the work of the philosophers Dickoff, James, and Wiedenbach (1968), who postulated a number of levels of theory for nursing practice, including factor-isolating, factor-relating, situation-relating, and situation-producing or prescriptive theory. Some of these forms of theory parallel those of traditional non-practice disciplines and some do not.

It is this wider view within which the place and value of concepts may be under-stood in nursing. In the applied field of forestry, for example, taxonomic work involving species classification (i.e., conceptually distinguishing species) has been described as "essential for the fundamental understanding of biodiversity and its conservation" (Sunderland, 2012, para. 1). For the African rattan species, "Taxonomic work of this kind is not purely an academic exercise . . . [It] is an essential basis for the conservation, development and management of the resource itself" (Sunderland, para. 6). Thus, even in sciences dealing with the physical world from an applied perspective, concepts that distinguish among physical phenomena are important. Similarly, we would argue that concepts that delineate the phenomena of nursing care and nursing practice are essential for providing, documenting, communicating about, and studying care processes.

Statements

A statement is the result of expressing such a relationship among concepts. Developing statements is an important aspect of theory development. Laws and empirical general-izations, both being forms of scientific statements, supply much of the working back-bone of science. In a practice discipline, many of the diagnoses, interventions, or outcomes of practice may be based on such scientific statements. For example, Yeh (2002) hypothesized that there would be gender differences in the levels of stress and psychological distress experienced by parents whose children had cancer. Mothers in her study showed significantly higher scores on both stress and distress than did fathers. Yeh suggests that appropriate counseling and other interventions may be dif-ferent for fathers and mothers. Thus, for practice, statement development can be a very important and useful level of theory development. It is especially relevant when a theorist wishes to go beyond the concept (naming) phase but does not need the com-prehensive perspectives offered by a theory.

Thus, in any attempt to build a scientific body of knowledge, a **statement** is an extremely important ingredient. It must be formulated before explanations or predictions can be made. A statement, in the context of theory building, can occur in two forms, rela-tional statements and nonrelational statements. A **relational statement** declares a rela-tionship of some kind between two or more concepts. A **nonrelational statement** may be either an existence statement that asserts the existence of the concept (Reynolds, 1971) or a definition, either theoretical or operational.

Relational statements assert either association (correlation) or causality (Reynolds, 1971). Associational statements are simply those that state which concepts occur together. They may even state the direction of the association between concepts, for example, positive, negative, or none. A positive association implies that as one concept occurs or changes, the other concept occurs or changes in the same direction. For example, a positive association is demonstrated by the statement, "Palmar sweating increases as anxiety increases." A negative association implies that as one concept occurs or changes, the other concept occurs or changes in the opposite direction. For example, the statement "As anxiety increases, concentration decreases" is a negative association. The "none" relationship implies that the occurrence of one concept tells us nothing about the occurrence of the other concept.

Causal statements demonstrate a cause-and-effect relationship. The concept that causes the change in the other concept may be referred to in research as the independent variable and the concept that is changed or affected, the dependent variable. An example of a causal statement might be, "The application of undiluted bleach (NaOH) to a colored cotton cloth will cause the color in the cloth to fade."

Adjuncts to relational statements are nonrelational statements. Nonrelational statements are the way by which the theorist clarifies meanings in the theory. **Existence statements** are usually simple statements of assertion about a concept. They are especially useful when the theorist is dealing with highly abstract material. For instance, the assertion "There is a phenomenon known as maternal attachment" is an existence statement. If little was known about the existence of such a phenomenon, it would be helpful to a reader for the theorist to name his or her concept and claim its existence as a starting place in the theory.

The means by which the theorist introduces the reader to the critical defining attributes of each concept is by using theoretical **definitions**. These definitions are usually abstract and may not be measurable. Operational definitions reflect the theoretical definitions, but they must have the measurement specifications included (Hardy, 1974). Theoretical and operational definitions are critical in theory building. Without them, there is no way to test and thus validate the theory in the real world.

Theories

Well-formulated theories provide an integrative understanding of phenomena by systematically organizing relevant concepts and statements. Thus, the generally accepted definition of a **theory** is an internally consistent group of relational statements that presents a systematic view about a phenomenon and that is useful for description, explanation, prediction, and prescription or control. Associated with the theory may be a set of definitions that are specific to concepts in the theory. Theory is usually constructed to express a new idea or a new insight into the nature of a phenomenon of interest. A theory, by virtue of its predictive and prescriptive potential, is the primary means of meeting the goals of the nursing profession concerned with a clearly defined body of knowledge (Meleis, 1997). That knowledge is a vital component in the human decision-making process involved in evidence-based clinical care and policy formation. Some authors have disagreed with the notion of prescription and control as valid purposes of theory in nursing positing that these contravene the holistic and humanistic nature of nursing. We continue to believe that these two functions of theory are still valid in a world where evidence-based practice is a prevailing paradigm in practice. However, we also believe that just because scientific theories may permit prediction or control of certain phenomena through relations posited, it does not follow that those theories provide sufficient grounds for using that knowledge as a means of control. It is human judgments about the goals, obligations, and rights of those with whom and for whom care is planned that are the final bases for nurses' use of theory in practice situations.

Description, explanation, prediction, and prescription represent different phases of theory development. The ideal theory would do all these things well and simultaneously. However, there is rarely, if ever, such a thing as an ideal theory in any discipline—one that accomplishes all four functions at the same time. Because science is evolutionary and because the human organism is intrinsically fallible, theories are always changing. At any point in time, theories in a discipline may be found at all stages of development. Some theories are specifically designed as explanations, such as the theory of evolution, without any intention of predictability. Others are designed specifically to yield predictability but do not provide prescription or control. Indeed, there are times when prescription or control might be impossible or unethical. For example, major earthquakes can be predicted but not yet controlled and, one hopes, never prescribed. We ought not to despair at this apparently imperfect world of theory building. Scientific thought grows through a self-correcting process. The submission of one's ideas to the critique and analysis of one's colleagues leads to a phenomenon of revision, validation, and extension of any given theory.

The graphic representation of a theory is called a model. As Baltes, Reese, and Nesselroade have noted, a model is "any device used to represent something other than itself" (1977, p. 17). The parts of a model should correspond to, or be isomorphic to, the parts of the theory they represent (Brodbeck, 1968, p. 583). A model may be drawn mathematically, as an equation, for instance, or it may be drawn schematically using symbols and arrows. A mathematical model might look something like this:

$$Y = {}_{a1}X^{(1)} + {}_{a2}X^{(2)} + {}_{a3}X^{(3)} + E$$

In this equation, Y represents a dependent criterion variable, X represents an independent (predictor) variable, each a represents the mathematical weighting applied to the respective Xs, and E represents an error term (unexplained variance). A schematic model might look more like Figure 3–1.

In Figure 3–1, the boxes represent different concepts A, B, C, and D. The arrows in the model represent the direction of the relationships (concept A is related to concept B). The + or − over the arrows represents the valence of the relationship (concept A

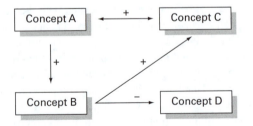

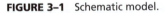

FIGURE 3–1   Schematic model.

is positively related to concept B). Models can be developed either pretheoretically or posttheoretically. The pretheoretical model acts either as a heuristic device or as an attempt by the theorist to discover missing linkages in early theorizing. The posttheoretical model is developed after the theory to lay bare the internal and formal structure of the theory—the system of interrelationships among the concepts.

For the purposes of this book, the term *model* will be used only in its mathematical or schematic sense. This stipulated usage of *model* is necessary to quantify and clarify the relationships between concepts in any theoretical discussions in this book. In some nursing literature, however, *model* may be given a specialized meaning: "the image of the entire field and concepts of all its major units—the goal, patiency, and so forth" (Riehl & Roy, 1980, p. 7). In selected nursing literature, the term *model* is reserved for what we have called the "grand theories." For further clarification of levels and types of models, see "Additional Readings" at the end of this chapter.

INTERRELATEDNESS OF ELEMENTS

Theory development may begin at the level of concepts and statements. For example, in the simplified, complete process of theory development, a theorist might start with concept development. As this is accomplished, the goals of statement development and ultimately theory development would be pursued. For example, in their development of a theory of patient advocacy, Bu and Jezewski (2007) began at the concept level (using concept analysis to be described later in this chapter) and progressed to the middle-range theory level.

Only when one has a unified account of a set of relationships, as theories provide, can the goals of description, explanation, and/or prediction in science be achieved (Hempel, 1966). Theories, of course, need to be tested or validated through research and practice. Testing may in turn highlight areas within theories where revision is needed. At this point, the process of theory development is begun again. These phases of theory development are graphically shown in Figure 3–2. Thus, theory

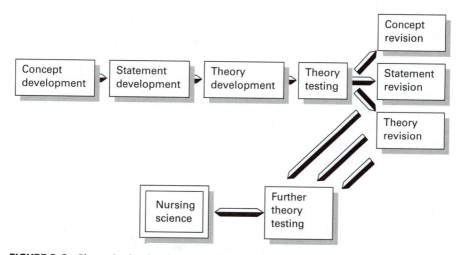

FIGURE 3–2   Phases in the development of nursing science.

development, research, and practice are part of the larger process of the scientific development of a discipline, not separate processes that are ends in themselves. Whereas this book will focus on theory development, readers should keep in mind the interdependence of theory with research and practice. As we have discussed in Chapter 2, none is complete without the others in interrelationship.

APPROACHES TO THEORY BUILDING

Derivation, synthesis, and analysis are the three basic approaches to theory building we use in this book. A theory builder may move back and forth among these approaches; however, we will present them separately to aid the beginner in getting a better picture of each one.

Derivation

Analogy or metaphor is the basis of **derivation**. Derivation allows the theorist to transpose and redefine a concept, statement, or theory from one context or field to another. Our strategy of derivation is heavily influenced by the work of Maccia and Maccia (1966) on educational theory models. This approach to theory building can be applied to areas in which no theory base exists. Derivation may also be used in fields in which existing theories have become outmoded and new, innovative perspectives are needed. Derivation provides a means of theory building through shifting the terminology or the structure from one field or context to another. For example, one might take a concept from chemistry, such as chemical equilibrium, and, by analogy, use it to derive a description of how information exchange occurs within a group of professionals.

Synthesis

In synthesis, information based on observation is used to construct a new concept, a new statement, or a new theory. Synthesis allows the theorist to combine isolated pieces of information that are, as yet, theoretically unconnected (Bloom, 1956, p. 206). Synthesis works well where a theorist is collecting data or trying to interpret data without an explicit theoretical framework. Much descriptive clinical research consists of collecting large amounts of data in the hope of sifting out important factors and relationships. Synthesis can aid in this sifting process. For example, nurses in school settings might use academic and family information to try to identify factors associated with teenage drug abuse or pregnancy. A researcher might use synthesis to name the clusters in a factor structure or to name the themes in a qualitative data analysis. As data mining of large databases has become one of the informatics procedures for producing practice-based evidence (Horn & Gassaway, 2007), synthesis will be the primary strategy needed to make sense of the data mined.

Analysis

Using **analysis** allows the theorist to dissect a whole into its component parts so that they can be better understood (Bloom, 1956, p. 205). As Newman has so elegantly put it (Newman, Smith, Pharris, & Jones, 2008), it is often through the part that the whole can be encountered. Thus, in analysis the theorist examines the relationship of each of the parts to each of the other parts and to the whole. Analysis is especially useful in areas in which there is an existing body of theoretical literature. Analysis allows one to clarify, refine, or sharpen concepts, statements, or theories. Analysis allows the theorist to examine and reexamine existing knowledge about phenomena, as a means to improve the accuracy, currency, or relevance of the knowledge.

STRATEGY SELECTION

We have superimposed the three approaches to theory building over the three elements of theory. Nine *strategies* for theory building result from this cross-classification of elements and approaches. The strategies and their specific uses in theory building are presented in Table 3–1. By carefully determining the elements of theory desired and the nature of available literature and information on a topic, the theorist may use Table 3–1 as a guide to strategy selection. To determine a suitable theory-building strategy, first of all, the theory builder must be clear about his or her area of interest. Next, a theorist must decide whether to focus on concepts, statements, or the overall

TABLE 3–1   Strategies of Theory Building Resulting from Cross-Classification of Elements of Theory with Approaches to Theory Building

| Elements of Theory | Approaches to Theory Building | | |
	Derivation	Synthesis	Analysis
Concept	Strategy: Concept derivation (Chapter 4)	Strategy: Concept synthesis (Chapter 7)	Strategy: Concept analysis (Chapter 10)
	Use: To shift and redefine concept(s) from one field to another.	Use: To extract or pull together concept(s) from a body of data or set of observations.	Use: To clarify or redefine an existing concept.
Statement	Strategy: Statement derivation (Chapter 5)	Strategy: Statement synthesis (Chapter 8)	Strategy: Statement analysis (Chapter 11)
	Use: To shift and reformulate the content or structure of statements from one field to another.	Use: To extract or pull together one or more statements from a body of data or set of observations.	Use: To clarify or refine an existing body of statements.
Theory	Strategy: Theory derivation (Chapter 6)	Strategy: Theory synthesis (Chapter 9)	Strategy: Theory analysis (Chapter 12)
	Use: To shift and reformulate the content or structure of theories from one field to another.	Use: To pull together a theory from a body of data, set of observations, or set of empirical statements.	Use: To clarify or refine an existing theory.

theory. This will depend on the quality of concept, statement, and theory development that already exists in the area of interest. To determine which element best fits their needs, theorists may ask themselves several questions.

1. What is the existing extent of theory development on the topic of interest?
2. How adequate is the existing theory development?
3. In which element is the available theory the weakest: concepts, statements, or the overall theory?
4. What do review articles suggest about the kind of theory development needed next on the topic?
5. What is my personal judgment about the element of theory development that would be the most productive for me to pursue now on my topic of interest?

Carefully consider these questions. Your answers should help you clarify where you should begin theory building: with concepts, statements, or the whole theory.

Selecting the approach to be used depends a lot on the extent and type of literature and data available on a topic. Here the theorist may ask another set of questions.

1. Is there any existing literature on the topic?
2. If literature exists, is it research based or purely speculative (untested)?
3. Is the literature tied together by any common conceptual or theoretical frameworks?
4. What do "state of the art/science" articles suggest about the adequacy of existing theoretical work on the topic? Are new perspectives, organization, or refinement needed?
5. What types of information or data do I have direct access to: clinical observations, field notes, computerized data files, de-identified electronic patient data?
6. What unique resources do I, as theory builder, have access to that would facilitate my theory-building efforts: extensive library collection, computer facilities, access to several databases, or clinical research projects with ready access to subjects?
7. What is my personal judgment about the approach to theory building that would be the most productive for me to pursue now on my topic of interest?

Carefully examine your answers to these questions. Although more than one approach may be possible, the approach that is the most workable overall should get your first consideration. If the first choice becomes unsatisfactory at a later date, an alternative approach may be considered. It is also possible that simultaneously using two or more strategies may be helpful.

By putting together the decision about the element of theory and the approach most suited to the topic of interest, the choice of a specific strategy for theory building should be clear. For example, assume that "hopelessness" is a topic of interest that showed a need for further work at the concept level to differentiate it from the concept of "depression." Moreover, assume that analysis appeared best suited for dealing with the extensive literature on this concept (Dunn, 2005). Concept analysis would then be a reasonable strategy for further theory building on hopelessness.

Each of the strategies is described more fully in the subsequent chapters. One of these strategies, concept analysis, has been a subject of debate, and we address that debate in Chapter 10.

INTERRELATEDNESS OF STRATEGIES

Limiting yourself to only one approach or strategy may not be conducive to successful theory development. As a theory is being constructed, using one strategy may lead you directly to a second strategy that further develops the new theory. We have proposed nine strategies here: concept, statement, and theory derivation; concept, statement, and theory synthesis; and concept, statement, and theory analysis. These nine are not all inclusive of the possible strategies available for use, although they are inherent within most of them (see classic approaches to theory development in Aldous [1970], Burr [1973], Hage [1972], and Zetterberg [1965]). They are our conception of the best strategies to use in nursing theory development in its present state.

No one strategy is going to supply all the needs for theory construction that may arise within one's purview or indeed within the discipline. The theorist will need to determine what the current status of the knowledge base is before selecting a strategy to use. Once the strategy is selected, it should be used until it fails to yield additional information about the topic of interest. When the limits of one strategy are reached, it is time to turn to another strategy. For example, the sequential use of different strategies in the evolution of a theory is exemplified in the development of the theory of unpleasant symptoms (Lenz, Suppe, Gift, Pugh, & Milligan, 1995) and in the theory of wisdom in practice (Matney, Avant, & Staggers, 2015).

Theory building is iterative. That is, the theorist must continue to use and repeat strategies until the level of desired sophistication in the theory is reached. Hanson (1958) called this iterative process "retroduction." He described the process as using both induction and deduction sequentially to arrive at an adequate theoretical formulation. In effect, Hanson proposed that first the theorist identify several propositions that are fairly specific and induce from them one more general proposition. The second phase of retroduction is to use the new proposition to deduce some new, more specific propositions. This process adds considerably to the body of theoretical knowledge. It is, in fact, the way theory develops in the real world.

We have not attempted to classify these strategies as either inductive or deductive. It seems to us that the only pure inductive strategies are the synthesis ones because they are clearly data based. The other strategies, derivation and analysis, may involve theorizing both inductively and deductively. Although it may seem to some that we emphasize quantitative methods in our approach to theory development, that is not the case. Many of these strategies are distinctly qualitative in nature and involve creative judgment and, in many cases, require retroductive thinking. We have preferred to de-emphasize the notions of induction and deduction in the strategy chapters, however, in order to keep the strategies as clear and practical as possible. The idea of retroduction makes a great deal more sense to us given the state of the art and the nature of theory in nursing. Similarly, distinctions between qualitative and quantitative methods, while useful in some situations (e.g., see Chapters 7 and 8 on concept synthesis and statement synthesis, respectively), are not our main focus.

Perhaps using some examples here might demonstrate how the strategies can be used interdependently. Let us assume that a theorist reads an article that presents a new theory. A theory analysis helps the theorist understand that the concepts in the theory do not have any operational definitions. The theorist decides to use concept analysis to develop better operational definitions. While using these two analysis strategies, the theorist begins to see possibilities for new relationships among some of the concepts. When he finally decides to formulate statements reflecting those new relationships, the statement synthesis strategy is used.

A second example might be a doctoral student who, during his/her studies, begins developing a concept he/she hopes to use in his/her dissertation. The beginning interest in the concept occurred during the student's clinical practice. After several small field studies, the concept was synthesized. Later, when other concepts needed to be linked to the new one, a statement derivation strategy was used to provide an appropriate structure for the concepts. Finally, after the student graduated, a theory synthesis strategy was ultimately completed. Another theorist, reading the student's discussion of the theory, decided to use it in another discipline, and so theory derivation was used.

A final real-world example is from the Lenz et al. (1995) study mentioned above. Working separately, Pugh and Milligan investigated fatigue in the intrapartum and postpartum periods, respectively. Pugh's study was deductive. Milligan's study was inductive. In discussions, they began to realize that there were many similarities in the two phenomena. They subsequently synthesized the two sets of data plus data from the literature to develop a single framework for studying fatigue in childbearing. In the meantime, Gift and Cahill (Lenz et al., 1995) were studying dyspnea in chronic obstructive pulmonary disease (COPD). Dyspnea and fatigue were found to coexist. Realizing that there was analogic similarity between the concepts of fatigue in childbearing and fatigue in COPD, the investigators analyzed their conceptualizations of fatigue and systematically compared the similarities and differences. Subsequently, after considerable work, they were able to synthesize a theory of unpleasant symptoms from the three data sets, their analyses, and their combined reviews of literature. Thus, in the development of the theory of unpleasant symptoms, all three approaches to theory development were used—synthesis, derivation, and analysis.

As you can see from this example, each strategy stands alone, and yet each is interdependent with the others. Each strategy provides the theorist with unique information, and yet all of them yield productive ideas for further theory development.

The hallmark of successful theorists is that they allow themselves the freedom to play with ideas or strategies until those ideas or strategies fit the needs of the theorist. As you work with the various strategies, you will become more comfortable with their use. You may even modify some of them or develop new strategies for your theory construction repertoire.

Summary

In this chapter, we have dealt with the elements, approaches, and strategies of theory building. The elements of a theory are concepts, statements, and theories. Derivation, synthesis, and analysis are the approaches to theory building. By combining the elements with the approaches, we have constructed a nine-cell matrix of theory-building strategies. Multiple strategies may often be employed before the theory development process is complete.

References

Aldous J. Strategies for developing family theory. *J Marriage Fam.* 1970;32:250–257.

Baltes PB, Reese HW, Nesselroade JR. *Life-Span Developmental Psychology: Introduction to Research Methods.* Monterey, CA: Brooks/Cole; 1977.

Bergdahl E, Berterö CM. Concept analysis and the building blocks of theory: Misconceptions regarding theory development. *J Adv Nurs.* 2016;72(10):2558–2566.

Bloom BS, ed. *Taxonomy of Educational Objectives. Handbook 1: Cognitive Domain.* New York, NY: McKay; 1956.

Brodbeck M. Models, meaning, and theories. In: Brodbeck M, ed. *Readings in the Philosophy of the Social Sciences.* New York, NY: Macmillan; 1968, pp. 597–600.

Bu X, Jezewski MA. Developing a mid-range theory of patient advocacy through concept analysis. *J Adv Nurs.* 2007;57(1):101–110.

Burr JW. *Theory Construction in Sociology of the Family.* New York, NY: Wiley; 1973.

Cox CL. An interaction model of client health behavior: Theoretical prescription for nursing. *Adv Nurs Sci.* 1982;5(1):41–56.

Dickoff J, James P, Wiedenbach E. Theory in a practice discipline, part I. *Nurs Res.* 1968;17:415–435.

Dunn SL. Hopelessness as a response to physical illness. *J Nurs Scholarsh.* 2005;37(2):148–154.

Fawcett J. Criteria for evaluation of theory. *Nurs Sci Q.* 2005;18:131–135.

Hage J. *Techniques and Problems of Theory Construction in Sociology.* New York, NY: Wiley; 1972.

Hanson NR. *Patterns of Discovery.* Cambridge, England: Cambridge University Press; 1958.

Hardy ME. Theories: Components, development, evaluation. *Nurs Res.* 1974;23:100–107.

Hardy ME. Perspectives on nursing theory. *Adv Nurs Sci.* 1978;1(1):37–48.

Hempel CG. *Philosophy of Natural Science.* Englewood Cliffs, NJ: Prentice Hall; 1966.

Horn SD, Gassaway J. Practice based evidence design for comparative effectiveness research. *Med Care.* 2007;45(10):S50–S57.

Kaplan A. *The Conduct of Inquiry.* San Francisco, CA: Chandler; 1964.

Lenz ER, Suppe F, Gift AG, Pugh LC, Milligan RA. Collaborative development of middle-range nursing theories: Toward a theory of unpleasant symptoms. *Adv Nurs Sci.* 1995;17(3):1–13.

Maccia ES, Maccia GS. *Development of Educational Theory Derived from Three Educational Theory Models.* Project No. 5-0638. Columbus, OH: Ohio State University; 1966.

Matney SA, Avant K, Staggers N. Toward an understanding of wisdom in nursing. *Online J Issues Nurs.* 2015;21(1):9.

Meleis AI. Theoretical nursing: Definitions and interpretations. In: King I, Fawcett J, eds. *The Language of Nursing Theory and Metatheory.* Indianapolis, IN: Sigma Theta Tau Honor Society in Nursing; 1997.

Newman M, Smith M, Pharris M, Jones D. The focus of the discipline revisited. *Adv Nurs Sci.* 2008;31(1):E16–E27.

Parse RR. Parse's criteria for evaluation of theory with a comparison of Fawcett's and Parse's approaches. *Nurs Sci Q.* 2005;18:135–137.

Reynolds P. *A Primer in Theory Construction.* Indianapolis, IN: Bobbs-Merrill; 1971.

Riehl JP, Roy C. Theory and models. In: Riehl JP, Roy C, eds. *Conceptual Models for Nursing Practice.* 2nd ed. New York, NY: Appleton-Century-Crofts; 1980.

Sunderland T. Why taxonomy is important for biodiversity-based science. *Forest News.* 2012. Accessed at http://blog.cifor.org/8746/why-taxonomy-is-important-for-biodiversity-based-science?fnl=en

Yeh C. Gender differences of parental distress in children with cancer. *J Adv Nurs.* 2002;38(6):598–606.

Zandi M, Vanaki Z, Shiva M, Mohammadi E, Bagheri-Lankarani N. Security giving in surrogacy motherhood process as a caring model for commissioning mothers: A theory synthesis. *Jpn J Nurs Sci.* 2016;13(3):331–344.

Zetterberg HL. *On Theory and Verification in Sociology.* Totowa, NJ: Bedminster Press; 1965.

Additional Readings

Readers who wish to do additional reading about theory and approaches to theory development may find the sources below, many of which are classics, to be of interest. (An asterisk indicates a reference for the advanced reader.)

*Blalock HM. *Theory Construction: From Verbal to Mathematical Formulations.* Englewood Cliffs, NJ: Prentice Hall; 1969.

*Broudy H, Ennis R, Krimerman L, eds. *The Philosophy of Educational Research.* New York, NY: Wiley; 1973.

Chinn PL, ed. *Advances in Nursing Theory Development.* Rockville, MD: Aspen; 1983.

Chinn PL, Kramer MK. *Integrated Theory and Knowledge Development in Nursing.* 7th ed. St. Louis, MO: Mosby; 2008.

Dubin R. *Theory Building.* 2nd ed. New York, NY: Free Press; 1978.

Fawcett J. The relationship between theory and research: A double helix. *Adv Nurs Sci.* 1978;1(1):49–62.

Fawcett J. A framework for analysis and evaluation of conceptual models of nursing. *Nurs Educ.* 1980;5:10–14.

Hardy ME. Perspectives on knowledge and role theory. In: Hardy ME, Conway ME, eds. *Role Theory.* New York, NY: Appleton-Century-Crofts; 1978:1–15.

Jacox A. Theory construction in nursing: An overview. *Nurs Res.* 1974;23:4–13.

King I, Fawcett J. *The Language of Theory and Metatheory.* Indianapolis, IN: Sigma Theta Tau International Honor Society of Nursing; 1997.

*Kuhn TS. *The Structure of Scientific Revolutions.* 2nd ed. Chicago, IL: University of Chicago; 1970.

*Lakatos I, Musgrave A, eds. *Criticism and the Growth of Knowledge.* Cambridge, England: Cambridge University Press; 1970.

Meleis AI. *Theoretical Nursing: Development and Progress.* 5th ed. Philadelphia, PA: Lippincott Williams & Wilkins; 2012.

Newman M. *Theory Development in Nursing.* Philadelphia, PA: Davis; 1979.

Newman MA. *Health as Expanding Consciousness.* 2nd ed. New York, NY: National League for Nursing; 1994.

Suppe F. *The Semantic Conception of Theories and Scientific Realism.* Urbana, IL: University of Illinois Press; 1989.

Suppe F, Jacox AK. Philosophy of science and the development of nursing theory. In: Werley HH, Fitzpatrick JJ, eds. *Annual Review of Nursing Research.* 1985;3:241–267.

Wallace WL. *The Logic of Science in Sociology.* Chicago, IL: Aldine-Atherton; 1971.

PART

2

Derivation
Strategies

This part presents an approach to developing concepts, statements, and theories using the strategies of derivation. These strategies facilitate development of new concepts, statements, or theories. As a group, they may be well suited to situations where theoretical work does not yet exist or where it is outmoded. For the derivation strategies, we draw on the insightful methodological work of Elizabeth Maccia and her colleagues (Maccia, 1963; Maccia & Maccia, 1963), but we place that work in a nursing context. At the heart of the derivation approach is the use of analogy to foster a new way of thinking about a phenomenon—whether at the level of concept, statement, or theory. Seeing that the phenomenon of interest is like something already known may come in a flash. Aha! In each chapter, we present the mechanics of derivation at its respective levels of concept, statement, and theory to make explicit how theoretical work on one domain of scholarship may serve as a vehicle for generating theoretical work in yet another domain.

Use of a derivation strategy, such as concept derivation, is always done for a purpose. Newly coined concepts enable us to point to previously unrecognized or poorly understood events. For example, when it was introduced, the concept of "social capital" drew attention to resources and clout that certain individuals possessed that enhanced their connections with others (Coleman, 1988). By contrast, individuals lacking in social capital were seen as isolated from resources and connections that might be especially important, for example, in overcoming socially conditioned barriers to health and well-being. Although the derivation of the concept of social capital from the parent (source) concept of *capital* in the field of finance and economics is readily apparent, in many cases of concept derivation the formal explication of the derivation is omitted. As a result, if one judges by formal citations in the nursing literature, concept derivation and the related strategies of statement and theory derivation appear to be among the lesser-used strategies in nursing theory development. Nonetheless, informal use of derivation is no doubt more widespread.

Careful concept, statement, and theory development is the basis of any attempt to describe or explain phenomena. It is also prerequisite to any adequate theory. In general, use of derivation may be useful when a theorist has some familiarity with an area of interest at the practice level, but deems that there is a paucity of language to represent the phenomenon in practice or scientific discourse. If you are trying to determine whether the derivation approach is suited to the phenomenon you are seeking to describe or explain, it might help to consider several questions such as those listed in the "Strategy Selection" section in Chapter 3. Appraising issues such as the level of theory development, the type of available literature, and the direction of the literature in the focal area of interest will help you determine whether use of a derivation approach is suitable for your project.

On the other hand, if you have already determined that derivation is an appropriate approach, then take some time to reflect on whether your goal is to

- propose one or more concepts about phenomena that you want to study in more depth,
- link two or more concepts in statements, or
- construct a more comprehensive and theoretical picture of a phenomenon.

Depending on your goal, you may focus on concept (see Chapter 4), statement (see Chapter 5), or theory derivation (see Chapter 6), respectively.

REFERENCES

Coleman JS. Social capital in the creation of human capital. *Am J Sociol.* 1988;94:S95–S120.

Maccia ES. Ways of inquiring. In: Maccia ES, Maccia GS, Jewett RS, eds. *Construction of Educational Theory Models.* Cooperative Research Project No. 1632. Washington, DC: Office of Education, U.S. Department of Health, Education, and Welfare; 1963, pp. 1–13.

Maccia ES, Maccia GS. The way of educational theorizing through models. In: Maccia ES, Maccia GS, Jewett RE, eds. *Construction of Educational Theory Models.* Cooperative Research Project No. 1632. Washington, DC: Office of Education, U.S. Department of Health, Education, and Welfare; 1963, pp. 30–45.

4

■ ■ ■

Concept Derivation

Questions to consider before you get started reading this chapter:

▶ Are you interested in finding a way to express a new idea about a research problem or clinical phenomenon?

▶ Are you interested in looking outside your own field of study to see how others may have expressed similar ideas?

Introductory Note: Reasoning by analogy or metaphor is a powerful experience during creative work. It is commonplace when trying to express novel ideas to look to other areas of inquiry for insight and inspiration. In presenting this chapter on concept derivation, we attempt to give the reader some explicit guidance in how to derive concepts that may enrich their theorizing within practice, teaching, or research. Readers are encouraged to read Chapters 4, 5, and 6 in tandem in order to grasp the overall derivation process.

DEFINITION AND DESCRIPTION

The basis of concept derivation lies in an analogy between phenomena in two fields or areas of inquiry. The process of concept derivation builds on the earlier work of Maccia (1963) and Maccia and Maccia (1963). By looking to a defined *source* or *parent field* for an analog to aid in developing a new field of interest, concepts in the new field may be derived. Further, by redefining concepts from the parent field to fit the new field, a new set of concepts is created. Thus, the newly defined concepts no longer rely on the parent field for meaning. The parent field may reside either within the broader discipline of nursing or in other disciplines.

The strategy of concept derivation is applicable where a meaningful analogy can be made between one field that is conceptually defined and another that is not. Expressed more precisely, concept derivation consists of moving a concept (*Concept* 1) from one field of inquiry (*Field* 1) to another field (*Field* 2). In the process of transposing a concept, it is necessary that the concept (*Concept* 1) be redefined as a new concept (*Concept* 2) that fits the new field of inquiry (*Field* 2). This process is diagrammed in Figure 4–1. Thus, *Concept* 1 leads to *Concept* 2, but *Field* 1 and *Field* 2 are *not* the same. Redefinition of *Concept* 1 results in a concept (*Concept* 2) that is based on but different from *Concept* 1. (Note that the concept redefinitions in the

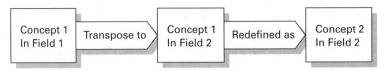

FIGURE 4–1   Process of concept derivation.

strategy of concept derivation are usually at the theoretical level and not to be confused with operationally defining concepts in a research study.)

At first glance, concept derivation might appear to be a mechanical process. Nonetheless, creativity and imagination are required. First of all, a theorist must select a parent field (*Field* 1) with concepts that bear an analogy to the new field or area of inquiry. To grasp the analogous nature of the two fields may require first taking the time for immersion in the potential parent field of inquiry. In some cases, concepts from the natural sciences have been extended into the social and behavioral sciences. For example, concepts such as "system" from biology and "energy" from physics (the source or parent fields) are common in both the social and behavioral sciences and nursing (fields using the derived concepts). There is no rule, however, about where one may find a rich conceptual perspective for concept derivation. Insight of the theorist is needed.

Creativity and imagination are needed for a second reason: meaningful redefinition of the concepts when they are transposed into the new field of inquiry. Redefining is more than merely assigning a slightly modified definition to a word. The type of redefinition that occurs in productive concept derivation requires that the derived concepts be linked to the new field (*Field* 2) by definitions that result in truly innovative ways of looking at phenomena in *Field* 2. One of the most productive uses of concept derivation results when a new taxonomy or typology of phenomena in *Field* 2 is derived. A new taxonomy or typology provides not only a new vocabulary for classifying phenomena in *Field* 2 but, more importantly, new ways of looking at *Field* 2. The theoretical work of Roy and Roberts (1981, p. 55) provides a classic example of a typology introduced into nursing. Using Helson's concepts of focal, contextual, and residual stimuli from psychophysics, Roy redefined these concepts within nursing to form a typology of factors related to adaptation levels of persons (pp. 53–55). This derivation process is presented in Figure 4–2.

Concept derivation is more than simply applying a concept in unchanged form to a phenomenon where it has not been previously used. The meaning of the concept must be

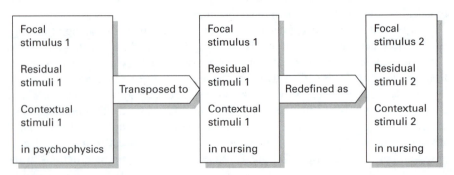

FIGURE 4–2   Concept derivation from Helson's to Roy's concepts.

developed and changed to fit a new phenomenon. For example, assume that the concept "role change" has not been previously applied to the transition from in-hospital patient to outpatient status. Assume further that role change may be applied to the transition in patient status without any change in the meaning of the concept of role change. Although the application of that concept to transition in patient status may be scientifically interesting, it is not a true case of concept derivation because role change was simply linked to a new phenomenon to which it already had relevance and meaning. Role change thus was not used as a metaphor or analogy, but rather its meaning was left intact.

PURPOSE AND USES

The purpose of concept derivation is to generate new ways of thinking about and looking at some phenomenon. It provides a new vocabulary for an area of inquiry by relying on an analogous or metaphorical relationship between two phenomena: one defined and known and one undefined and under exploration. By relying on a parent field (*Field* 1) for ways of talking about and understanding another (*Field* 2), the concept development process can be accelerated compared to slower methods such as concept synthesis, which relies on analysis of observations and data in concept development.

There are two situations in which concept derivation may be particularly useful: (1) in potential fields or areas where no concept development has yet taken place and (2) in fields in which currently existing concepts have contributed little to advancing inquiry about the phenomenon of interest, in either practical or theoretical terms. In other words, the field is stuck and needs a new perspective.

Regarding the first situation, it is not uncommon for nurses to encounter new situations in which little existing conceptual work has been done, for example, dealing with patients in their 10th decade without living relatives except for grandchildren and great-grandchildren. Existing concepts about parent–child relationships may simply not apply to understanding these skipped-generational family relationships. In such situations, concept derivation may be useful.

In regard to the second situation, existing concepts may simply have become outmoded; hence, more innovative ways of classifying the phenomena in a field may be needed. For example, the traditional concepts that divided areas of nursing practice into medical, surgical, obstetrical, pediatric, and psychiatric nursing are less relevant today than in the past. These divisions are less useful now as more and more is known about how developmental, environmental, and genetic factors interact to produce health or disease in people across the life span. Thus, a new perspective for classifying nursing specialties and their respective knowledge domains is needed. Concept derivation may be helpful in constructing a more relevant classification system.

PROCEDURES FOR CONCEPT DERIVATION

Four basic steps or phases comprise the concept derivation strategy. Whereas some of these steps in actual practice may occur simultaneously, we present them in logical sequence to facilitate clarity. Furthermore, users of this strategy may find as they proceed that they need to return to preceding steps to clarify or validate their work at an earlier step. This is especially likely to happen as users move from an orientation phase (getting familiar with their topic of interest) to the intense working phase. We underscore these points so that readers are not misled. Concept derivation is an efficient strategy for concept development, but to carry it out adequately is not necessarily a quick, mechanical process.

1. The concept developer needs to become thoroughly familiar with existing literature related to the topic of interest. This involves not only reading the literature but also critiquing the level and usefulness of existing concept development found there. If the existing literature on your topic of interest is lacking in relevant concepts, or if concepts exist but they have ceased to stimulate growth of understanding about the topic, then concept derivation may be suitable as a theory development strategy.

2. Examine other fields for new ways of looking at the topic of interest. Read widely in both related and dissimilar fields. Because you cannot know in advance exactly where the most fruitful analogies will be found, it is advisable to begin by casting a broad net. From a practical standpoint, it is important not to rush this step; frequently, the analogies surface or become apparent at unexpected times and places. Because this step relies to some extent on creative insight, it can be facilitated by maintaining a relaxed, patient attitude and not trying to force an immediate solution.

3. Choose a parent concept or set of concepts from another field to use in the derivation process. The parent–field concepts should offer a new and insightful way of viewing the topic of interest. For example, suppose you were puzzled by some unexpected findings about inconsistencies within hospital workers under stress. You might turn to the field of submarine design for an analogy to understand the compartmentalizing that seemed to be occurring. The choice of a parent field may come in a flash or may be the result of a careful fitting process between the new and the parent field (Lenz, Suppe, Gift, Pugh, & Milligan, 1995).

4. Finally, the concept developer needs to redefine the concept or set of concepts from the parent field in terms of the topic of interest. In the example mentioned in step 3, the hospital workers' inconsistencies were conceptualized as the "submarine syndrome," which was defined as closing off areas in which an employee was experiencing stress so that these did not interfere with other areas of functioning—analogous to efforts to prevent sinking the submarine. Furthermore, if a set of concepts is being redefined in terms of the topic of interest, it can provide a preliminary taxonomy for describing the basic types that comprise the topic of interest. Once a preliminary set of definitions has been made, check these out with colleagues familiar with the topic of interest. Any constructive criticism received, even though momentarily painful, can be very helpful in further refining the initial work. Be sure to give yourself a pat on the back at this point!

A classic illustration of the process of concept derivation is contained in Sameroff's work on levels of parental thinking about the parent–child relationship (Sameroff, 1980, pp. 348–352). Sameroff, an expert in child development, began with a working familiarity of literature on human development and family relationships. Sameroff was searching for a new way of understanding parental thought processes that might explain differences in parental childrearing behaviors. He reviewed existing concepts relevant to understanding parental thinking: parental attitudes and expectations and social norms. These concepts in themselves provided only limited ways of understanding parental thinking. In sum, a new perspective was needed. Sameroff was interested in "the level of abstraction utilized by parents to understand development" (p. 349). He turned to the groundbreaking work of the French psychologist Piaget (1963), in which stages of cognitive development in children were elaborated. Sameroff identified an analogy between cognitive development in children and parental thinking:

> Research on the cognitive development of the child has shown that the infant must go through a number of stages before achieving the logical thought processes that characterize adulthood. Similarly, parents may use different levels in thinking about their relationship with the child. (p. 349)

Based on Piaget's four stages of cognitive development (sensorimotor, preoperational, concrete operational, and formal operational), Sameroff proposed by analogy four levels of parental thinking. Briefly, in Piaget's classic work on the sensorimotor stage, the advent of language marks a stage in which cognition is tied to actions, with learning rooted in the senses and manipulation. With passage into the next stage, the preoperational stage, the child uses images and symbols in addition to actions in cognitive processes, but objects are understood in terms of single methods of classification, for example, size. Advancing to the concrete operational stage allows the child to think in terms of logical operations or rules, such as equivalence and serialization—for example, grouping objects in a series by size. In Piaget's final stage of formal operations, the child's logical operations move beyond concrete realities to abstract possibilities that may be proposed and evaluated (Biehler, 1971; Mussen, Conger, & Kagan, 1980; Piaget, 1963).

In his work, Sameroff proposed four analogous levels of parental thinking: symbiotic, categorical, compensatory, and perspectivistic (see Figure 4–3). Parents who respond to the child from the symbiotic level act on a here-and-now basis. Parents do not separate the child's or infant's responses from their own actions. At the

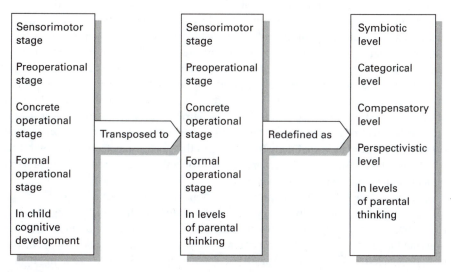

FIGURE 4–3 Concept derivation from Piaget's to Sameroff's concepts.

categorical level, parents see themselves as separate from the child. The child's behavior stems from traits or characteristics of the child; for example, the child is stubborn. Parents who view the child from a compensatory level see the child's behavior as age related—for instance, the child is stubborn because he or she is a toddler. At the perspectivistic level, parents see the child's behavior "as stemming from individual experiences in specific environments. If those experiences had been different, the child's characteristics would be different" (Sameroff, 1980, p. 352). Interestingly, Sameroff found that the majority of parents he studied functioned at the categorical level.

Looking back at Sameroff's process, his expertise in the child development field allowed him to complete the first two steps of concept derivation with ease. He knew the literature and was able to critique the utility of existing concepts in the field. This expertise also made readily available to him alternative perspectives needed in deriving concepts about parental thinking levels and also led to selecting Piaget's work as most promising. He then proceeded to flesh out the parental levels of thinking that were analogous to Piaget's stages. In the final step of concept derivation, Sameroff transposed Piaget's concepts and redefined them in ways relevant to parental thinking. He also created new labels for his four stages so that the terms in his new framework better fit the parenting phenomenon.

APPLICATION OF CONCEPT DERIVATION TO NURSING

An example of concept derivation in nursing may be found in the work of Braun, Wykle, and Cowling (1988), who derived the concept of "failure to thrive in older persons." Noting the phenomenon of weight loss among some institutionalized elderly, they proposed that "failure to thrive among elderly persons may, perhaps, mirror the [already established] pediatric phenomenon" of failure to thrive (p. 809). To further develop the concept of failure to thrive with the elderly, a careful review of literature was done to identify similarities and differences between pediatric and geriatric symptoms and origins. They concluded that pediatric failure to thrive is "a global concept with multiple possible . . . etiologies" and includes weight loss and developmental and depressive symptoms (p. 811). In elderly people, the concept may be "viewed as a broad symptom complex originating, perhaps, from varied physiological, psychological, or combined sources" manifested in weight loss, physical and cognitive decline, and depressive symptoms such as hopelessness (p. 812).

Braun et al.'s (1988) derivation builds on the similarity between some of the manifestations of weight loss noted across these two developmental stages. Although not identical phenomena, the parent field (pediatric literature) was used to structure the development of the concept of failure to thrive among the elderly. However, the concepts are different in that pediatric failure to thrive is associated with growth and developmental retardation, whereas in elderly people the concept represents a process of decline in weight and functioning.

Lillekroken's (2014) derivation of "slow nursing" from the ideas of the Slow Movement in the field of sociology is another example. Lillekroken suggests that, "the Slow Movement opens up certain questions of time and space, promoting a way of living that emphasizes quality rather than quantity" (p. 42). Being deliberately slow in a fast-paced environment is the basic idea from the Slow Movement. In her derivation, she defines her new concept as follows: "slow nursing is a perspective that focuses on respect for the patient as a person, emphasizing quality, by paying attention to and reflecting on patient's needs and resources, using theoretical and practical knowledge, commitment, creativity, and intuition to know when, why and how to be in the world of nursing" (p. 43).

Several things should be kept in mind in applying concept derivation to nursing. First, because the concerns of nurses may overlap with those of other health professions, the first step of concept derivation need not be limited to nursing literature. Medical, educational, developmental, and social work literature, to mention only a few, may be relevant to developing a sense of extant concepts about the topic of interest. Should concepts from these related fields seem adequate, there is no need to proceed any further. In turn, if an extensive search of literature shows that related fields have not attended to the topic of interest, or if the conceptual work elsewhere seems limited, then concept derivation in nursing may benefit these other fields as well.

Second, as noted earlier, there is no rule about where to look for rich analogies or metaphors for nursing phenomena. In addition to fields of inquiry in nursing, the natural sciences (physics, zoology, and chemistry) and behavioral sciences as well as applied areas such as law, engineering, and education may be considered. Discussions with nursing colleagues as well as experts in other fields may be useful in identifying potentially useful parent fields from which to derive concepts.

Third, theorists should not be impatient in selecting a promising set of concepts from which to derive concepts for nursing phenomena. Frequently, assimilation or incubation time is needed to see the fit between two fields of study. This type of insight typically comes in a flash that may be preceded by a period of frustrating lack of progress.

Fourth, the final step of concept derivation, redefining the concepts in terms of the phenomena in the field of interest, may be laborious. Definitions may need to be redone several times before a final satisfactory outcome is achieved. Setting aside the work for brief periods may be helpful in producing the new and creative perspective desired. Critically judging the merits of one's work prematurely may also stifle creativity. The theorist should remain patient but persistent.

Several examples of concept derivation reported in the nursing literature are presented in Table 4–1. In one of these cases, the concept of *nurse dose* was derived to better understand "nursing care as an intervention" (Manojlovich & Sidani, 2008, p. 310). In another case, the concepts of nursing human capital and nursing structural capital were derived as part of a larger program in which a theory of nursing intellectual capital was derived (Covell, 2008).

ADVANTAGES AND LIMITATIONS

Concept derivation as a strategy has the advantage of letting the theorist avoid beginning from scratch. The use of concepts from another field speeds along the creative process. Indeed, Maccia (1963) has suggested that the perspective that concept derivation employs may underlie sources of theory development in general. Having newly derived concepts to express new underlying ideas can trigger new approaches to assessment or tool development for practice. New derived concepts also can lead to new directions for research.

TABLE 4–1   Examples of Studies Using Concept Derivation

Author(s)	Application of Concept Derivation
Lenz et al. (1995)	The concept of pain was used to "redefine" dyspnea as a subjective sensation (p. 6)
Brauer (2001)	Holistic patterns of function were derived for persons with rheumatoid arthritis
Manojlovich and Sidani (2008)	The multidisciplinary concept of dose was used to derive the concept of nurse dose, which had the attributes of purity, amount, frequency, and duration
Covell (2008)	Concepts from business were used to derive the concepts of nursing human capital and nursing structural capital
Lillekroken (2014)	The concept of slow movement was used to derive the concept of slow nursing

Two limitations to concept derivation as a theory development strategy should be borne in mind. First, although the derived concepts may provide useful labels, concepts alone are limited in their scientific usefulness. In themselves, concepts do not provide explanations, predictions, or control of phenomena. Only relational statements and theories have this potential (see Chapter 3). Development of concepts, however, can be the first stage in development of statements and theories. Concepts may label the dimensions of a phenomenon, but more is needed to achieve the larger goals of science and practice.

Second, despite the fact that a concept (*Concept* 1) from the parent field (*Field* 1) has been useful in that field, a concept derived from it (*Concept* 2) may not automatically be equally so. Unfortunately, being wellborn does not guarantee success. Thus, the scientific utility of a derived concept is unknown until it is tested in practice and research (see Chapter 13). Uncertainty about the scientific usefulness of new ideas is not limited to concept derivation as a strategy. There is risk endemic in proposing any new idea. Until ideas are tested, their value remains unknown.

UTILIZING THE RESULTS OF CONCEPT DERIVATION

Concepts developed through the derivation strategy may be used in at least two ways in research and theory development: (1) derived concepts can provide working concepts for use in clinical work such as nursing diagnosis development; and (2) derived concepts can provide preliminary classification schemes of nursing phenomena for use in further research, theory development, and clinical practice. In these uses, it is important to determine whether the concepts derived have empirical validity in the new field.

To test the validity of derived diagnostic concepts, readers are referred to the classic methodology literature in the field of nursing diagnosis (e.g., Gordon & Sweeney, 1979) and the "Concept Testing" section in Chapter 13. In research and theory development, derived concepts should be reassessed for their utility in describing phenomena in ways that further the aims of a field of study and that pull together the findings of relevant research. Where derived concepts delineate new phenomena in need of systematic measurement, they may be used as the base for tool development (see Waltz, Strickland, & Lenz [2005] on operationalizing nursing concepts).

Moreover, concept derivation can be used as an instructional heuristic in the teaching–learning process. When introducing unfamiliar concepts to students, analogs can facilitate concept introduction. Such application of concept derivation requires that useful analogs be available and already understood by students.

Summary

The strategy of concept derivation employs an analogy or metaphor to transpose concepts from one field of inquiry to another. There are no exact rules for selecting a field from which to derive concepts. Concept derivation is suited to topics of interest in which there is no extant concept development or in which existing concepts have become stagnant. The steps in concept derivation include becoming familiar with and critiquing existing literature on a topic, searching other fields for conceptual perspectives, choosing a promising set of concepts from which to derive new concepts, and then generating new concepts by analogy from the parent field. The strategy of concept derivation may speed up the concept development process. The strategy is limited by the level of theory achieved and the uncertainty about the ultimate usefulness of the derived concepts.

Practice Exercise

You may try out the steps of the concept derivation process using the practice exercise that follows. Because it is not feasible to do each step completely, we will assume that preparatory steps have been completed already to facilitate the exercise.

First, let's start by assuming that you are interested in a new way of understanding nurse–patient communication in primary care settings. Let's also assume that after an extensive review of literature on nurse–patient communication, your suspicion is confirmed that the literature lacks innovative concepts relevant to nurse–patient communication in primary care settings. After searching the behavioral sciences and finding little that seems promising, you happen to talk with a geographer at a social function. He is discussing the concepts that underlie the design and uses of maps. During the course of the conversation, you see a striking analogy between the map concepts and idea of nurse–patient communication in primary care. You see the patient as a "traveler" and the nurse as a source of "travel information" in getting to a "destination."

In this exercise, take out a map of your state. List the kinds of information the map provides to a traveler. List how you use a map as you travel between two cities in your state. List the different reasons you might be traveling and how this might affect what you refer to on the map. Review these lists thoroughly. Now select the key ideas from these lists that seem to you to describe the ways a traveler uses a map to get to a destination. Now think of the patient and nurse in a primary care setting. Transfer your key ideas (i.e., concepts) about the ways a traveler uses a map to the primary care setting. Use these key ideas to think about nurse–patient communication. After you get a feel for these key ideas in the primary care setting, then you may jot down short definitions that describe the concepts in terms of nurse–patient communication. Do not worry yet about whether your definitions and concepts make sense. Set aside your work for a while. Look at your key concepts and definitions again. Clarify any fuzzy wording or ideas. Now try out your ideas on some colleagues who will give constructive criticism. From their reactions, further refine your concepts and definitions.

Bear in mind, there is no one right set of concepts or definitions that you should have derived. If you had had a colleague simultaneously do this same exercise, that person's concepts and definitions would probably be somewhat different from yours. For comparison purposes, two examples of concepts that we derived by this exercise are presented in Table 4–2. In Example 2, the defining characteristics of the derived concepts are also provided. You may find that the concepts and definitions that you derived are more interesting than the ones we presented!

TABLE 4–2   Two Examples of Derived Concepts

Parent Field: Informational Functions of Maps for Travelers	New Field of Interest: Informational Functions of Primary Care Nurses
Example 1. Parent Concepts	**Example 1. Derived Concepts**
1. Direction	1. Orientation
2. Points of interest	2. Facilities available
3. Alternate routes	3. Alternates for diagnosis and treatment
4. Mileage estimates	4. Duration of care
5. Geographic reference points	5. Reference points for progress
6. Destination	6. Goal of care
Example 2. Parent Concepts and Defining Qualities	**Example 2. Derived Concepts and Defining Qualities**
1. Business travel—for a specific purpose	1. Focused care—care of a specific problem
1.1 Efficient travel pace	1.1 Rapid attention to presenting problem
1.2 Direct route on main thoroughfares	1.2 Focus of attention on presenting problem
1.3 Specific information on access points on route	1.3 Specific information about time and place of treatments
1.4 Reliable accommodations	1.4 Reliable personnel and facilities
1.5 Time frame limited to specific business objective	1.5 Time frame for care determined by presenting problem
2. Pleasure travel—travel for recreation and growth	2. Revitalization care—care for health promotion
2.1 Leisurely pace of travel	2.1 Careful consideration to patient concerns and questions
2.2 Scenic routes	2.2 Attention to overall health status
2.3 Alternate access points for possible side trips	2.3 Information about health promotion alternatives
2.4 Pleasurable accommodations	2.4 Competent and humanistic care
2.5 Time frame negotiable based on wishes	2.5 Time frame negotiated based on health promotion needs and wants

References

Biehler RF. *Psychology Applied to Teaching*. Boston, MA: Houghton Mifflin; 1971.

Brauer DJ. Common patterns of person–environment interaction in persons with rheumatoid arthritis. *West J Nurs Res*. 2001;23:414–430.

Braun JV, Wykle MH, Cowling WR. Failure to thrive in older persons. *Gerontologist*. 1988;28:809–812.

Covell CL. The middle-range theory of nursing intellectual capital. *J Adv Nurs*. 2008;63:94–103.

Gordon M, Sweeney MA. Methodological problems and issues in identifying and standardizing nursing diagnoses. *Adv Nurs Sci*. 1979;2(1):1–15.

Lenz ER, Suppe F, Gift AG, Pugh LC, Milligan RA. Collaborative development of middle-range nursing theories: Toward a theory of unpleasant symptoms. *Adv Nurs Sci*. 1995;17(3):1–13.

Lillekroken D. Slow nursing—The concept inventing process. *Int J Hum Caring*. 2014;18(4):40–44.

Maccia ES. Ways of inquiring. In: Maccia ES, Maccia GS, Jewett RS, eds. *Construction of Educational Theory Models*. Cooperative Research Project No. 1632. Washington, DC: Office of Education, U.S. Department of Health, Education, and Welfare; 1963, pp. 1–13.

Maccia ES, Maccia GS. The way of educational theorizing through models. In: Maccia ES, Maccia GS, Jewett RE, eds. *Construction of Educational Theory Models*. Cooperative Research Project No. 1632. Washington, DC: Office of Education, U.S. Department of Health, Education, and Welfare; 1963, pp. 30–45.

Manojlovich M, Sidani S. Nurse dose: What's in a concept? *Res Nurs Health*. 2008;31:310–319.

Mussen PH, Conger JJ, Kagan J. *Essentials of Child Development and Personality*. Philadelphia, PA: Harper & Row; 1980.

Piaget J. *Psychology of Intelligence*. Paterson, NJ: Littlefield, Adams & Co.; 1963.

Roy C, Roberts SL. *Theory Construction in Nursing: An Adaptation Model*. Englewood Cliffs, NJ: Prentice Hall; 1981.

Sameroff AJ. Issues in early reproductive and caretaking risk: Review and current status. In: Sawin DB, Hawkins RCB, Walker LO, Penticuff JH, eds. *Exceptional Infant*. Vol. 4. *Psychosocial Risks in Infant–Environment Transactions*. New York, NY: Brunner/Mazel; 1980, pp. 343–359.

Waltz CF, Strickland OL, Lenz ER. *Measurement in Nursing Research*. 3rd ed. New York, NY: Springer/Davis; 2005.

5

■ ■ ■

Statement Derivation

Questions to consider before you get started reading this chapter:

▶ Are you seeking a way to generate new ideas and connections about a research problem or clinical phenomenon?

▶ Are you interested in looking outside your immediate area of interest to see how others may have ideas that may inspire you?

▶ Are you particularly interested in developing statements about a phenomenon of interest?

Introductory Note: If you have answered "yes" to any of the above three questions, then statement derivation may fit your needs. Statement derivation builds on an analogy between a parent statement in a source field and one in a new area of inquiry. The analogous nature of the two statements may be grasped as an "Aha," or in the course of methodical inquiry. Like concept derivation, statement derivation is foundational in the larger process of theory derivation, a more frequently used strategy. A firm grasp of statement derivation as a strategy is useful to readers who wish to pursue theory derivation activities, or who wish simply to understand the process of statement formulation with greater clarity. As a result, readers are encouraged to read Chapters 4, 5, and 6 in tandem in order to grasp the overall derivation process. One note of caution: theorists may sometimes use the terminology of *statement derivation* when they simply mean *statement development*. In this book, we reserve the terminology of *statement derivation* for statements that are developed by use of analogy.

DEFINITION AND DESCRIPTION

Statement derivation is a strategy for developing a statement or set of statements about a phenomenon by use of an underlying analogy between two fields of inquiry. A statement in the context of statement derivation takes the form of a declarative sentence in which a relationship is posited between two or more concepts. That relationship may also be expressed schematically.

Statement derivation draws on the earlier work of Maccia and Maccia (1963) on educational theorizing through models. A statement (*Statement* 1) from one field of interest (*Field* 1) is used to derive the content or structure of a second statement

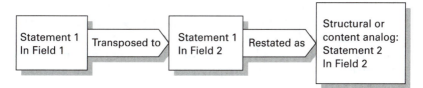

FIGURE 5–1 Process of statement derivation.

(*Statement* 2) for a second field (*Field* 2). Thus, a new statement (or new set of statements) is created that shares some common structural or content features with an existing statement (or set of statements). Despite similar structure or terminology, the new and existing statements are distinct because each refers to a separate field of interest (see Figure 5–1).

Identifying an analogy (or likeness) between phenomena in two different fields is the basis of statement derivation. The form of that analogy may be either *content* or *structural*.

- In a *content analogy*, the likeness rests in the content or concepts in two fields. For example, the concept of *mental health literacy* recently served as a model for proposing the concept of *gestational-weight-gain health literacy* (Champlin, Walker, & Mackert, 2016).
- In a *structural analogy*, the likeness rests in the logical structure by which concepts are linked together within statements; the parent statement serves by analogy as the structure for relating concepts within the statement in the second field. Consider the following fictitious statement: When a critical threshold is reached, further coaching of a learner leads to reduced performance. Structurally, this statement could be understood as follows: When _____ is reached, further _____ leads to reduced _____.

On the surface, the two fields of interest do not necessarily have to appear similar. What is required is the presence of analogous dimensions between phenomena in the two fields. For example, let us assume the following statement holds true in physical science:

For any two objects in motion close to each other, there are forces that attract the objects to each other as well as forces that repel them.

By analogy, we might theorize:

For any two persons who are in close physical contact with each other, there are forces that attract the persons to each other as well as forces that repel them.

Despite gross differences in the phenomena in the two fields, these two statements bear a structural and content similarity to each other.

The processes for deriving the content and structure of statements are crucial to understanding statement derivation. Deriving the content and structure of a new statement from an existing source or parent statement involves two logically separate derivations. Whereas a theorist would no doubt carry out simultaneously the content and structural derivations of a statement, we will carry these out separately to more clearly illustrate them.

Derivation of the content of a new statement is akin to concept derivation (see Chapter 4): A theorist specifies the terms or concepts to be included in a new statement and their accompanying definitions within the new field. Derivation of the structure of the new statements entails specifying the type of linkage between the newly derived concepts or terms. The linkage may be a unidirectional causal relationship, a simple positive relationship, a negative association, or a more complex algebraic relationship. (See Chapter 11 on *statement analysis* for the types of linkages that may obtain between the concepts in statements.) It is the theorist's specific goals for and intended usage of derived statements that determine whether they are endpoints or part of a larger program of theory development. In the latter case, statement derivation may be done to set the stage for a program of theory development that incorporates theory derivation.

Let's look at the following sample statement that will be used to derive a statement about family interaction.

When the volume of a gas is held constant, the temperature and pressure are positively related.

Content derivation focuses on specifying family terminology to parallel the key chemical concepts or terms in this statement: *gas*, *volume*, *temperature*, and *pressure*. For example, the terms *family*, *amount of interaction*, *amount of comments*, and *amount of responses* might be defined as respective analogs of the chemical terminology.

In looking at the structural derivation of a new statement, content terms that refer to the properties of the phenomenon, for example, *pressure*, may be eliminated and replaced by simple place-holding symbols such as A, B, and C. Thus, our beginning statement may be rewritten as follows:

When the A of B is held constant, the C and D are positively related.

This noncontent statement presents only the skeleton or structure of relationships among our unspecified concepts or terms A, B, C, and D. As written, the statement makes logical sense, but does not have any meaning in terms of real phenomena. That is, until A–D are given substance by specifying terms linked to reality, the statement is not empirically interpretable. To specify meanings for A–D, let us substitute the terms developed earlier for family interaction.

When the amount of interaction of a family is held constant, the amount of comments and the amount of responses are positively related.

Although most cases of statement derivation entail both content and structural derivation, this need not always be the case. If a theorist has already delineated relevant concepts describing a phenomenon and lacks only a clear mode of interrelating them, only the structural aspect of statement derivation may be needed.

Analogies in the structure or content of statements across fields are derived as the theorist grasps implicit similarities between two fields of interest. As a result, a large measure of the success of statement derivation hinges on the theorist's insightful selection of an existing field that contains rich parallels with the theorist's field of interest. There is no set rule for selecting timely and fruitful sources or parent fields from which to begin statement derivation. A theorist's sense or awareness of phenomena in the field of interest is certainly an important ingredient. Consequently, reading in fields that are related as well as unrelated to the theorist's interests can establish a range of alternate fields from which to begin statement derivation. The heuristic value of a parent field can be determined only as a theorist attempts to actually derive statements from a parent field.

PURPOSE AND USES

The purpose of statement derivation is to formulate one or more statements about a phenomenon that is currently not well understood. Statement derivation is especially suited to situations in which (1) no available database or body of literature exists, (2) current thinking is becoming outmoded, or (3) existing statements do not sufficiently capture the phenomenon of interest. Thus, new perspectives are needed.

Analogy is one of the bases of formulating innovative hypotheses. Statement derivation is broadly based on the use of analogy, that is, recognition of an underlying similarity in the structure of relationships in two disparate phenomena. It is this recognition or use of analogy that may underlie development of new and interesting relationships expressed as hypotheses. For example, William McGuire reported how he used the idea of biological inoculation to formulate by analogy his hypotheses about "inducing resistance to persuasion" in the psychological domain (1976, p. 41).

Statement derivation is especially relevant when a theorist wishes to clarify how two or more concepts about a phenomenon are related or wants a derived set of statements about a phenomenon from which to then build an integrated theoretical model of it. For example, suppose a theorist wished to clarify how telephone support from a clinical nurse specialist (CNS) affects men's coping after surgery for prostate cancer. An initial literature search of CINAHL showed the theorist that there were articles about the role of the CNS and care of patients with prostate cancer (e.g., Higgins, 2000; McGlynn et al., 2014; Ream et al., 2009). Furthermore, further search showed only a few studies focused specifically on telephone support from clinical nurse specialists for men with prostate cancer (Anderson, 2010; Lynch, 2012). The nurse theorist decided that further attention to this important area of cancer care was needed. Statement derivation appeared to be the most reasonable and rapid means of developing one or more statements about telephone support from a CNS and resultant coping of men with prostate cancer. We will continue with the example of CNS telephone support in the next section.

PROCEDURES FOR STATEMENT DERIVATION

Statement derivation may be broken down into several steps. In actual practice, a theorist may move through several steps almost simultaneously or occasionally repeat steps to improve the final results. The steps are, thus, guideposts rather than rigid lockstep maneuvers in statement building. Bearing this in mind, we list below the steps in statement derivation.

1. Become thoroughly familiar with any existing literature on a topic of interest. This should involve not only reading but also critically evaluating the level of usefulness of statements about the topic of interest. This step should determine the need to use the statement derivation strategy. If a need for a new perspective is evident, or a paucity of relevant literature is available, then statement derivation may be appropriate.

2. Search other fields for new ways of looking at the topic of interest. Read literature from several fields, both fields similar to and dissimilar from the topic and field of interest. Be alert to those aspects of the literature that specifically express the major relational statements of each field.

3. Select the source or parent field to be used in the derivation process, and carefully identify the structural and content features of the parent statements to be used in derivations. Be sure to separately consider both the structural suitability and the content suitability of statements in the parent field. Because derivation is not a mechanical process, the theorist is free to modify statements in the parent field to increase their suitability to the derivation process. Thus, statements from the parent field may be restated to enhance their clarity and to more sharply display the structure of relationships between concepts.

4. Develop new statements about the topic of interest from the content and structure of statements in the parent field. This step, simply stated, consists of restating the parent statements in terms of the subject matter of the new field, that is, the theorist's topic of interest.

5. Redefine any new concepts or terms in the derived statements to fit the specific subject matter of the topic of interest. If statement derivation is used only to provide the structure for interrelating concepts that already exist in the field of interest, much of this step may already be done. Even so, it is prudent to reassess the suitability of definitions of terms when they are placed within the structure of new statements. Adaptations in meaning may be needed.

APPLICATION OF STATEMENT DERIVATION TO NURSING

To illustrate these steps in operation, we will continue to explore the hypothetical case of the nurse theorist interested in CNS telephone support and its relationship to men's coping with prostate cancer. For this illustration, the theorist had already identified the two concepts of *CNS telephone support* and *coping* as the concepts of interest. Thus, only a structural linkage between the two concepts needs to be specified in the statement derivation. In searching other fields for analogous ways of viewing the CNS–patient telephone interaction, the theorist located literature on the inverted *U* function. In psychological literature, independent variables such as anxiety are related to outcomes such as performance in a curvilinear or inverted U form. Thus, high and low levels of anxiety are related to less effective performance, whereas moderate levels of anxiety are associated with high levels of performance. The inverted U function has proven to be useful in other fields such as interactions between mothers and high-risk infants (Field, 1980). The nurse theorist therefore chose the inverted U function as the structure for a statement about CNS telephone support and coping with prostate cancer. The nurse's rationale for this choice was that low support was likely to be insufficient to enhance coping and high support might stifle emerging coping capabilities, whereas moderate support was likely to optimally promote coping. In applying the inverted U function to the concepts of interest, the following statement was derived:

> *CNS telephone support is related to patient coping with prostate cancer as an inverted U function: high and low levels of CNS telephone support are related to low patient coping, whereas moderate levels of CNS telephone support are related to high levels of patient coping.*

The inverted U function between CNS telephone support and patient coping is depicted in Figure 5–2.

To complete the statement development process, the theorist then prepared definitions of CNS telephone support and patient coping with prostate cancer. The theorist also operationally defined high, medium, and low levels of CNS telephone support based on the literature.

The theorist in our illustration of CNS telephone support utilized only the structural aspect of statement derivation. Because the content concepts were already identified, only a structure for interrelating them was needed. This was provided by the inverted U function. When theorists are deriving both the content and structure of a new statement, the derivation process will more closely resemble the example of family-interaction patterns presented earlier in this chapter.

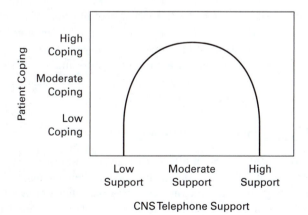

FIGURE 5–2 Hypothetical relationship of CNS telephone support to patient coping with prostate cancer.

The derived statement about CNS telephone support predicts how support is related to patient coping. However, the empirical validity of this or any other derived statements cannot be known before testing. Testing the accuracy of derived statements is quite important to the practice of nursing. Testing is needed to see if indeed low, moderate, and high levels of CNS telephone support are related to patient coping as an inverted *U* function. If confirmed by research, the statement is relevant to evidence-based approaches to practice. (*Note:* The example of CNS telephone support for postoperative patients with prostate cancer is presented for illustrative purposes and should not be construed as a definitive or comprehensive review on this topic.)

An initial way of assessing the potential plausibility of derived statements is to examine existing research literature for supporting evidence. Perhaps studies not directly aimed at testing the effects of CNS telephone support contain data that are relevant to the statement in question. Perhaps related research has been done in other areas of cancer care. Although such data are not a direct test of the CNS telephone support–coping statement, they add to its plausibility or implausibility. Finally, if highly regarded theories are found to predict the inverted *U* function between CNS telephone support and coping, a further measure of support is given to the statement. None of these methods outlined here is a substitute for definitive testing of a derived statement, but each aids in making a provisional estimate of the plausibility of the statement.

Ultimately, derived statements must be tested to determine their credibility. Such testing is essential before derived statements can be applied to practice. A lengthy discussion of statement testing is outside the focus of this chapter. Readers may consult research methods texts for information about appropriate research designs for testing interventions and related clinical questions (Pedhazur & Schmelkin, 2013; Polit & Beck, 2012). Statement testing is also briefly covered in Chapter 13.

Finally, theorists should not begin evaluating the empirical support for a statement before they have come to closure on the derivation process. Even in the early stages of derivation when a theorist is selecting parent statements, these should not be stringently judged, but simply examined and toyed with. Sometimes seemingly unlikely candidates may prove to be winners in the long run. We are reminded of Maccia and Maccia's (1963) use of the physiology of eyeblinking as a framework for deriving statements about student learning. After the derivation process is initially completed, it is a good idea to set it aside for a few days and then review it again. If the theorist is satisfied that the work is clear and lucid, then evaluating empirical support for a derived statement may be in order.

ADVANTAGES AND LIMITATIONS

As a strategy, statement derivation offers advantages. The strategy is an economical and expeditious way of developing statements about a phenomenon. Unlike statement synthesis, the strategy does not require research data collection as a starting point. Armed with an idea of the phenomenon of interest, reference materials from other fields, and a measure of creative ability, a theorist may commence statement derivation. The strategy is not limited to any discipline or phenomenon. It may be used with whatever subject matter a theorist chooses. Statement derivation also has limitations. Derivation of new statements from credible statements in another field does not lend support directly to the newly derived statements. Even though derivation may facilitate development of interesting new scientific statements, independent empirical support of derived statements is still required ultimately.

UTILIZING THE RESULTS OF STATEMENT DERIVATION

Statements constructed through the derivation process are essentially untested; thus, their most suitable application is in directing research efforts to test them. We see several noteworthy areas of research particularly suited for testing derived statements: (1) correlational studies to assess the relationship of an antecedent to a clinical phenomenon, and (2) studies to test the usefulness of a nursing intervention to ameliorate a clinical problem. Derived statements may also be useful in developing innovative frameworks for programs of research.

Research methods texts that may be helpful in statement testing are cited earlier in this chapter. To estimate the provisional empirical support for a derived statement, existing research findings often offer clues. For example, correlational data from other studies can sometimes provide information about whether proposed antecedents of clinical phenomena really hold true. By examining existing data tables in published research, such provisional evidence can often be located. If such evidence is found, it supports the need for a research study to directly test the derived statements.

Statement derivation also may serve as a useful instructional strategy. As a classroom exercise for students, it can be used as the means of generating research hypotheses when students are beginning to learn the research process. Often students get caught up in the details of each specific research topic. Statement derivation offers a means of involving students in joint classroom exercises that free them to think more broadly about phenomena that concern nursing.

Summary

Statement derivation employs an analogy as a basis for constructing new statements about a phenomenon. The theorist selects a parent field as the base for statement development. Analog statements are identified. These may occur in the content or structure of derived statements. There are no exact rules for locating fruitful parent fields to use in derivation.

Statement derivation involves becoming familiar with and critiquing literature on the topic of interest, searching for a parent field, identifying content and structural features in parent statements, developing analogous content and structure for derived statements, and redefining new concepts within the new field of interest. Derived statements require independent testing to establish their empirical validity. As a strategy, statement derivation is economical and expeditious.

Practice Exercises

To practice statement derivation, we have selected source or parent statements from a variety of fields. Included among these are some classic statements from the fields of learning and biology. Before trying to do any derivations with them, identify the phenomenon you would like to derive new statements about. Select one or more of the statements below as a parent statement. Identify the content and structural aspects of the parent statement. Develop the content and structural analogs of the derived statement. Redefine, if needed, any new concepts in the derived statements. If you want a guide to getting started on the Practice Exercise, see two worked out examples at the end of this section.

STATEMENTS FROM SEVERAL DISCIPLINES

1. "Adaptation to life with a chronic illness is facilitated by a network of interpersonal relationships" (Chrisler & O'Hea, 2000, p. 330).
2. "The more frequently we have made a given response to a given stimulus, the more likely we are to make that response to that stimulus again" (Hill, 1985, pp. 30–31).
3. "Organisms are surviving because they are adapted, and they are adapted because they are surviving" (Burnett & Eisner, 1964, p. v).
4. "Neutral events that accompany or precede established negative reinforcements become negatively reinforcing" (Skinner, 1953, p. 173).
5. "Change occurs in little explosions in which matter is created and destroyed" (Wheeler, 2001, p. 41).
6. "By the preservation of constancy of the internal environment, warm-blooded animals are freed from the influence of vicissitudes in the external environment" (Cannon, 1963, p. 178).
7. "Blinking functions to protect the eye from contact and to rest the retina and the ocular muscles" (Maccia & Maccia, 1963, p. 34).
8. "The constant bombing of the pancreas by . . . huge hits of sugars and fats can eventually wear out the organ's insulin-producing 'islets' . . ." (Critser, 2001, p. 146).

Here are two worked out examples to aid readers in getting started on the Practice Exercise. Below, words in *italics* constitute content derivations, whereas words not italicized represent derived structural forms within which content concepts are located.

In the first worked out example, Maccia and Maccia (1963) began with statement 7 from which they derived the following statement about educational processes:

Distraction functions to protect from *mental stress* and to rest from *mental effort.* (p. 34)

For our second worked out example, we started with statement 6. Our wish was to describe the individual's strengths in a social context. We defined the structure of statement 6 as follows:

By the preservation of constancy of A, Bs are freed from the influence of Cs.

We defined the content terms *A–C* as follows: *A* is self-esteem, *B*s are human beings, and *C*s are social stressors. By inserting our content terms within the structural form, the following new statement was derived:

By the preservation of constancy of self-esteem, human beings are freed from the influence of social stressors.

If you chose to use statement 6 in your derivations, your content concepts may be quite different from the ones we used. Still, you should be able to identify the content and structural aspects of your derivations and see if they parallel the example here. If your derived statements look plausible, try to find literature that supports the statements. If you wish, map out a plan for empirically testing your statements.

References

Anderson B. The benefits to nurse-led telephone follow-up for prostate cancer. *Br J Nurs.* 2010;19(17):1085–1090.

Burnett AL, Eisner T. *Animal Adaptation.* New York, NY: Holt, Rinehart & Winston; 1964.

Cannon WB. *The Wisdom of the Body.* New York, NY: Norton; 1963.

Champlin S, Walker LO, Mackert M. Gestational weight gain through a health literacy lens: A scoping review. *J Perinat Educ.* 2016;25(4):242–256.

Chrisler JC, O'Hea EL. Gender, culture, and autoimmune disorders. In: Eisler RM, Hersen M, eds. *Handbook of Gender, Culture, and Health.* Mahwah, NJ: Erlbaum; 2000, pp. 321–342.

Critser G. Let them eat fat. In: Ferris T, ed. *The Best American Science Writing 2001.* New York, NY: HarperCollins; 2001, pp. 143–153.

Field TM. Interactions of high-risk infants: Quantitative and qualitative differences. In: Sawin DB, Hawkins RC, Walker LO, Penticuff JH, eds. *Exceptional Infant.* Vol. 4. *Psychosocial Risks in Infant–Environment Transactions.* New York, NY: Brunner/Mazel; 1980, pp. 120–143.

Higgins D. The role of the prostate cancer nurse specialist. *Prof Nurse.* 2000;15:539–542.

Hill WF. *Learning: A Survey of Psychological Interpretations.* 4th ed. New York, NY: Harper & Row; 1985.

Lynch T. Telephone helpline supports patients with prostate cancer. *Cancer Nurs Pract.* 2012;11(3):30–34.

Maccia ES, Maccia GS. The way of educational theorizing through models. In: Maccia ES, Maccia GS, Jewett RE, eds. *Construction of Educational Theory Models.* Cooperative Research Project No. 1632. Washington, DC: Office of Education, U.S. Department of Health, Education, and Welfare; 1963, pp. 30–45.

McGlynn B, White L, Smith K, Hollins G, Gurun M, Little B, et al. A service evaluation describing a nurse-led prostate cancer service in NHS, Ayrshire and Arran. *Int J Urol Nurs.* 2014;8(3):166–180.

McGuire WJ. The yin and yang of progress in social psychology: Seven koan. In: Strickland H, Aboud FE, Gergen KJ, eds. *Social Psychology in Transition.* New York: Plenum Press; 1976, pp. 33–50.

Pedhazur EJ, Schmelkin LP. *Measurement, Design, and Analysis: An Integrated Approach.* New York, NY: Psychology Press; 2013.

Polit DF, Beck CT. *Nursing Research: Generating and Assessing Evidence for Nursing Practice.* 9th ed. Philadelphia, PA: Lippincott Williams & Wilkins; 2012.

Ream E, Wilson-Barnett J, Faithfull S, Fincham L, Khoo V, Richardson A. Working patterns and perceived contribution of prostate cancer clinical nurse specialists: A mixed method investigation. *Int J Nurs Stud.* 2009;46:1345–1354.

Skinner BF. *Science and Human Behavior.* New York, NY: Free Press; 1953.

Wheeler JA. How come the quantum? In: Ferris T, ed. *The Best American Science Writing 2001.* New York, NY: HarperCollins; 2001, pp. 41–43.

Additional Readings

Maccia ES, Maccia GS. *Development of Educational Theory Derived from Three Educational Theory Models*. Project No. 5-0638. Washington, DC: Office of Education, U.S. Department of Health, Education, and Welfare; 1966.

Maccia ES, Maccia GS, Jewett RE, eds. *Construction of Educational Theory Models*. Cooperative Research Project No. 1632. Washington, DC: Office of Education, U.S. Department of Health, Education, and Welfare; 1963.

6

■ ■ ■

Theory Derivation

Questions to consider before you get started reading this chapter:

▶ Are you seeking a way to generate a new organizing framework or theory about a research problem or clinical phenomenon?

▶ Are you interested in looking outside your immediate area of interest to see others who may have ideas that may inspire you?

Introductory Note: If you have answered "yes" to the above two questions, then theory derivation may fit your needs. In theory derivation, the theorist creates a new theory by use of analogy to an existing theory. This strategy may be easy for nurses and other health care workers to grasp because analogy and metaphor frequently are employed in their teaching of patients and their families. Thus, the derivation strategies are very popular with our students because the strategies are intuitive and easy for them to grasp. A firm grasp of concept and statement derivation is useful to readers who wish to pursue theory derivation. As a result, readers are encouraged to read Chapters 4, 5, and 6 in tandem in order to grasp the overall derivation process. One note of caution: theorists may sometimes use the terminology of *theory derivation* when they simply mean *theory development*. In this book, we reserve the terminology of *theory derivation* for theories or models that are developed by use of analogy.

DEFINITION AND DESCRIPTION

Some of the earliest foundations of derivation occurred in the 1960s in the field of education (Maccia, Maccia, & Jewett, 1963). We have drawn heavily on that work. Using analogy to obtain explanations or predictions about a phenomenon in one field from the explanations or predictions in another field is the basis for theory derivation (Maccia et al., 1963). Thus, a theory (*Theory* 1) from one field of interest (*Field* 1) offers some new insights to a theorist who then moves certain content or structural features into his or her own field of interest (*Field* 2) to form a new theory (*Theory* 2). Theory derivation is a creative and focused way to develop theory in a new field in that what is required is (1) the ability to see analogous dimensions of phenomena in two distinct fields of interest and (2) the ability to redefine and transpose the content and/or structure from *Field* 1 to *Field* 2 in a manner that adds significant insights

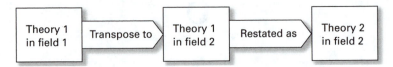

FIGURE 6–1   Process of theory derivation.

about some phenomenon in *Field* 2 (Figure 6–1). In one of the most legendary examples of use of analogy, Hempel (1966) describes Kekulé's insight into the structure of benzene as a hexagon. As Kekulé dreams in front of the fire, he envisions the atoms gyrating in a snakelike fashion. Next, as Hempel describes it, "Suddenly, one of the snakes formed a ring by seizing hold of its own tail and whirled mocking before him. Kekulé awoke in a flash: he had hit upon the now famous and familiar idea of representing the molecular structure of benzene by a hexagonal ring" (p. 16). While in this example the source of the analogy came from Kekulé's own mind, it nonetheless exemplifies the role that analogy can play in advancing theoretical understanding.

Seeing an analogy requires imagination and creativity; it is not a mechanical exercise. Theory derivation requires the theorist to be able to redefine networks of concepts and statements so that they are meaningful in the new field, but theory derivation goes beyond statement derivation. First, in theory derivation a whole network of interrelated concepts or a whole structure is moved from one field to another and modified to fit the new field. Second, in statement derivation you move only individual isolated statements from one field to another and modify them. Statement derivation is thus on a smaller scale than theory derivation, but understanding the process of transposing concepts and the structural forms that link them in statements (see Chapter 5) is essential to theory derivation. In addition, we wish to aid readers in distinguishing theory derivation from theory adaptation and theory substruction (Bekhet & Zauszniewski, 2008; McQuiston & Campbell, 1997), with which it is sometimes confused (see Table 6–1 for these distinctions).

PURPOSE AND USES

Theory derivation is particularly useful where no data are available or where new insights about a phenomenon are needed to inspire research and testing. Theory derivation is also useful when a theorist has a set of concepts that are somehow related to each other, but has no structural way to represent those relationships. (See Chapter 5 on statement derivation for more detailed description of structure derivation.) In this case, the theorist might find that some other field of interest has a structure in one of its theories that is analogous to the relationships of the concepts in which he or she is interested. The theorist may use the derivation strategy by transposing the structure to his or her field to systematically organize the concepts being considered. This adds to the body of knowledge in the theorist's field in a significant and rapid way that might not have happened for some time without the derivation strategy. A classic example of this is Nierenberg's (1968, 1973) use of Maslow's hierarchical structure of needs to derive a theory of negotiation.

TABLE 6–1   Comparison of Theory Derivation, Adaptation, and Substruction

Theory Derivation	Theory Adaptation	Theory Substruction
Aim: to create a new theory by use of analogy to an existing theory in another field	Aim: to make a minor change in an existing theory to better fit the research focus	Aim: to specify links from "constructs" or "concepts" in the theory to "empirical indicators" in a situational focus
Moves laterally: from the theoretical level in one field to the theoretical level in another field	"Level" of the theory is unchanged: for example, may add or redefine a term (concept); modify a relationship	Moves "downward": from very abstract theoretical level to ultimately the operational level
Example: using a biological theory of adaptation to, by analogy, develop a theory of maternal psychological adaptation	Example: adding the concept of "Internet support" to a theory of social support and coping in order to update the theory	Example: concretizing the concept of "support" in a general theory by identifying progressively more specific concepts that lead to a valid scale for measurement in a pediatric research situation

When a theorist has some ideas about the basic structure of a phenomenon but is struggling with articulating concepts to describe it, theory derivation is also very useful. Another theory in a different field may provide the theorist with a set of analogous concepts that can help describe the phenomenon, if suitably redefined for the field of interest. Again, this procedure creatively adds to the body of knowledge in the theorist's own field. We used one example of this strategy in Chapter 4, where Roy and Roberts (1981) developed the concepts of focal, contextual, and residual stimuli in patient assessment from a psychophysics theory by Helson.

Several examples of theory derivation come quickly to mind when we consider systems theory (e.g., Miller, 1978). Many of our nursing models in their original form have been direct derivations from systems theory—Roy and Roberts (1981); Neuman (1980); Erickson, Tomlin, and Swain (1983); and others have significant aspects of theory derivation in them.

PROCEDURES FOR THEORY DERIVATION

Although the actual process may not occur sequentially, theory derivation can be discussed as a series of sequential steps. However, theory derivation is really more of an iterative process. That is, the theorist goes back and forth between some or all of the steps until the level of sophistication of the theory is acceptable.

TABLE 6–2	**Steps or Phases of Theory Derivation**

Step or Phase	Step-Related Activity
1	Read widely on the topic of interest
2	Look for analogies in other fields
3	Choose "parent" theory
4	Identify concepts and structure of parent theory
5	Develop new statements and define "new" concepts in derived theory

There are several steps or phases in theory derivation, which are summarized in Table 6–2.

1. Be cognizant of the level of theory development in your own field of interest and evaluate the scientific usefulness of any such development. This implies that you are or will arrange to be thoroughly familiar with the literature on the topic of interest. If your evaluation leads you to believe that none of the current theories is suitable or useful, then theory derivation can proceed.
2. Read widely in nursing and in other fields for ideas while allowing imagination and creativity free rein. Reading widely enables you to understand ways of putting theory together and gives insight into new concepts and structures you may not have thought about before. Allowing your imagination and creativity free rein opens your mind to possible analogies. Discovering analogies is often done accidentally or as a creative intuitive leap rather than systematically.
3. Select a parent theory to use for derivation. The parent theory should be chosen because it offers a new and insightful way of explaining or predicting about a phenomenon in the theorist's field of interest. The parent theory may be, and often is, from another field or discipline, but a nursing theory may also be used. Any theory that provides you with a useful analogy can be chosen. However, just any theory won't do. Many theories will shed no light at all on the concepts of interest or fail to provide useful structure for the concepts and are therefore worthless to the theorist. Keep in mind here that the whole parent theory may not be needed to form the new theory. Only those portions that are analogous and therefore relevant need to be used.
4. Identify what content and/or structure from the parent theory is to be used. Perhaps only the concepts or only the statements are analogous, but not the overall structure. Or perhaps the structure is perfect but the parent concepts and statements are not. Perhaps the theorist needs concepts and statements as well as structure. In the derivation strategy, the theorist is free to choose what best fits the needs of the situation.
5. Develop or redefine any new concepts or statements from the content or structure of the parent theory in terms of the phenomenon of interest to the theorist. This is not only the hardest part of theory derivation but also the most fun. It requires creativity and thoughtfulness on the part of the theorist. Basically, the concepts or structure that is borrowed from the parent field is modified in such

TABLE 6–3 Examples of Theory Derivations

Author	Theory Derivation
Condon (1986)	A theory of development of caring in the nurse was derived from a parent theory of moral development
Wewers and Lenz (1987)	Derived a theory of relapse among ex-smokers from a theory of posttreatment functioning of alcoholics
Mishel (1990)	Uncertainty of illness theory (revised based on chaos theory)
Jones (2001)	Derived a theory about nursing time based on alternatives to clock/calendar time
Covell (2008)	Intellectual capital theory was used to derive a theory of nursing intellectual capital
Pedro (2010)	Health-related quality of life in rural cancer survivors
	(*Note:* Pedro used a combination of theory derivation and theory adaptation)

a way that it becomes meaningful in the theorist's field. Sometimes the modifications are small, but occasionally they will be substantial before the theory makes sense in the new setting.

Table 6–3 presents examples of theories developed or modified using the strategy of theory derivation. The selected examples draw on a wide range of parent theories and are applied to a variety of phenomena. This diversity indicates the potential range of applications of theory derivation.

EXAMPLES OF THEORY DERIVATION

Illustrations are often clearer than verbal explanations of theory derivation, so we provide several brief examples of theory derivation. Let us begin with a classic example. Maccia et al. (1963) used both concepts and structure of a theory of eyeblinks to derive a theory of education. Because they were some of the first scholars to explicitly use derivation for theory development, we have included an example from their work. Listed below are a few of the principles and their derivations from Maccia et al. (see Table 6–4).

While the preceding illustration presents the derivation process as a set of interrelated statements, the strategy may also be applied to parent theories or theoretical models that are captured in diagrammatic form. To illustrate this, in Figure 6–2, we have presented our rendering of a (fictitious) simple theoretical model of plant tropism. (The material for this model is based on the material on the website of Indiana University [2009].) The model we constructed of plant tropism indicates that when conditions for growth are suboptimal, plants may use directional stimuli to alter their responses and thereby achieve more favorable conditions for growth. The common illustration of this response is when plants are placed in windows and growth becomes oriented toward the outdoors where light is more abundant.

TABLE 6–4 Example of Theory Derivations

Parent Theory Statements*	Maccia et al.'s Derivation*
1. Either the eyes are or are not covered by lids.	1. The student is either distracted or attentive.
2. Blinking functions to protect the eyes from contact and to rest the retina and the ocular muscles.	2. Distraction functions to protect the student from mental stress and to rest from mental effort.
3. Blinking may be either reflexive or nonreflexive.	3. Distraction may be either voluntary or involuntary.
4. Reflex blinking may be inhibited by a fixation object or by drugs.	4. Involuntary distraction may be inhibited by attention cues or by drugs.
5. Nonreflexive blinking may occur if seeing is unwanted.	5. Voluntary distraction may occur if learning is unwanted.

*Except for minor modifications, the above are direct quotations from Maccia et al. (1963, p. 34). For ease of illustration, we have omitted quotation marks, but acknowledge the quoted nature of this material here.

The focus of our derived theory is one that is sometimes seen in community and public health nursing: the surprising health of some individuals despite challenging environments. The derived theory that we have created (see Figure 6–3) deals with the phenomenon of positive deviance in which some individuals living in low-resource situations still find ways to thrive despite their adverse circumstances (Marsh, Schroeder, Dearden, Sternin, & Sternin, 2004). For illustrative purposes, we have used the plant tropic response as an analogy to aid us in constructing a theoretical model of the phenomenon of positive deviance. (Note that our model is presented primarily to illustrate the process of theory derivation and is not intended to represent the full complexity of positive deviance.)

In the derived model, we have used the same structural form of the parent model with one modification. We have added bidirectional arrows between *uncommon retrieval of thriving requisites* and *nontraditional source of requisites*. We have done this to show the active role of positive deviants in thriving efforts in low-resource

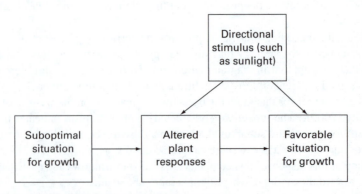

FIGURE 6–2 Model of tropic plant growth responses.

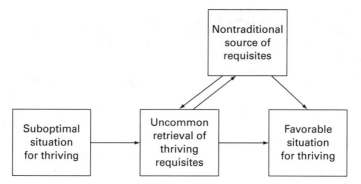

FIGURE 6–3 [Fictitious] Derived model of positive deviants' responses to low-resource environments.

environments. Thus, the model indicates that positive deviants, despite finding themselves in suboptimal situations for thriving, are able to seek and use uncommon methods to attain thriving requisites and thereby create more favorable situations for thriving. A classic example of this is consuming available plants that are not typically included in the diet of the local low-resource community.

APPLICATION OF THEORY DERIVATION TO NURSING

In an early nursing example of derivation, Wewers and Lenz (1987) derived a theory of relapse among ex-smokers from Cronkite and Moos's (1980) theory of posttreatment functioning of alcoholics (see Table 6–5). Wewers and Lenz not only primarily used content derivation but also derived a simplified structure. Table 6–5 lists three propositions from Cronkite and Moos with the derivations made by Wewers and Lenz.

TABLE 6–5 Example of Theory Derivations

Parent Theory Statements (Cronkite & Moos, 1980)	Wewers and Lenz's (1987) Derivation
1. Pretreatment symptoms such as alcohol consumption, type of drinker, depression, and occupational functioning are related to alcohol treatment outcomes (p. 48).	1. Pretreatment symptoms such as cigarette consumption and type of smoker are related to smoking relapse (p. 48).
2. "Stressful life events were negatively associated with some aspects of recovery" (p. 49).	2. "Both the social contextual stressor of major life events and the internal stressor of craving" are associated with smoking relapse (p. 49).
3. Family environment is "weakly related to alcohol recovery" (p. 49).	3. "Long term smoking cessation is associated with having family members who are nonsmokers or who had previously been able to quit smoking" (p. 49).

TABLE 6–6 Example of Theory Derivations	
Parent Theory Statements (Mishel, 1990)	**Mishel's (1990) Derivation**
1. "In far-from equilibrium conditions, the sensitivity of the initial condition is such that small changes yield huge effects, and the system reorganizes itself in multiple ways" (p. 259).	1. "Abiding uncertainty can dismantle the existing cognitive structures that give meaning to everyday events. . . . This loss of meaning throws the person into a state of confusion and disorganization" (p. 260).
2. "Fluctuations in the system can become so powerful . . . that they shatter the preexisting organization" (p. 259).	2. If the uncertainty factors of disease or illness multiply rapidly past a critical value, the stability of the personal system can no longer be taken for granted (paraphrase, p. 259).
3. "Auto-catalytic processes result in a product whose presence encourages further production of itself" producing disorder (p. 259).	3. "The existence of uncertainty in one area of illness often feeds back on itself and generates further uncertainty in other illness-related events" (p. 260).

In some cases, we have adapted the wording of the propositions to show the derivations more clearly. Because there was already a large amount of literature available on smoking, Wewers and Lenz adopted propositions in their derivation that fit knowledge specifically about smoking. This is an excellent example of how to use the strategy flexibly in theory-building efforts.

Theory derivation can happen using two closely related fields as in the preceding example of Wewers and Lenz's (1987) derivations. Or insight can come from widely disparate fields. It is the theorist's creativity and intuition that provide the insight into the analogy. Mishel's (1990) reconceptualization of the uncertainty of illness theory provides an example of derivations between widely disparate fields. Mishel used the content and structure of chaos theory to help her describe more clearly the outcome portion of her theory of uncertainty in illness (see Table 6–6). We have selected three statements to illustrate how the derivation was made. In an effort to be as clear and succinct as possible, we have at times restated the propositions to make the analogies more obvious. Note that the derivations presented below do not follow the direct symmetrical form of the parent theory, but the analogous translation is relatively clear.

A theorist does not have to derive both concepts and structure. Derivation can be used only for concepts or only for structure. Let us examine one example in which only concepts were used. Jones (2001) used concepts to derive a theory about nursing time based on Adam's (1995) alternatives to clock/calendar time. See Table 6–7 for Adam's parent theory concepts with definitions and Jones's derivation. For other examples, see those in Table 6–3 and the references under "Additional Readings" at the end of this chapter.

TABLE 6–7 Example of Theory Derivations

Parent Theory Statements (Adam, 1995)	Jones's (2001) Derivation on Nursing Time
1. Temporality—"the cycle of life and death that occurs against the backdrop of unidirectional time" (p. 155).	1. Temporality—"There are unlimited amounts of parallel and cyclical time frames within which nurses exist simultaneously and within each frame we organize, plan, and regulate our lives" (p. 154).
2. Timing—is "when" time but clock and calendar times are not the only points of reference in determining "when" for scheduling, synchronization, allocation of resources, etc.	2. Timing—"Timing in . . . nursing is dependent on multiple considerations, based on past, present, and future times" (p. 156).
3. Tempo—Time may seem to advance at varying speeds, for example, "when we speak of time moving quickly or slowly" (p. 156).	3. Tempo—"Processes in the health services are mutually implicated in how much is achieved within a given timeframe in the timing of actions and in the temporality of existence" (p. 156).

ADVANTAGES AND LIMITATIONS

Theory derivation is a focused and creative way to develop theory in new areas of interest. It is an exciting exercise in that it requires the theorist to use imagination in seeing analogies from one field and modifying them for use in a new field. In addition, theory derivation provides a way of arriving at explanation and prediction about a phenomenon where there may be little or no information, literature, or formal studies available.

One disadvantage is that the theorist must be familiar with a number of fields of interest other than his or her own field of interest. This implies reading widely and being constantly on the alert for new and profitable analogies. In addition, the theorist must be thoroughly familiar with the literature and current thinking about his or her particular area of interest. Otherwise, when the time comes to draw an analogy, the theorist will have difficulty choosing appropriate boundaries for the new theory.

Derived theories are constructed in the context of discovery (Rudner, 1966). As a result, the theories thus developed lack evidence of validity until they are subjected to empirical testing in the context of theory validation and testing. Even if the theory is extremely relevant to practice or research, it must first be validated before it can be used. Methods that may be used to test theories are presented in Chapter 13.

Novice theorists often become so excited about their new generalizations that they fail to take into account any dissimilarities, or disanalogies, present in the parent theory. These disanalogies should at least be considered for any valuable information that they might provide in the new theory. The disanalogies may give further insight into the phenomenon or may provide useful red flags of trouble ahead.

Finally, theory derivation is only the first step in a program of research. To be useful and credible for application to practice, a theory developed by derivation needs testing through research.

UTILIZING THE RESULTS OF THEORY DERIVATION

The uses of theory derivation are to provide structure when only concepts are available, to provide concepts when only structure is available, or to provide both concepts and structure as an efficient way to begin theory development. The results of theory derivation are easily used in nursing education, practice, research, and theory development.

Theory derivation is an excellent way to obtain a theoretical framework for curriculum building in education. In addition, it can be used as a teaching tool with graduate students as a way to introduce them to theorizing in general. It is relatively easy to learn and fun to do as a group exercise. (To make the idea of theory building less scary for beginning students, we often ask them first to derive a new theory that has to do with their daily lives rather than nursing. When they are successful at this, we then ask them to derive a nursing theory.)

Theory derivation can provide significant new insights for clinical practice. Clinicians can provide themselves with a useful theoretical framework to guide their practice by using the results of theory derivation.

Theory derivation is also a means of designing a conceptual model for a research program. Moving concepts and/or structure from the parent field with appropriate changes yields a rich source of potential hypotheses for study, as Wewers and Lenz (1987) demonstrated. It is an efficient strategy for achieving a body of knowledge about a phenomenon.

Summary

Theory derivation is a means of adding new theory development to a field. In using it, the theorist employs analogy to obtain explanations or predictions about a phenomenon in one field from explanations or predictions in another field. Both concepts and structure can be moved from the parent field to the new one, undergoing modifications along the way.

There are five steps to theory derivation: (1) become thoroughly familiar with the topic of interest; (2) read widely in other fields, allowing your imagination to help you find useful analogies; (3) select a parent theory to use for derivation; (4) identify what content and/or structure from the parent theory is to be used; and (5) modify or redefine new concepts and/or statements in terms of the phenomenon of interest. Once the new theory has been formulated, it must be tested empirically to validate that the new concepts and structure actually reflect reality in the new field.

Theory derivation is a creative means of constructing new theories. One disadvantage is that the theorist must be widely read in several fields as well as his or her own field. In addition, the theorist must remember to consider the dissimilarities as well as the similarities between the parent field and the new field.

At this point in our development of a nursing knowledge base, theory derivation is a highly workable strategy for nursing. It provides a means of developing a theory with innovative content. If carefully done and carefully tested, derived theories could play an immediate role in the development of scientific knowledge in nursing.

Practice Exercises

EXERCISE 1

Use the theoretical statements about eyeblinks in Table 6–4 to construct a set of statements about patient education for nursing in your own particular area of clinical interest. Feel free to use the derived statements in the table as a guide.

EXERCISE 2

Use the diagram in Figure 6–2 on tropic plant growth responses to derive a model of dealing with equipment shortages in health emergencies in field settings. Since this is an exercise, focus mainly on working out the parallel concepts that best fit the parent model. After this is done, you may wish to make some further modifications so that it has the feel of a realistic model.

References

Adam B. *Timewatch: The Social Analysis of Time*. Cambridge, England: Polity Press; 1995.

Bekhet AK, Zauszniewski JA. Theoretical substruction illustrated by the Theory of Learned Resourcefulness. *Res Theory Nurs Pract*. 2008;22(3):205–214.

Condon EH. Theory derivation: Application to nursing . . . the caring perspective within professional nurse role development. *J Nurs Educ*. 1986;25(4):156–159.

Covell CL. The middle-range theory of nursing intellectual capital. *J Adv Nurs*. 2008;63:94–103.

Cronkite RC, Moos RH. Determinants of the post-treatment functioning of alcoholic patients: A conceptual framework. *J Consult Clin Psychol*. 1980;48:305–316.

Erickson HC, Tomlin EM, Swain MAP. *Modeling and Role Modeling: A Theory and Paradigm of Nursing*. Englewood Cliffs, NJ: Prentice Hall; 1983.

Hempel CG. *Philosophy of Natural Science*. Englewood Cliffs, NJ: Prentice Hall; 1966.

Indiana University. Plant tropic responses. Accessed online on November 26, 2009, at http://plantsinmotion.bio.indiana.edu/plantmotion/movements/tropism/tropisms.html.

Jones AR. Time to think: Temporal considerations in nursing practice and research. *J Adv Nurs*. 2001;33(2):150–158.

Maccia ES, Maccia GS, Jewett RE. *Construction of Educational Theory Models*. Cooperative Research Project #1632. Columbus, OH: Ohio State University Research Foundation; 1963.

Marsh DR, Schroeder DG, Dearden KA, Sternin J, Sternin M. The power of positive deviance. *Br Med J*. 2004;329:1177–1179.

McQuiston CM, Campbell JC. Theoretical substruction: A guide for theory testing research. *Nurs Sci Q*. 1997;10(3):117–123.

Miller JG. *Living Systems*. New York, NY: McGraw-Hill; 1978.

Mishel MH. Reconceptualization of the uncertainty of illness theory. *Image*. 1990;22(4):256–262.

Neuman B. The Betty Neuman health care systems model: A total person approach to patient problems. In: Riehl JP, Roy C, eds. *Conceptual Models for Nursing Practice*. 2nd ed. New York, NY: Appleton-Century-Crofts; 1980.

Nierenberg GI. *The Art of Negotiating*. New York, NY: Hawthorne; 1968.

Nierenberg GI. *Fundamentals of Negotiating*. New York, NY: Hawthorne; 1973.

Pedro L. Theory derivation: Adaptation of a contextual model of health related quality of life to rural cancer survivors. *Online J Rural Nurs Health Care*. 2010;10(1):80–95.

Roy C, Roberts SL. *Theory Construction in Nursing: An Adaptation Model*. Englewood Cliffs, NJ: Prentice Hall; 1981.

Rudner R. *Philosophy of Social Science*. Englewood Cliffs, NJ: Prentice Hall; 1966.

Wewers ME, Lenz E. Relapse among ex-smokers: An example of theory derivation. *Adv Nurs Sci*. 1987;9(2):44–53.

Additional Readings

Challey PS. Theory derivation in moral development. *Nurs Health Care*. 1990;11(6):302–306.

Comley AL, Beard MT. Toward a derived theory of patient satisfaction. *J Theory Construct Test*. 1998;2(2):44–50.

Henderson JS, Hamilton P, Vicenza AE. Chaos theory in nursing publications: Retrospective and prospective views. *Complexity Chaos Nurs*. 1995;2(1):36–40.

Olson RW. *The Art of Creative Thinking: A Practical Guide*. New York, NY: Barnes Noble; 1980.

Teel CS, Meek P, McNamara AM, Watson L. Perspectives unifying symptom interpretation. *Image*. 1997;29(2):175–181.

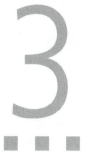

Synthesis Strategies

In this part, we present the synthesis strategies for forming concepts, statements, and theories. The next three chapters will focus on ways to systematically develop these various levels of theory. At their heart, the synthesis strategies involve observations or findings of observations already captured in the literature as a foundation for concept, statement, or theory development. Deciding which synthesis strategy will be most useful depends on considering questions about the level of theory development, the type of literature available on the topic, and the quality and completeness of the existing literature. Readers are encouraged to read Chapter 3 as a further guide to strategy selection.

When gathering of new observations is needed to fuel understanding of a phenomenon, either qualitative or quantitative methods, or both, may be used depending on the theory builder's purposes. New concepts (Chapter 7), statements (Chapter 8), or theories (Chapter 9) may be formed through synthesis of such observations. Synthesis strategies may also be applied to existing data or literature that is in need of consolidation. Depending on the state of knowledge about a phenomenon and the theory builder's purpose, synthesis strategies may be directed toward concept, statement, or theory development (Chapters 7, 8, or 9, respectively). Although we present the three synthesis strategies as separate entities, their subject matter is interrelated. Thus, readers who choose a synthesis strategy are encouraged to read the three as a set for a better orientation to the synthesis strategy. If you are unsure of the synthesis strategy (i.e., concept, statement, or theory) best suited to the phenomenon you are seeking to describe or explain, it might help to consider several questions such as those listed in the "Strategy Selection" section in Chapter 3 or those that are presented at the beginning of each chapter.

The presentation of synthesis strategies in relation to qualitative or quantitative methods is primarily intended to locate such methods within a synthesis-based program of theory development. It is not our aim to provide an exposition of qualitative or quantitative methods. Readers are referred to qualitative (Corbin & Strauss, 2015; Denzin & Lincoln, 2018) or quantitative (Hebel & McCarter, 2011; Plichta & Kelvin, 2013; Polit, 2010; Polit & Beck, 2017; Tabachnick & Fidell, 2014; Warner, 2013) methods texts for a full exposition of these respective methods.

REFERENCES

Corbin J, Strauss AC. *Basics of Qualitative Research: Techniques and Procedures for Developing Grounded Theory.* 4th ed. Thousand Oaks, CA: Sage Publications; 2015.

Denzin NK, Lincoln YS. *The Sage Handbook of Qualitative Research.* 5th ed. Thousand Oaks, CA: Sage Publications; 2018.

Hebel JR, McCarter RJ. *A Study Guide to Epidemiology and Biostatistics.* 7th ed. Gaithersburg, MD: Aspen; 2011.

Plichta SB, Kelvin E. *Munro's Statistical Methods for Health Care Research.* 6th ed. Philadelphia, PA: Lippincott Williams and Wilkins; 2013.

Polit DF. *Data Analysis and Statistics for Nursing Research.* 2nd ed. Boston, MA: Pearson; 2010.

Polit DF, Beck CT. *Nursing Research: Generating and Assessing Evidence for Nursing Practice.* 10th ed. Philadelphia, PA: Lippincott Williams & Wilkins; 2017.

Tabachnick BG, Fidell LS. *Using Multivariate Statistics.* 6th ed. Boston, MA: Pearson, Allen & Bacon; 2014.

Warner RM. *Applied Statistics: From Bivariate to Multivariate Techniques.* 2nd ed. Los Angeles, CA: Sage Publications; 2013.

7

■ ■ ■

Concept Synthesis

Questions to consider before you get started reading this chapter:

▶ Are you observing a clinical phenomenon but have no way to name it?

▶ Do you have clusters of related data but no way to summarize them?

▶ Are you confronted with a need to explain a phenomenon but the current explanations are inadequate or confusing?

If any of these situations are what you are facing, then concept synthesis may be the method to help you resolve it. Concept synthesis is a means of combining disparate data or observations into something new and giving it a name that makes it possible to communicate clearly about it. It is particularly useful in naming and describing phenomena in practice.

Introductory Note: There are increasingly urgent demands for evidence on which to base nursing practice. However, evidence has to be about something. What is that something? The phenomena about which nurses are concerned are the things they deal with on an everyday basis in their work. However, describing, explaining, and predicting about those phenomena has been limited by the inability to name the concepts that represent or capture those phenomena in a way that is easily communicated, or documented. As we can describe how we think, what we do, and how effective what we do is, we can avoid finding ourselves on the defensive related to the evidence about our practice. Concept synthesis is an extremely useful strategy for developing a standard language about our practice.

DEFINITION AND DESCRIPTION

As in all synthesis strategies, concept synthesis is based on observation or empirical evidence. The data may come from direct observation, qualitative or quantitative evidence, literature, or some combination. The process of concept synthesis is one of the most exciting ways of beginning theory building. It permits the theorist to use clinical experience as one place to begin.

In a very real sense, you must start from scratch when doing concept synthesis. Concepts are ordered information about the attributes of one or more things that enables us to differentiate among them (Wilson, 1963). Therefore, the theorist using this strategy must invent a new way of grouping, or ordering, information about some event or phenomenon, when the relevant dimensions are unclear or unknown.

Everyone actually does concept synthesis. New concepts often develop from very ordinary activities. Creation of a new concept does not require genius. In fact, all of us who think form new concepts, or categories, as our experiences in the world broaden and increase. When children learn that things have names, they begin to place things into categories. These are not always logical categories at first, but they become so as the child learns to associate things that are similar in some way. As the child's experience increases, he or she begins to compare new information with the already-learned concepts, or categories, of things. If the new information fits one of the previously existing concepts, or categories, it is easily assimilated. If the new information does not fit any previously existing concept or category, then the child must develop a strategy for dealing with the new information. He or she has one of three choices: (1) misname the information by putting it in an old category; (2) deny the new information altogether; or (3) develop a new concept (Breen, 2002; Hunt, 1962; Spitzer, 1977; Stevenson, 1972).

A parent, teacher, or someone else in the child's environment may help in this effort. If a child has always categorized animals with four legs and a tail as "doggie" and then encounters an animal with four legs, a tail, and an udder, that goes "moo," and is 4 feet tall, there will be some discrepancy between the new animal and the familiar doggie. The parent may help the child solve the problem by saying, "That is a cow." We, as adults, are not always so lucky. When we encounter a new phenomenon in our own experience, there is not always someone around to tell us what the new concept is. We must invent our own name to explain the new phenomenon. This, in effect, is concept formation, the precursor of concept synthesis.

There are several ways to synthesize concepts: (1) by discovering new dimensions of old or existing concepts; (2) by examining sets of related concepts for similarities or discrepancies; or (3) by observing new phenomena or clusters of phenomena that have not been described previously. When the discovery of a new concept has been made, a name is chosen or invented that will demonstrate the meaning and allow for pertinent communication about it. The new concept should be defined and its defining attributes delineated so that the reader or user of the new concept can determine what is and what is not intended by the new concept.

PURPOSE AND USES

Concept synthesis is used to generate new ideas. It provides a method of examining data for new insights that can add to theoretical development. New concepts enrich our vocabulary and point to new areas for study.

Historically, Dray's (1959) classic idea of "explanatory generalizations" is very similar to concept synthesis. He speaks of these explanatory generalizations as occurring in a process of synthesis that "allows us to refer to x, y, and z collectively as 'a so and so.'" It is, in effect, explaining by finding an appropriate classification for the phenomenon under investigation and naming it. Gordon (1982) has called this same process "pattern recognition." This is a particularly useful strategy for developing nursing diagnoses. In fact, almost any new diagnosis, new syndrome, or new taxonomy represents an attempt at concept synthesis. Whenever a new phenomenon or cluster of phenomena are described empirically or generated from data, the process of concept synthesis has already begun.

Concept synthesis is useful in several areas: (1) in areas where there is little or no concept development; (2) in areas where concept development is present but has had no real impact on theory or practice; and (3) in areas where observations of phenomena are available but not yet classified or named. Concept synthesis also may be used in conjunction with other strategies as part of a larger program of theory development. Such a multi-strategy approach is shown in the development of the middle-range theory of unpleasant symptoms (Lenz, Suppe, Gift, Pugh, & Milligan, 1995).

APPROACHES TO CONCEPT SYNTHESIS

Qualitative, quantitative, and literary approaches may be used either alone or together to do concept synthesis. Each approach to concept synthesis requires the use of data—qualitative, quantitative, or literary. We will describe each approach and give some relevant examples. Then we will outline the steps of concept synthesis. The steps are the same regardless of the kind of data you use.

Qualitative Synthesis

Qualitative synthesis requires using sensory data such as that gained from listening or observing to obtain information. It speaks to properties of things without assigning a numerical value to the amount of the property present. As the data are collected, they are examined for similarities and differences much as one would in using a grounded theory approach (Benoliel, 1996; Corbin & Strauss, 2015; Eaves, 2001; Glaser, 1978, 1992; Glaser & Strauss, 1967; Kirk & Miller, 1986; Mullen, 1994; Stern, 1994). Basically, qualitative synthesis involves recognizing patterns among observations. (For further discussion of qualitative methods, see Chapter 8 on statement synthesis.)

Denham's (2002) research on family routines is an excellent example of qualitative synthesis. Three ethnographic studies of family routines and rituals were conducted in Appalachia. The first study, of families with preschoolers, yielded seven categories of health routines: dietary practices, sleep and rest patterns, activity patterns, avoidance behaviors, dependent care activities, medical consultations, and health recovery activities. The second study, of families who had lost a family member, yielded five categories: self-care routines, member caregiving, medical consultation, habitual high-risk behaviors, and mental health behaviors. The third study, of disadvantaged families, yielded six categories: self-care routines, dietary practices, mental health, family care, preventive care, and illness care. From these three sets of categories, Denham synthesized six new concepts that described family health routines. The six new concepts were self-care routines, safety and prevention, mental health behaviors, family care, illness care, and member caregiving.

Kolanowski's (1995) study is an older but still good example of qualitative synthesis. Kolanowski used qualitative data to extract meaningful clusters of disturbing behaviors manifested by persons with dementia. Five distinct clusters emerged from the study. Kolanowski named the five clusters aggressive psychomotor behavior, non-aggressive psychomotor behavior, verbally aggressive behavior, passive behavior, and functionally impaired behavior.

Finally, Elo and Calltorp (2002) used concept synthesis to develop a "classification of healthcare services used in public health nursing practice" (p. 201). Health care services rendered by public health nurses as documented in Swedish patient records served as the data source for the concept synthesis project. The larger goal of the project was to develop a model for public health nursing services. Their multistep process of concept synthesis included first extracting "nouns and verb phrases" (p. 202), then generating 186 labels for nursing actions, searching for new actions in additional records, and finally developing "main categories in a tentative classification system" (p. 202) that was organized hierarchically. Subsequent steps included confirming and revising the categories by reference to literature and expert review. The outcome was six service categories: health promotive, health protective, diagnostic, therapeutic, rehabilitative, and terminal health care (p. 204).

Quantitative Synthesis

Numerical or statistical data are necessary for **quantitative synthesis**. You may use any studies—experimental or nonexperimental, single case or group designs—as long as they provide quantitative data about the phenomenon of interest. Statistical methods may be employed to extract clusters of attributes comprising a new concept as well as depicting those attributes that do not belong to the concept. Measures such as Q sorts, factor analysis, and Delphi techniques are especially helpful for generating meaningful clusters. Oldaker's (1986) study of normal adolescents' psychological symptomatology is a good example of a quantitative concept synthesis. From several indices of psychological symptoms and personality, Oldaker used principal axis factor analysis to synthesize four concepts related to identity confusion: intimacy, negative identity, diffusion of time perspective, and diffusion of industry.

A classic quantitative study of concept synthesis is that of Kobasa (1979a, 1979b), who studied the effects of life stress on middle- and upper-echelon managers. What she discovered surprised her—of the managers who were identified by high stress levels as at risk for illness, about one-third had not had any or at least few illnesses. What made these executives different? Everything Kobasa knew about stress suggested that they should be sick. Was it something in the executives' responses to stressful events that protected them from illness? As a result of these questions, Kobasa set up several studies to collect data on the categories of openness to change, involvement, and control over events. As the data were analyzed, the categories were reduced slightly to challenge, commitment, and control. Finally, the concept name "hardiness" was used to accurately reflect the three combined categories. Additional studies have since validated the concept for some occupations but not entirely for others. However, the concept has made a major impact on theorizing about stress (Cataldo, 1993; Kobasa, 1979a, 1979b; Kobasa, Hiker, & Maddi, 1979; Lambert & Lambert, 1987; Nichols & Webster, 1993; Pietrzak et al., 2010; Pines, 1980; Wagnild & Young, 1991).

Literary Synthesis

The careful examination of literature is required in **literary synthesis** in order to acquire new insights about phenomena of interest. This examination may yield previously unrecognized concepts for study. Particular to literary concept synthesis is the idea that the literature itself becomes the database. Colling's (2000) study of passive behaviors in people with Alzheimer's disease is an example of literary synthesis. Fifteen studies yielded a total of 82 behaviors. The 82 behaviors were then clustered into six initial groupings: diminution of cognition, diminution of psychomotor activity, diminution in feeling emotions, diminution of responding to emotions, diminution of interactions with people, and diminution of interactions with the environment. Next, Colling constructed an instrument using the six categories and with all categories and behaviors defined. She asked a panel of experts in gerontology to sort the behaviors into the categories. The categories were refined and reduced based on results of the analysis of the panel responses. The same six experts then participated in a second round of independent ratings. The final analyses yielded a taxonomy of five independent categories: diminution of cognition, diminution of psychomotor activity, diminution of emotions, diminution of interaction with people, and diminution of interactions with the environment. Finally, the new concepts or categories were evaluated for consistency of use across raters, and for consistency with the need-driven dementia-compromised behavior framework (Algase et al., 1996).

A second example is Smith, Swallow, and Coyne's (2015) synthesis of two frameworks of care for pediatric families, family-centered care and partnership in care. Using 30 studies published between 1999 and 2014 related to both concepts, the authors formulated a novel framework related to working with parents whose children have long-term, chronic conditions. Their synthesis resulted in three new concepts in a framework they named "parent—professional collaboration—a framework for involvement" (p. 20). The three concepts were "valuing parents' knowledge and experiences," "supporting parents in their role as caregiver," and "incorporating parents' expertise into clinical and psychosocial care" (p. 20). The authors provide a table that allows the reader an overview of the 30 studies selected for the synthesis, thus providing the reader with a way to follow the process. In addition, the authors delineate both the collaborative processes underpinning each of the three new concepts and also suggest the nursing actions needed to achieve those processes. For someone new to the process of synthesis, this article is a good example to review.

A final example of a literary synthesis is Finfgeld-Connett's (2008) study of the art of nursing. Using literature from 1982 to 2006, she constructed a comprehensive definition of the concept. Antecedents of the art of nursing were found to be empirical and metaphysical knowledge. The attributes of artful nursing were found to be relationship centered and expert practice and creativity. Outcomes were beneficent actions aimed at improving health and easing distress. Both patients and nurses benefit as a result of artful nursing. Finfgeld-Connett's final theoretical definition was the following: "The art of nursing appears to consist of expert use and adaptation of empirical and metaphysical knowledge and values. It is relationship-centered and involves sensitively adapting care to meet the needs of individual patients. In the face of uncertainty, creativity is employed in a discretionary manner. Artful nursing promotes beneficent practice and results in enhanced mental and physical well-being among patients. It also appears to result in professional satisfaction and personal growth among nurses" (p. 383).

Mixed Methods

Any of the three approaches to concept synthesis may be used alone or together. There is no hard-and-fast rule about how or when they may be used. Thus, the needs of the theorist and the state of the science are what drive decisions and choices of method. Several studies used either single or mixed methods of concept synthesis (Anderson & Oinhausen, 1999; Beitz, 1998; Bunting, Russell, & Gregory, 1998; Colling, 2000; Goldberg, 1998; Kolanowski, 1995; Polk, 1997; Wendler, 1999). The following examples will show how various approaches can be used sequentially or combined to render useful new concepts.

Goldberg (1998) explored the meanings of spirituality using two approaches to concept synthesis. The attributes that arose from the literature on spirituality were meaning, presencing, empathy, compassion, giving hope, love, religion or transcendence, touch, and healing. First, these attributes were clustered into fewer categories. Goldberg then looked at overarching similarities—all implied relationships, either physical or emotional or both. Reviewing the three clusters helped Goldberg realize that a psyche—soma dichotomy was not helpful. The three clusters were thus collapsed into one concept and named "connection."

In a classic study, Clunn (1984) used grounded theory combined with questionnaires to study the cues nurses used to formulate a nursing diagnosis of potential for violence and whether the nurses discriminated between degrees of violent behavior. Using interviews, literature, and scales, 11 concepts were synthesized from Clunn's study: medical history, content of verbalizations, peer relationships, social history, background factors, purposeful motor actions, nonpurposeful motor actions, intensity or emotionality of verbalizations, pervasive affective state, labile emotional reactions, and cognitive indicators of disequilibrium. From these 11 concepts, Clunn synthesized three major factors—interaction, action, and awareness—as the cue categories most used in diagnosing potential for violence. These three factors emerged in both the qualitative and the quantitative portions of the study. Her findings indicated that the actual cues and categories of cues nurses used in assessing the client's potential for violence were similar but the patterns that were salient for some groups of nurses (e.g., emergency room) were not the same as those for other groups (e.g., state hospital).

Finally, Burke, Kaufmann, Costello, and Dillon (1991) provided an excellent example of concept synthesis using data from several sources. In their study of the stress of parenting a chronically ill child with repeated hospitalizations, they formed two new concepts. The first was "hazardous secrets," which reflects the parents' perceptions of the parent–health care worker interaction. The parents saw these secrets (e.g., faulty information, gaps in care, and inexperience of the worker) as potentially hazardous to their child. The second concept reflected the process by which the parents managed the stress and was named "reluctantly taking charge" and encompassed vigilance, negotiating rules, calling a halt, and persistent information seeking.

PROCEDURES FOR CONCEPT SYNTHESIS

We will discuss the steps of concept synthesis sequentially but, as in most of the strategies, they are really iterative. That is, you do not always progress from step to step but may cycle through steps several times or go back and forth between steps. Glaser and Strauss (1967) refer to the aim of this process as reaching theoretical saturation. To do this, you must become thoroughly familiar with the area of interest by using many resources, including literature reviews and case studies. All provide potential sources of usable data.

During the time you are becoming theoretically saturated, begin to classify the data you acquire. The system of classification need not be rigorous. Indeed, it is better if the system stays fairly loose at this stage. While you are classifying the data, look for clusters of phenomena that seem to relate closely to each other or overlap considerably and combine them. To do this, clustering requires only that each classification category be compared to every other category. This can be done using factor analysis on a computer but is not really difficult when done by the theorist using visual inspection.

Once you are satisfied that all the clusters have been discovered and combined where possible, examine the clusters for any hierarchical structure. If there are clusters that appear very similar but one is of a broader nature than the other, it may be helpful to reduce the two clusters into one higher-order concept. When the new concept has been reduced as much as possible, a name should be chosen for it that accurately describes it and that facilitates communication about it.

Once the concept is named, the next step is to verify the new concept empirically and modify it as necessary. Verification involves a return to literature, field studies, data collection, and colleagues to discover if the concept is empirically supported. That is, do any of these data sources provide additional information that will expand, clarify, negate, or limit the concept? This process continues until the theorist is satisfied that no new information is being received. At this point, the process stops and the new concept is considered adequate. The new concept should then be described in a theoretical definition that includes its defining attributes.

Finally, determine, if possible, where the new concept fits into existing theory in the area. Consideration should be given to the distinctive insights and potential approaches to research and practice the new concept makes possible. There may even be times when a concept is so radically different from current theoretical positions that a whole new field of study emerges. A good example of this effect was the discovery of microbes that generated the field of bacteriology. Sometimes an existing system of thinking is completely changed, as when the concept of relativity completely changed the orientation of the field of physics or when the human genome mapping revolutionized the study of human health and illness.

Keeping your working memory updated on current thinking about the phenomena of concern to you is a critical factor that facilitates concept synthesis. It is very important to be thoroughly familiar with one's own field of interest. It is equally important to be able to retain a significant amount of that knowledge in your memory. Keeping notes of your thinking and using concentrated periods of work can help to keep your mind alert. In this way, phenomena that don't compute with existing ways of thinking become more obvious.

However, because memory is fallible, it is very useful for theorists to develop a notebook or electronic file of memos to themselves. In these memos, observations should be carefully recorded. These may be directly observed phenomena, statistical findings, or information summaries from literature. Both at the time of writing the memo and at the time the theorist reviews the file of memos, insights and interpretations of the data should be added. These interpretive notes form the basis for developing classifications in initial concept synthesis efforts and in efforts to develop higher concepts at a later time (Schatzman & Strauss, 1973).

The ability to observe is another critical factor that facilitates concept synthesis. Obviously, a keen observer is more likely to see new phenomena than one who never looks. This skill is not inborn. It is acquired with practice. Observing clinical practices, for example, may cause you to discover new phenomena. Asking questions about practices may allow you to formulate new ideas about interventions, for example. (If you feel you are not a careful observer, try Practice Exercise 1 at the end of this chapter.)

The skill of evaluating evidence is a corollary to the skill of observation. This ability to look at data, determine their value, and extract new ideas can also be learned. The literature on evidence-based practice is replete with examples of how to evaluate evidence. Refer also to "Additional Readings" on evaluating research at the end of this chapter or any good research text for honing such perceptions.

Openness to new ideas is the last critical factor that influences concept synthesis. This implies, at least, a freedom from the fear of discovering something new. Many nurses practice nursing precisely as they were taught and have little inclination to question or experiment with new ways of doing or thinking about things. Change for many people is very threatening, and certainly synthesizing a new concept will initiate some change, if only in thinking. Therefore, before concept synthesis can occur, the nurse must be willing to allow the possibility of new ideas.

New ideas come to us from all our senses. Most of us are verbally and mathematically trained but have little practice relying on taste, smell, vision, or touch to help us arrive at new ideas. It is often helpful to think divergently by forcing ourselves to use other than our verbal or mathematics skills to arrive at new ideas about phenomena.

Coupled with the idea of using all our senses to help us generate new concepts is the admonition to take plenty of time. The process of synthesis is creating something new; it cannot be accomplished quickly. Ideas take time to develop or incubate. Relax and don't push yourself.

ADVANTAGES AND LIMITATIONS

Concept synthesis provides a mechanism for creating something new from data already available. It provides new insights and adds texture and richness to the fabric of developing theory. Given the growing use of electronic patient records and nursing informatics, the naming of nursing phenomena and nursing activities makes concept synthesis especially pertinent. The process of concept synthesis is especially useful as a means of generating and naming potential nursing diagnoses, interventions, and outcomes.

Concept synthesis does take time and requires the theorist to be open to risk taking. The theorist must begin with raw data and attempt to conceive a new idea from it. Sometimes this happens quickly. More often, it happens only after considerable time and thought.

Verifying concepts also takes time. This is when the theorist feels most uncomfortable. What if the new concept can't be verified? The fear of being wrong is powerful, especially when the theorist may view the new concept as a brainchild and is very attached to it. The necessity here is for the theorist to remain objective and scientific. If the concept is truly data based, it should come through the verification with only minor revisions.

Finally, concepts in themselves are only useful to describe a phenomenon. They do not provide for explanation, prediction, or prescription. It is only when concepts are connected to each other through relational statements that we have the possibility of a hypothesis or a theory.

UTILIZING THE RESULTS OF CONCEPT SYNTHESIS

Concept synthesis is useful when there is a need to explain something by classifying it, or when we need wholly new concepts or new uses for old ones. But what do you do with a new concept once you've synthesized it?

Several things can and should be done. The first of these is to verify, support, or validate the new concept (see Chapter 13). This is very much like establishing content validity or transferability in research, and the same methods can be used for either task. Once the concept has attained an adequate degree of support, a good theoretical definition containing the defining attributes should be written. When this is accomplished, the new concept should be shared by publishing it.

Knowledge development in the nursing discipline requires valid new concepts. New concepts are useful in both our science and our practice. In education, the new concept could be used to describe nursing phenomena to students in a meaningful way or to classify patient needs or nursing actions. In practice, the new concept may give clinicians fresh insights into patient problems, new nursing diagnoses, and possible new nursing interventions. In research and theory building, the new concept may provide fruitful new hypotheses or induce a change in thinking about some phenomenon of concern that in turn will generate more research.

Summary

Concept synthesis employs pulling together various elements of data into a pattern or relationship not clearly seen before to form a new concept. The steps of concept synthesis include becoming thoroughly familiar with an area of interest, loosely classifying the data you have acquired about the area of interest, looking for and combining clusters of classified phenomena that seem to relate closely or overlap, choosing a name for the cluster that accurately represents the phenomenon and that will facilitate communication about it, verifying the new concept empirically, and determining whether or where the new concept fits into current theory and practice.

Concept synthesis is a highly creative activity and may add significant new information to a given area of interest. The strategy is limited by the length of time needed for full concept development and by the fact that concepts alone do not provide predictive potential.

Practice Exercises

EXERCISE 1. OBSERVING

Choose an object in your environment, such as a piece of equipment you use frequently or an object you handle every day. Spend 10 minutes observing the object. Make a list of everything you see about it. How long was your list? If you saw only a few things, go back and spend 10 more minutes observing it. Is your list longer? Did you take apart the object and describe each piece separately? If not, why not? Now, go back and look again. Spend 10 minutes listing all possible uses of the item. How long was the list? Did you describe uses for each part of the item as well as for the whole? If not, why not? Learning to be a keen observer requires that our stereotypes be disposed of and that we keep an open and creative mind when we really look at something familiar.

EXERCISE 2. MEMORY

Without looking at one, draw a telephone keypad. Put in the letters and numbers where they belong (Adams, 1979).

Very few people can do this right the first time. The exercise demonstrates how we may think we have all the data we need because we use the phone every day after all, but are so familiar with the object we no longer really *see* it. Try this exercise again with an object you use every day at work or at home. First, draw it without looking, then go back and draw it again while you look at it. How did the two differ?

EXERCISE 3. CONCEPT CLUSTERING

Below are 28 names of concepts. Make at least two concept clusters from the list.

soap	car	volcano	duck
tennis racket	desk	hat	deodorant
dog	vote	fish	bus
toothbrush	disk	grass	mop
policy	elephant	guidelines	orange
frog	avocado	melody	panpipe
umbrella	basket	bucket	turnip

EXERCISE 4. CONCEPT SYNTHESIS

In order to facilitate your practice of the steps in concept synthesis, we have structured this exercise more than will be the case in reality. In fact, what we have done here is to present a kind of matrix used in morphological analysis to help get you started (Adams, 1979).

Let us assume that you and your staff are frustrated at the inefficient ways patients are transported from place to place in your hospital. You decide to discover a new concept of

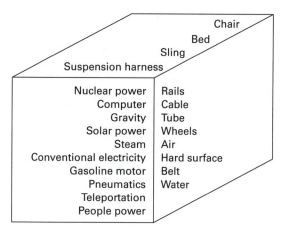

FIGURE 7–1   Three-way matrix.

patient transportation. To construct the matrix you need at least three parameters. Let us assume you choose (1) the power source to be used, (2) the devices into which the patient will be put, and (3) the medium in or on which the device will move. Figure 7–1 is the matrix we constructed. Feel free to add additional columns.

Now pick one item at random from each of the three axes and combine them. If, for instance, you got a bed with wheels that ran on people power, you have the conventional gurney—not too helpful. But what if you got a bed on a track that was run by a computer? That is a new idea. Now try it several times. List the combinations. Then choose the two most likely new ideas. Choose a name that describes the new phenomenon. Let your imagination work here. If you got a combination of sling, pneumatic power, and tube, for instance, what could you call it? How about Pneuma-port? or Pneuma-sling? Sling-a-Pat? There are many possibilities.

The next two steps are to verify the concept empirically. In this exercise, verification would need to explore whether or not the technology and the administrative and economic support were available to construct a prototype model. Once the model was constructed, pilot testing would demonstrate its feasibility, efficiency, and effectiveness. The last step is to determine whether the prototype fits into existing systems of hospital care or whether it requires a whole new system.

This brief exercise may seem very artificial, and it is; but it is one example of concept synthesis and should demonstrate the basic steps for you. Remember, practice makes perfect!

References

Adams JL. *Conceptual Blockbusting: A Guide to Better Ideas.* 2nd ed. New York, NY: W.W. Norton; 1979.

Algase DL, Beck C, Kolanowski A, Berent SK, Richards K, Beattie E. Need-driven dementia-compromised behavior: An alternative view of disruptive behavior. *Am J Alzheimer's Dis.* 1996;11(6):10–19.

Anderson JA, Oinhausen KS. Adolescent self-esteem: A foundational disposition. *Nurs Sci Q.* 1999;12(1):62–67.

Beitz JM. Concept mapping: Navigating the learning process. *Nurse Educ.* 1998;23(5):35–41.

Benoliel JQ. Grounded theory and nursing knowledge. *Qual Health Res.* 1996;6:406–428.

Breen J. Transitions in the concept of chronic pain. *Adv Nurs Sci.* 2002;24(4):48–59.

Bunting SM, Russell CK, Gregory DM. Computer monitor. Use of electronic mail (email) for concept synthesis: An international collaborative project. *Qual Health Res.* 1998;8(1):128–135.

Burke SO, Kaufmann, E, Costello EA, Dillon MC. Hazardous secrets and reluctantly taking charge: Parenting a child with repeated hospitalizations. *Image.* 1991;23(1):39–45.

Cataldo JK. Hardiness and depression in the institutionalized elderly. *Appl Nurs Res.* 1993;6(2):89–91.

Clunn P. Nurses' assessment of a person's potential for violence: Use of grounded theory in developing a nursing diagnosis. In: Kim MJ, McFarland GR, McLane AM, eds. *Classification of Nursing Diagnoses: Proceedings of the Fifth National Conference.* St. Louis, MO: Mosby; 1984, pp. 376–393.

Colling KB. A taxonomy of passive behaviors in people with Alzheimer's disease. *J Nurs Scholarsh.* 2000;32(3):239–244.

Corbin J, Strauss AC. *Basics of Qualitative Research: Techniques and Procedures for Developing Grounded Theory.* 4th ed. Thousand Oaks, CA: Sage Publications; 2015.

Denham SA. Family routines: A structural perspective for viewing family health. *Adv Nurs Sci.* 2002;24(4):60–74.

Dray W. "Explaining what" in history. In: Gardiner P, ed. *Theories of History.* New York, NY: Free Press; 1959.

Eaves YD. A synthesis technique for grounded theory data analysis. *J Adv Nurs.* 2001;35(5):644–653.

Elo SL, Calltorp JB. Health promotive action and preventive action model (HPA model) for the classification of health care services in public health nursing. *Scand J Public Health.* 2002;30:200–208.

Finfgeld-Connett D. Concept synthesis of the art of nursing. *J Adv Nurs.* 2008;62(3):381–388.

Glaser BG. *Theoretical Sensitivity.* Mill Valley, CA: Sociology Press; 1978.

Glaser BG. *Basics of Grounded Theory Analysis.* Mill Valley, CA: Sociology Press; 1992.

Glaser BG, Strauss AL. *The Discovery of Grounded Theory: Strategies for Qualitative Research.* Chicago, IL: Aldine; 1967.

Goldberg B. Connection: An exploration of spirituality in nursing care. *J Adv Nurs.* 1998;27(4):836–842.

Gordon M. *Nursing Diagnosis: Process and Application.* New York, NY: McGraw-Hill; 1982.

Hunt EB. *Concept Learning.* New York, NY: Wiley; 1962.

Kirk J, Miller ML. *Reliability and Validity in Qualitative Research.* Beverly Hills, CA: Sage Publications; 1986.

Kobasa SC. Personality and resistance to illness. *Am J Commun Psychol.* 1979a;7:413–423.

Kobasa SC. Stressful life events, personality, and health: An inquiry into hardiness. *J Pers Soc Psychol.* 1979b;37:1–11.

Kobasa SC, Hiker RRJ, Maddi SR. Who stays healthy under stress? *J Occup Med.* 1979;21:595–598.

Kolanowski AM. Disturbing behaviors in demented elders: A concept synthesis. *Arch Psychiatr Nurs.* 1995;9(4):188–194.

Lambert CE, Lambert VA. Hardiness: Its development and relevance to nursing. *Image.* 1987;19(2):92–95.

Lenz ER, Suppe F, Gift AG, Pugh LC, Milligan RA. Collaborative development of middle-range nursing theories: Toward a theory of unpleasant symptoms. *Adv Nurs Sci.* 1995;17(3):1–13.

Mullen PD. The potential for grounded theory for health education. In: Glaser BG, ed. *More Grounded Theory Methodology: A Reader.* Mill Valley, CA: Sociology Press; 1994, pp. 127–145.

Nichols PK, Webster A. Hardiness and social support in human immunodeficiency virus. *Appl Nurs Res.* 1993;6(3):132–136.

Oldaker S. Nursing diagnoses among adolescents. In: Hurley ME, ed. *Classification of Nursing Diagnoses: Proceedings of the Sixth National Conference.* St. Louis, MO: Mosby; 1986, pp. 311–318.

Pietrzak RH, Johnson DC, Goldstein MB, Malley JC, Rivers AJ, Morgan CA, et al. Psychosocial buffers of traumatic stress, depressive symptoms, and psychosocial difficulties in veterans of Operation Enduring Freedom and Iraqi Freedom: The role of resilience, unit support, and postdeployment social support. *J Affect Disord.* 2010;120(1–3):188–192.

Pines M. Psychological hardiness: The role of challenge in health. *Psychol Today.* 1980;14(7): 34–42, 98.

Polk LV. Toward a middle-range theory of resilience. *Adv Nurs Sci.* 1997;19(3):1–13.

Schatzman L, Strauss AL. *Field Research: Strategies for a Natural Sociology.* New York, NY: Prentice Hall; 1973.

Smith J, Swallow V, Coyne I. Involving parents in managing their child's long-term condition: A concept synthesis of family-centered care and partnership-in-care. *J Pediatr Nurs.* 2015;30(1):143–159.

Spitzer DR. *Concept Formation and Learning in Early Childhood.* Columbus, OH: Merrill; 1977.

Stern PN. The grounded theory method: Its uses and processes. In: Glaser BG, ed. *More Grounded Theory Methodology: A Reader.* Mill Valley, CA: Sociology Press; 1994, pp. 116–126.

Stevenson HW. Concept learning. In: Stevenson HW, ed. *Children's Learning.* New York, NY: Appleton-Century-Crofts; 1972, pp. 308–322.

Wagnild G, Young M. Another look at hardiness. *Image.* 1991;23(4):257–259.

Wendler MC. Using metaphor to explore concept synthesis. *Int J Hum Caring.* 1999;3(1):31–36.

Wilson J. *Thinking with Concepts.* New York, NY: Cambridge University Press; 1963.

Additional Readings

Eakes GC, Burke ML, Hainsworth MA. Middle-range theory of chronic sorrow. *Image.* 1998;30(2):179–184.

Harris CC. Cultural values and the decision to circumcise. *Image.* 1986;18(3):98–104.

Hurley ME, ed. *Classification of Nursing Diagnoses: Proceedings of the Sixth National Conference.* St. Louis, MO: Mosby; 1986.

Klausmeier H. The nature of uses of concepts. In: *Learning and Human Abilities: Educational Psychology.* 4th ed. New York, NY: Harper & Row; 1975, pp. 268–298.

Kleinmuntz B, ed. *Concepts and the Structure of Memory.* New York, NY: Wiley; 1967.

Long KA, Weinert C. Rural nursing: Developing the theory base. *Sch Inq Nurs Pract.* 1989;3(2):113–127.

Moch SD. Health-within-illness: Concept development through research and practice. *J Adv Nurs.* 1998;28(2):305–310.

Rogge MM. *Development of a Taxonomy of Nursing Interventions: An Analysis of Nursing Care in the American Civil War.* Unpublished doctoral dissertation. Austin, TX: University of Texas; April 1985.

Rosenbaum JN. Self-caring: Concept development in nursing. *Recent Adv Nurs.* 1989;24:18–31.

Ryan-Wenger NM. A taxonomy of children's coping strategies: A step toward theory development. *Am J Orthopsychiatry.* 1992;62(2):256–263.

Sandelowski M, Docherty S, Emden C. Qualitative metasynthesis: Issues and techniques. *Res Nurs Health.* 1997;20:365–371.

Whittemore R, Roy C. Adapting to diabetes mellitus: A theory synthesis. *Nurs Sci Q.* 2002;15:311–317.

Williams A. A literature review on the concept of intimacy in nursing. *J Adv Nurs.* 2001;33:660–667.

8

■ ■ ■

Statement Synthesis

Questions to consider before you get started reading this chapter:

▶ Are you seeking a means to pull together from existing data one or more statements of relationships about a research problem or clinical practice area?

▶ Do you have access to databases that can aid you in identifying and retrieving existing studies for the statements you are hoping to construct?

Introductory Note: If you have answered "yes" to the above two questions, then statement synthesis may be a strategy to achieve your goal. Unlike other statement development strategies, statement synthesis requires evidence in some form as a beginning point. In using evidence to develop statements of relationships between concepts, the theorist increases understanding of the phenomena of interest. Statement synthesis may contribute to knowledge about simple two- or three-factor relationships. Synthesized statements about risk factor associations and intervention outcomes are the backbone of evidence-based practice guidelines for risk factor assessment and intervention. Statement synthesis also may be an incremental phase essential to the larger goal of theory synthesis. Thus, statement synthesis is part of the incremental process of theory development, especially when one moves from observations or data to general statements. Like the lowly spoon, though, statement synthesis may be underappreciated, but a vital tool for the feast of practice and research. (*Note:* Readers may find it helpful to review the material on the nature of statements in Chapter 3 before proceeding further in this chapter.)

DEFINITION AND DESCRIPTION

As a strategy, statement synthesis is aimed at specifying relationships between two or more concepts based on evidence. The evidence may come from various sources: (1) qualitative or quantitative methods applied to observations or interviews of individuals or groups; or (2) literature-based sources such as literature reviews, conclusions extracted from interrelated studies, standards of practice, or practice guidelines.

Logically, statement synthesis involves two operations: (1) moving from evidence to inferences, and (2) then generalizing from specific inferences to more abstract ones (see Figure 8–1).

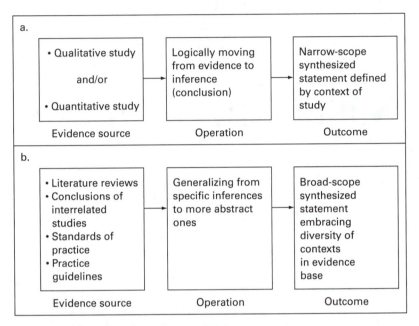

FIGURE 8–1   Evidence-based statement synthesis.

In moving from evidence to inferences, evidence comprises a thoughtful series of observations that are the basis of interrelating concepts. For example, a nurse may interview caregivers of persons with dementia in nursing homes about the experience of caring for them. From qualitative analysis of the interview transcripts, clusters of related ideas about the social experience of caring for persons with dementia are constructed. The nurse then links related clusters into relational statements such as:

> *Caregivers of persons with dementia in nursing homes relate more fully to them when they have a sense of a person's life story before coming to the nursing home (see Figure 8–1a).*

As a second source of evidence for statement synthesis, a nurse may use statistical methods to compress many individual observations or measurements. Quantitative indices, such as correlation coefficients, can describe the presence and strength of a relationship between two variables. In this situation, statement synthesis permits relationships expressed in numerical form to be translated into verbal or linguistic form. For example, suppose a nurse gathers data about two variables, acculturation and emotional eating, and finds the correlation between them as $r = .35, p < .05$. One way this statistical information could be expressed is:

> *As acculturation increases, emotional eating increases.*

Statistically based statement synthesis can be extracted from both descriptive (nonexperimental) research and experimental research studies.

In the third source of evidence, a theorist undertakes statement synthesis about a topic for which much research already exists in published documents (see Figure 8–1b). For example, you might do an electronic search of research literature to locate institutional and communication factors that increase or reduce violence against nurses in hospitals. The process of synthesis might begin by cataloging relationships among variables that you found reported in the literature. Relationships would then be further organized and combined to obtain clear and general statements of relationships of various institutional and communication factors that increase or reduce violence against nurses. Because some relationships may be found repeatedly in studies, whereas others may be found in only one or two studies, statements may be grouped according to how much evidence is available for each one. The result of this work would ideally be several statements that capture the broad patterns of relationships among variables that are evident in the literature. Such sorting as well as weighing of support (evidence) for statements is the foundation of systematic reviews and evidence-based approaches to health care.

These introductory illustrations of statement synthesis show that this strategy consists of multiple and varied methods. The desired outcome of these diverse methods, however, is the same: the clear statement of relationships between two or more concepts. Furthermore, the theorist using statement synthesis pulls together, organizes, or extracts patterns of relationships from information gathered in reality—the outside world. Thus, observations and other methods of scientific measurement, for example, interviews and equipment readings, are essential to the process of statement synthesis.

For interested readers, a *self-assessment test* of introductory statistics is located at the end of this chapter. Obtaining maximum benefit from quantitative methods presented in this chapter may be enhanced by knowledge of introductory statistics. Readers may use this self-assessment to assess or refresh their knowledge of statistics. Several helpful statistical texts also are listed at the end of this chapter for interested readers.

Nevertheless, mastery of statistics is not essential for every method of statement synthesis. Familiarity with statistical methods, however, is an indispensable tool when large amounts of quantitative information are collected. Statistical methods may be useful in consolidating large amounts of collected information into a more interpretable form. Nonetheless, readers should not confuse statistics with statement synthesis. Statistical methods are only adjuncts to the process of specifying relationships among concepts in the field of interest.

PURPOSE AND USES

The purpose of statement synthesis is to develop from observations of phenomena one or more statements about relationships that exist among those phenomena. As indicated earlier, observations may be made directly by the theorist or may be drawn from the literature. Further, where large numbers of quantitative observations or measurements are made, these may be treated statistically to compress the information into a more interpretable form. When considering statement synthesis as a strategy, theorists should verify that one or more of three conditions in Box 8–1 hold true.

BOX 8–1   Three Conditions When Statement Synthesis May Be a
            Suitable Strategy

Condition 1: There is no conceptual or empirical work done to describe a topic of interest, but a series of observations can be made readily to establish some of the parameters (empirical qualities) of the phenomenon.

Condition 2: There are several concepts in use in an area of interest, and evidence is available or could be easily gathered to clarify how the concepts may be interrelated.

Condition 3: There are several published research studies on a phenomenon of interest, but the information contained in them has not yet been organized into meaningful conclusions that cross studies.

Because researchers and statisticians often draw a line between findings that are hypothesis-based versus those that are serendipitous, we next provide a few comments about some of the foundations of such an evidentiary line. Only readers interested in this issue need read this and the following paragraph. Although data or observations may be used to develop or test hypotheses, these two uses are logically distinct (Rudner, 1966). However, similar techniques may be employed for each of these two purposes. This similarity may lead to confusions. Theorists may needlessly apply rules for hypothesis testing to a statement development/synthesis context. For example, statistical results with a probability level slightly greater than .05 might be appropriate in some exploratory analyses so that promising findings are not disregarded. Conversely, theorists may discover certain relationships among phenomena using a flexible exploratory design, but then treat the discovery as if it were a tested conclusion. It is preferable, as a general rule, to treat the contexts of discovery and justification (i.e., testing) as distinct. That is, where data are used to extract relational statements (context of discovery), these same data should not be used again to claim the statements have been tested (context of justification). As a general rule, another independent data set should be used to cross-validate the original findings. Similarly, rigorous testing of hypotheses (context of justification) may be followed by further atheoretical analyses or massaging of the data (context of discovery). The latter, although important, does not carry the same evidential status as the former type of analysis.

Evidence used for statement synthesis (context of discovery) should be analyzed in ways that facilitate discovery. This may necessitate altering conventions such as traditional probability levels or using exploratory approaches such as bivariate statistical descriptions (Polit, 2010) to construct statements that meaningfully reflect relationships inherent in data or observations. Such flexibility may be wise and appropriate to maximally make use of information collected about a phenomenon in a discovery context. More rigorous approaches would be needed in a justificatory context. For example, improvements in measurement and conceptualization may occur that permit preliminary discovery observations to be more suitably and rigorously tested in a later stage of scientific refinement.

PROCEDURES FOR STATEMENT SYNTHESIS

Statement synthesis involves two basic logical operations: moving from observations to inferences and then generalizing from specific inferences to more abstract ones (see Figure 8–1). Two broad classes of methods exist for moving from observations to inferences: qualitative methods and quantitative methods. Generalizing from specific inferences to more general ones, the second operation, is facilitated by a process we have termed literary methods. In actual statement development, a theorist may of course move back and forth between these logical operations.

The complex and voluminous information about qualitative and quantitative methods makes a comprehensive exposition of each beyond the scope of this chapter. Instead, we focus on strategic aspects of these two methods and must necessarily be selective in our presentation of them. Readers needing more in-depth information about qualitative methods are referred to methods texts devoted exclusively to this topic (e.g., Corbin & Strauss, 2008; Denzin & Lincoln, 2011; Schreiber & Stern, 2001). Similarly, for more information about quantitative methods, standard research textbooks are available on this topic (e.g., Pedhazur & Schmelkin, 2013; Polit & Beck, 2012). Keeping these limitations in mind, we present a treatment of qualitative, quantitative, and literary methods as they relate strategically to developing statements about a phenomenon of interest.

Although qualitative approaches as a group vary in their purpose and specific method, typically a flexible or modifiable approach is utilized in data collection. This permits the theorist to explore the emerging picture of a phenomenon. Qualitative methods typically rely on interview (listening and questioning) and observation (watching) as sources of data. Coding categories generally emerge from reading and preliminary coding of transcribed interviews supplemented by observational notes. Grounded theory, a qualitative method that may contribute to statement synthesis, is presented later.

In contrast, quantitative methods involve measurement of variables on numerical scales or other quantifiable methods. Quantitative methods may be applied to both experimental and nonexperimental (descriptive or correlational) designs. Quantitative methods may be used to examine relationships between two or more factors, or differing patterns of response to a common event. Translating statistical information into conclusions expressed in linguistic form is a vehicle for statement synthesis.

Last, literary methods are aimed at organizing extant research information on a topic of interest. Sources of evidence in literary methods rely heavily on published research. Literary methods involve sifting through available information and putting that information into more concise and general form. In some instances, the theorist's work of literary statement synthesis will be expedited by the availability of comprehensive literature reviews, well-articulated standards of practice, or practice guidelines on topics of concern. As an example, Hess and Insel (2007) completed an extensive and systematic review of literature related to cognitive changes associated with chemotherapy and synthesized findings in the following statement:

> Cognitive function . . . may be altered among individuals diagnosed with cancer along two distinct and interacting pathways: (a) cancer diagnosis . . . and (b) direct physiologic effects of cancer treatment. . . . (p. 990)

Qualitative Methods

Grounded theory was one of the early qualitative approaches that lent itself to statement development (Glaser, 1978; Glaser & Strauss, 1967). It was used by nurses to study, for example, patients who underwent mastectomies (Quint, 1967a, 1967b), stepparent families (Stern, 1980), and families across life-cycle stages (Knafl & Grace, 1978). In using grounded theory, the theorist gains understanding of social phenomena by beginning with an open mind, avoiding preconceived ideas about ways of classifying and interrelating data, and observing social phenomena in natural settings. Although a theorist may begin with some general ideas about the area of interest, these are abandoned as categories more relevant to the phenomenon emerge. The theorist moves back and forth between data collection and data analysis in order to validate emerging ideas and refine concepts and relationships as new data are collected.

The strength of grounded theory is that the theorist uses direct observation of the phenomenon as the starting point for concept and then statement formation (Corbin & Strauss, 2008; Glaser, 1978; Glaser & Strauss, 1967; Quint, 1967a; Schatzman & Strauss, 1973). Data are coded into categories, and categories are interrelated as an ongoing part of the data analysis. A theorist may make observations, code them, make interpretive notes or memos about coded observations, and then make further observations to refine or clarify an emerging idea. The theorist's creative ability to construct meaningful general concepts and relational statements is a crucial part of qualitative research. See Benoliel (1996) or Eaves (2001) for a fuller overview of grounded theory methods.

A classic example illustrating grounded theory is Stern's (1980) work with stepfather families. Stern began her study by noting that the process by which a stepfather was integrated into an existing family had not been studied before.

> I had no basis on which to test existing theory, nor could I utilize identified existing variables, because none were identified. In other words, it was first necessary to find out what was going on in these families. (p. 20)

In phase 1, the *collection of empirical data*, Stern conducted intensive interviews with 30 stepfather families from a variety of social classes and ethnic groups. Data collected by observation and interviews were coded according to their main substance, and similarly coded data were then clustered together in categories. Two categories that Stern developed, for example, focused on rules in the family and enforcement techniques.

During the second phase, *concept formation*, a conceptual framework was developed with an eye to representing the phenomenon from the subjects' point of view. In attempting to understand how families integrate a stepfather into the existing mother–child system, Stern selected the discipline of children in the family as the framework. This framework was selected because of the emotional responses the topic of discipline produced when discussed with families.

The third phase, *concept development*, involved several steps. Categories were linked together to define key variables. Thus, Stern combined the categories of teaching, accepting, and copying into a larger umbrella category of affiliating actions. Common to affiliating actions was bringing the stepfather and child closer together. Emerging ideas necessitated further review of literature at this point. Attention also turned to relationships between categories. In Stern's (1980) study, she asked, "Under what conditions do the variables discipline and integration coexist?" (p. 22). Data were selectively sampled to clarify the relationship of these variables. Stern found that discipline and integration occurred together only when affiliating actions were also present. This demonstrates statement synthesis. To further consolidate thinking, a core variable was proposed. Core variables pull together key ideas about a phenomenon. Stern proposed "integrative discipline" as the core variable to explain how stepfather families use the issue of discipline to strengthen family solidarity.

During the fourth phase, *concept modification and integration*, the emerging ideas were further integrated and delimited. Data were coded in terms of theoretical ideas. Memos or interpretive notes were made as data were coded to aid in systematizing the findings of the study. Memos were then reorganized in a manner that facilitated the fifth phase, *production of the research report*. In this final phase, theoretical outcomes of the study were presented, substantiated by examples from the data.

Stern's classic exposition of using grounded theory illustrates a flexible, yet sensitive means of constructing statements about a social phenomenon. This method permits categories and relationships among these to be constructed from direct and thoughtful interaction of the theorist and the social phenomenon being studied.

Quantitative Methods

OVERVIEW   In this chapter, quantitative methods are examined within the framework of experimental and nonexperimental research. In experimental designs, some change is introduced by the investigator to determine its impact on outcomes, whereas in nonexperimental quantitative designs variation is observed as it naturally occurs. Each of these designs for quantitative research involves the collection and analysis of numerical data. The analysis of data typically is facilitated by statistical calculations such as means, standard deviations, percentages, correlation coefficients, and t test and F ratio values. Each of these designs contains some special advantages and limitations for the construction of statements about phenomena. To begin, each design will be described briefly, and then the group nonexperimental design will be presented to illustrate its use in statistically based statement synthesis.

Interpreting statistical data from quantitative-based studies assumes that the measurements used are reliable (Nunnally & Bernstein, 1994; Urbina, 2004; Waltz, Strickland, & Lenz, 2010). Validity of measures, particularly construct validity, may be less clear, however, given the reciprocal relationship between theory development and establishment of construct validity (Smith, 2005). Whereas it is beyond the scope of this chapter to deal with psychometric concepts such as reliability and validity as these affect the interpretation of statistical data, we must acknowledge these issues to provide a complete and accurate picture of quantitative methods.

EXPERIMENTAL DESIGNS   These designs are used to document the effects of nursing interventions in diverse situations. For example, Table 8–1 and Figure 8–2 show

TABLE 8–1   Individual and Mean Anxiety Levels for Patients Prior to Exploratory Surgery (Fictitious Data)

Patient ID	Before Hospitalization	After Admission	After Preoperative Education
Patient A	50	20	20
Patient B	30	40	60
Patient C	30	50	30
Patient D	30	50	30
Group mean	35	40	35

fictitious data on four patients having exploratory surgery. A nursing intervention of preoperative education is tested for its impact on reducing patients' anxiety. Mean scores describe the level of anxiety in the group at each time point and estimate the impact of the intervention on reducing anxiety. Examining the group means (bottom row of data) for anxiety level before hospitalization, after admission, and then after preoperative education shows that hospital admission led to an increase in anxiety, which was then quelled by preoperative education. For subgroups of individuals, however, the mean gives a misleading estimate of the intervention impact on them.

Looking at individual patients' patterns (top four rows of data), hospital admission appeared to be a relief to Patient A and reduced his anxiety level to well below preadmission levels. For Patient B, admission did raise her anxiety level somewhat, but worse yet, the preoperative education backfired and raised her level of anxiety still higher. Only Patients C and D had individual patterns that generally conformed to those of the group mean. Thus, a second important goal in analyzing data for statement synthesis about nursing interventions is to determine who will benefit from an intervention and who will not. (Readers may recognize similarities here to moderator effects [Bennett, 2000].) Now, suppose we are able to look at the fictitious patients' data further and learn that Patient A was very worried about some family conflicts that resolved just as he was being admitted to the hospital. He saw the upcoming surgery

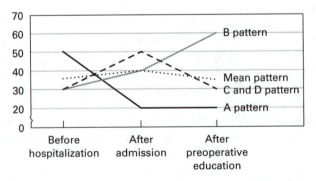

FIGURE 8–2 Individual and mean anxiety levels for patients prior to exploratory surgery (fictitious data).

as a "piece of cake" compared to the difficult family problems. Patient B, however, just had an important support person move out of town as she was being admitted. Patient B felt very fearful about going through the surgery alone, and this feeling increased after the preoperative intervention.

In our preoperative education example, patients were tested both before and after the experimental intervention so that change in anxiety could be compared on the same people across time points. In another variation of an experimental design, a control group whose members receive no intervention also may be included so that the effects of the experimental condition may be contrasted with the effects of the control condition. In any circumstances where it would be considered unethical to withhold some form of intervention, the control is converted to a usual care group so that there is no question of them receiving needed care. Comparisons made between groups are a way of determining the impact of the intervention in the experimental group using the control group as a reference point.

In these various types of experimental studies, statement synthesis occurs as the researcher translates numerical or statistical measures of impact into linguistic form. For our fictitious patients' data, we might develop the following statement:

Preoperative education led to a reduction in anxiety for 50% of preoperative patients; interpersonal changes in some patients' lives moderated the effectiveness of the intervention.

Most readers are already familiar with experimental studies and the type of conclusions that are reached about main effects. For example, *A support intervention was more successful in reducing depressive symptoms of new immigrants compared to an intervention involving referral to primary care.* We therefore also want to consider findings about differential benefit from an experimental intervention. In an actual example of testing for differential benefit, Kiernan, King, Kraemer, Stefanick, and Killen (1998) examined data from a weight-loss intervention. They used signal detection (involving chi-square tests) to determine which characteristics of participants affected successful weight loss (defined as loss of at least two body mass index units). Signal detection methods can aid in partitioning a larger group into successive subgroups that vary in rates of success on the key outcome. First, they found that the nature of the weight-loss program affected success rates, with those in a diet-only group being less successful than those in a diet-and-exercise-class group. Beyond this, Kiernan et al. identified subgroups within the diet-and-exercise-class group who were less or more successful. For example, persons who reported high body image dissatisfaction had difficulty being successful. Among those who were satisfied with their body image, further subgroups were found according to whether or not they had a history of multiple weight-loss attempts. Based on Kiernan et al.'s work, one statement of differential impact might be expressed as:

Persons with high body image dissatisfaction are less likely to benefit from a weight-loss intervention that includes exercise classes.

This synthesized statement points to the need for new ways to increase exercise in persons with high body image concerns, such as at home-based exercise that does not require exercising in a group context. (*Note:* Our presentation of the work of Kiernan et al. is offered for illustrative purposes. Because the findings reflect only one study, they should not be viewed as definitive.)

NONEXPERIMENTAL DESIGNS These designs often rely on correlation or regression techniques to interrelate variables. Data may be cross-sectional (collected at one time point) or longitudinal (collected over several time points). Sometimes such data sets may be considered as opportunities for "data mining." Although we will not discuss the variety of test statistics that may be used in nonexperimental (also called correlational or *ex post facto*) designs, we will discuss general strategies for the analysis and interpretation of nonexperimental data. Associated statistical and design issues are well treated in available research texts (e.g., Pedhazur & Schmelkin, 2013; Polit & Beck, 2012).

One of the most daunting problems that nonexperimental designs pose for a theorist is the risk of becoming buried in a sea of statistical information. The "shotgun" approach sometimes used in nonexperimental designs can result in every variable being tested for relationships to every other variable in the study. In a study of 10 variables (e.g., social class, age, gender, number of drugs, and number of hospital admissions), if each of these is correlated with every other variable, a total of 45 correlation coefficients will be generated. In a study of 100 variables, 4,950 variable relationships are possible. Immediately it becomes clear that strategies are needed to eliminate unnecessary statistical analyses and to organize those that are done into meaningful units of information. This is one of the most difficult tasks that faces a theorist using quantitative nonexperimental evidence for statement synthesis.

We recommend several suggestions to aid in organizing the process of data analysis and interpretation (see Box 8–2). These suggestions should not be interpreted as rules for data analysis. During data analysis, you may find that keeping a log of what was done and why is helpful in directing the analysis of data in new, but organized directions. Review the log frequently. Writing summaries of the results of completed data analyses may also be a useful reference point. Review these summaries, discuss them with colleagues, and compare them with results of published research. Occasionally, reading about research that is unrelated but similar in design can be helpful in organizing and guiding the data analysis in new and meaningful directions.

We next demonstrate the use of quantitative data in statement synthesis. We will present a small segment of data from a nonexperimental study that one of us completed. (Data were gathered with support from grant number NU 00677, Division of Nursing, U.S. Public Health Service.) In one part of the study, attitudes and beliefs of new mothers were investigated. Because the literature suggested that maternal parity and infant sex might influence attitudes and beliefs, data were analyzed separately according to parity (primiparas and multiparas) and infant sex (male and female) subgroups. Although this division reduced the number of subjects within groups, it provided a sharper picture of attitudes or belief patterns among new mothers. Table 8–2 presents the correlations among three attitudes and beliefs measured at the beginning and at the end of the neonatal period. The correlations are presented for each of the four subgroups of new mothers. The correlations of mothers' attitudes toward

BOX 8–2   Suggestions for Analysis of Nonexperimental Data in Statement Synthesis

1. Locate the most focal variables, those of greatest interest to you. Some variables are of interest for their own sake, for example, levels of adjustment or well-being before or after illness. Other variables are of interest only insofar as they may influence focal variables.
2. Examine the statistical indicators of central tendency and variability for the focal variables. If these variables are measured over several occasions, become familiar with changes that may occur in them.
3. Examine related literature for variables that have been found to covary with these focal variables.
4. Determine whether your focal variables are related as expected to these variables identified in the literature.
5. Reduce variables that seem to have a common orientation by such procedures as factor analysis (Tabachnick & Fidell, 2013), if possible. Social background variables can often be made more compact by this approach.
6. Pursue hunches that you may have about new variables in your data set that you suspect may be related to the focal variables.
7. Look for surprises in the data analysis results. These may be unanticipated relationships or unanticipated lack of relationships. Hypothesize about why these surprises may have occurred. Check out your hypotheses to the extent possible with your available data. These hypotheses, even though moving beyond statement synthesis itself, may be helpful for later theory synthesis.
8. You may have started out atheoretically (without any theory in mind to be tested), but you may find during the data analysis and interpretation phase that the results are consistent with available theories. These theories may in turn suggest new or previously unexplored areas for further analysis.
9. Discuss results obtained with colleagues knowledgeable in the area as well as with clinicians who know the area under study from a case-by-case perspective.

themselves as mothers are quite high for all four subgroups ($r = .62$ to $.77$). Thus, you might conclude that mothers' attitude toward themselves as mothers does not undergo major changes during the neonatal period, and assert that

> *Overall attitude toward oneself as mother was a relatively stable phenomenon across time regardless of parity or sex of infant.*

For beliefs about one's infant, however, this was not so. Beliefs about one's baby were significantly correlated across the neonatal period for primiparous mothers ($r = .35$ to $.41$), but not for multiparous mothers ($r = -.06$ to $-.12$). Thus, you might conclude:

> *Beliefs about one's baby are somewhat stable for first-time mothers; for mothers having other than a first baby, beliefs at the end of the neonatal period are unrelated to initial beliefs.*

TABLE 8–2   Correlations Between New Mothers' Attitudes or Beliefs at the Beginning and End of the Neonatal Period

	Attitude/Belief Correlations		
Maternal Parity/ Infant Sex	Beliefs About Baby	Attitude Toward Baby	Attitude Toward Self as Mother
Primiparous/female	.35[a] (28)	.44[b] (31)	.62[c] (31)
Primiparous/male	.41[b] (42)	.44[b] (43)	.66[c] (43)
Multiparous/female	−.06 (51)	.69[c] (51)	.67[c] (51)
Multiparous/male	−.12 (35)	.23 (38)	.77[c] (38)

Note: Numbers of subjects are in parentheses. These may vary within groups because of some missing data.

[a] $p < .05$.
[b] $p < .01$.
[c] $p < .001$.

This last finding was indeed surprising. Consequently, you might hypothesize underlying processes to explain these findings. For example, one hypothesis is that first-time mothers because of their inexperience with infants idealize them. Thus, when the infant's early behavior is different from expectations, these behaviors are ignored and the ideal maintained. Mothers who have already had at least one child may have learned that babies are very individual as they compared their earlier babies' growth and behavior with other babies. Thus, repeat mothers did not expect babies to conform to an ideal. As a result, repeat mothers change their initial beliefs about their later babies more readily than first-time mothers as they come to know their individual behaviors. Thus, unexpected findings can lead to new hypotheses for testing.

Now look at the column in Table 8–2 labeled "Attitude Toward Baby." Make a statement about how consistent across time mothers' attitudes toward their babies were for the four groups. In constructing your statement, you should have noted that mothers' attitudes toward their babies were significantly related across the neonatal period for all groups of mothers ($r = .44$ to .69) *except* for multiparous mothers of male infants ($r = .23$). Several hypotheses explaining this finding may be offered. For example, the data might be examined to determine whether male infants were indeed more variable than females in the neonatal period, and multiparous mothers were more likely to note this.

It is important to remember that although we have given a number of guidelines for the analysis and interpretation of quantitative nonexperimental data, we have not stated exact procedures for the application of this method. We have avoided stating procedures because we did not want to mislead readers into believing that statement synthesis is a mechanical process of inspecting data and then simply formulating statements from the data. A key strategic aspect of statistically based statement synthesis is in the organization of the data analysis. We have tried to emphasize this aspect, being assured that research methods texts amply cover procedural aspects of quantitative nonexperimental research (Pedhazur & Schmelkin, 2013; Polit & Beck, 2012). We believe that the information on strategic aspects of quantitative methods in a discovery context presented here is not addressed in conventional research texts.

Embedded in our presentation of quantitative methods has been a threefold process:

* approach data analysis in inventive yet organized ways,
* carefully describe results via systematic formulation of statements, and
* where possible, link statements derived from data with existing theories or hypothesized explanations.

Although the third phase moves beyond statement synthesis itself, it is meaningful to include it here to set the stage for other theoretical activities such as theory synthesis and theory testing.

Quantitative methods require the continuing and thoughtful attention of the theorist in the data analytic and interpretive processes, lest the theorist become lost in an array of numbers. Nonetheless, quantitative methods in general offer theorists the advantage of access to explicit numerical data about a phenomenon. Numbers may lack the flavor of reality but can aid in identifying relationships the naked eye may miss. Statements of relationships are in the end an abstraction about reality, not reality itself. Quantitative methods can facilitate the abstraction process in that their application to reality forces a theorist to think about reality in conceptual and quantitative dimensions.

Literary Methods

OVERVIEW OF LITERARY STATEMENT SYNTHESIS Literary methods of statement synthesis start out with statements derived from extant research. In contrast to statement analysis, literary methods of statement synthesis utilize only those statements in scientific literature that are derived or supported by evidence. Relationships that are conjectural on a theorist's part or that are not founded on research usually are not included. This criterion for statement inclusion does not necessarily mean that conjectures or unsupported statements are useless in theory construction. Rather, the criterion reflects the orientation of synthesis strategies: to begin theoretical work from evidence. Conjectural or unsupported statements fail to meet this criterion. Conjectural statements may be useful, however, in other types of strategies, such as statement derivation.

Literary statement synthesis, although time consuming, involves minimal cost and resources compared to other statement synthesis methods. Access to adequate library facilities is crucial to this method. Literary approaches to statement synthesis are especially useful in that statements generated are not limited to the findings of any one study. Access to findings of multiple studies on a topic of interest offers a richer database than any single study. Literary approaches will be only partly satisfactory, however, where the research on a topic is limited in amount and quality.

PROCESS OF LITERARY STATEMENT SYNTHESIS   To illustrate the process of statement synthesis, we examine a classic study conducted by Henthorn (1979). The following statement was empirically supported in Henthorn's study of disengagement and social reinforcement in adults who were 65 or older:

> *The greater the degree of disengagement [reported by older adults], the lower the level of reinforcement [of role behaviors by others] and the anticipated reinforcement [of role behaviors by others]. (p. 5)*

Often statements such as this need to be rewritten to clarify their meaning. In this example, the statement in fact describes two sets of relationships, which may be restated as follows:

> *The greater the degree of disengagement reported by older adults, the lower the level of reinforcement of role behaviors by others.*

and

> *The greater the degree of disengagement reported by older adults, the lower the anticipated reinforcement of role behaviors by others.*

There are several equivalent forms in which relational statements such as those above may be written:

> *The greater the X, the greater the Y.*
> *As X increases (or decreases), Y increases (or decreases).*
> *X and Y covary.*
> *X is positively (or negatively) related to Y.*

The form in which these preceding relational statements are written leaves open several questions:

- Is the relationship between X and Y reversible; that is, if an increase in X is related to an increase in Y, is an increase in Y also related to an increase in X?
- Is the relationship between the two variables X and Y causal or noncausal (simply associative)?

These questions can be answered only if the design of the research from which the statement was derived was aimed at disentangling these issues. Otherwise, the theorist must simply recognize the ambiguity and await further research that can clarify the answers to the reversibility and causality questions.

Experimental approaches, and in some cases longitudinal data, can help clarify questions left unclear by correlational or nonexperimental designs. Where answers to questions about causality and reversibility can be answered, the form in which statements may be written is more precise. For example,

Only if there is an increase in X, will there be an increase in Y, but the reverse is not true (nonreversible or unidirectional causality).

or

Only if there is an increase in X, will there be an increase in Y, and vice versa (reversibility or bidirectional causality).

Two techniques are involved in literary statement synthesis:

- making the meanings of the concepts included in a statement more general, or
- expanding the boundaries (scope of phenomena covered) to include a wider variety of situations.

The first may be done by merging less general concepts into a more abstract, general concept. The latter is done by reformulating the boundaries of a statement to increase the populations and situations to which it applies; for example, extending statements about small group-interaction patterns to all groups regardless of size. We will apply both of these techniques of literary synthesis. Our first revised statement taken from Henthorn will be the starting point:

The greater the degree of disengagement reported by older adults, the lower the level of reinforcement of role behaviors by others.

Now let us take a statement from Osofsky and Danzger's (1974) important research on early mother–infant interaction. They noted that:

The attentive mother tends to have a responsive baby and vice versa. (p. 124)

This early finding is supported by subsequent research showing that depressed mothers—who engage in less verbal speech with their infants—in turn have the infants who show less language development (Field, 2010). To synthesize the statements from Henthorn's (1979) and Osofsky and Danzger's (1974) studies, we first need to develop a broader concept from the concepts "degree of disengagement" and "attentive mother." Common to these two concepts is a more general concept: "amount of socially interactive behaviors that an individual displays." For the concepts, "level of reinforcement of role behaviors by others" and "responsive baby," a commonality exists in the higher-order concept "social reinforcement that accompanies socially interactive behaviors."

We further broaden the situational scope of our statement by shifting the boundaries from older adults or mothers and infants to an individual in social interaction with others. Thus, a synthesized statement drawn from Henthorn's and Osofsky and Danzger's studies may be made.

> *The amount of socially interactive behaviors that an individual displays is directly related to the amount of social reinforcement received from others.*

Finally, because we were unclear about the reversibility of Henthorn's statement, we chose a conservative interpretation of it and wrote the synthesized statement as nonreversible.

In the example of social interaction and reinforcement, we have tried to show how a general statement may be synthesized from two more narrowly focused statements. This was done to help the reader grasp the basic, and sometimes surprising, ways in which research outcomes can be pulled together into synthesized statements. Formulating a statement that generalizes to new and broader boundaries, of course, requires that additional data be sought to substantiate the new generalization. Nonetheless, an important move in theory construction may have been made as further evidence is being awaited.

APPLICATION OF LITERARY SYNTHESIS TO NURSING Now let's turn to actual examples of statement synthesis in nursing. This strategy has been shown to be useful in the process of building middle-range prescriptive theories in nursing. For example, statement synthesis has been cited as a component of prescriptive theory building related to the following clinical concerns: balance between analgesia and side effects in adults (Good & Moore, 1996); peaceful end of life (Ruland & Moore, 1998); and acute pain management in infants and children (Huth & Moore, 1998). In each of these three theory-building efforts, existing bodies of clinical knowledge gathered together in the form of either clinical guidelines or standards of practice were transformed into middle-range theories using the strategies of statement synthesis and then theory synthesis. An example of using statement synthesis to develop relational statements for such theories is well illustrated by Ruland and Moore's (1998) work in developing a statement related to patient comfort in end-of-life care.

First, Ruland and Moore (1998) examined 16 outcome criteria for standards of practice related to peaceful end of life developed by nursing experts in Norway. These 16 outcome criteria were then restated as five higher-order concepts (called "outcome indicators"), one of which was "the experience of comfort" (p. 172). Thirteen specific process criteria within the standards related to the experience of comfort were identified and restated in terms of three higher-order nursing interventions (called "prescriptors"). For example, one of three prescriptors was "preventing, monitoring, and relieving physical discomfort" (p. 173). The resulting synthesized statement including all three prescriptors was expressed as follows:

> Preventing, monitoring, and relieving physical discomfort, facilitating rest, relaxation, and contentment, and preventing complications contribute to the patient's experience of comfort. (p. 174)

Ruland and Moore synthesized a total of six relational statements that then served as the statemental components in their subsequent theory synthesis.

Yet another example of statement synthesis is reported by Mareno and Annesi (2016). Noting the need to better understand psychosocial factors that could have an impact on weight loss interventions, they undertook a statement synthesis related to the concepts related to one's "emotional state and feelings about one's body" (p. 1024). Using a systematic method to locate and identify research articles pertaining to these concepts, they applied the strategy of literary statement synthesis to formulate the following statement: "the amount of self-reported emotional eating . . . is directly related to an adult individual's recognition of her/his body size" (p. 1026). Their proposed next step is using this statement in hypothesis development and testing.

Finally, literary methods of statement synthesis may be given a still further level of precision. Where a series of statements has been synthesized from nursing research literature on a phenomenon, statements may be ranked or classified according to the level of support available to substantiate them, such as strong consistent support, moderate support, and low inconsistent support. Statements that have supporting evidence collected in multiple nursing studies using diverse populations would be ranked higher than those with a more limited base of evidence. Particularly where research findings are used as a basis for public policy formation or for application to practice, clear determination of the extent of support for synthesized statements is important. See examples of this in the section on Statement Testing in Chapter 13.

ADVANTAGES AND LIMITATIONS

Because methods of statement synthesis are so varied, we will speak to advantages and limitations in only the most general terms here. An evaluation of the advantages and limitations of statement synthesis methods as a group hinges on philosophical assumptions that are discussed here.

Statement synthesis as a method assumes that confrontation with reality is a useful and productive means of constructing theory. It assumes that without the aid of a clear guiding theory, a theorist can detect the dimensions of a phenomenon that are the most scientifically useful. In describing such atheoretical approaches to theory construction as "research-then-theory," Reynolds (1971) noted that these approaches assume there are real patterns that exist in nature. These patterns are then discovered by researchers using empirical methods. In this viewpoint, "research" is akin to "search." Reynolds further noted that the assumptions made about how scientific knowledge relates to the real world are philosophical and thus not amenable to resolution by scientific methods. We must leave our readers to decide for themselves if they find the assumptions of synthetic methods tenable. This issue goes beyond the scope of this book. We hope that readers will find these philosophical issues as intriguing as the more procedural ones treated in this book.

UTILIZING THE RESULTS OF STATEMENT SYNTHESIS

The aim of statement synthesis is to formulate statements about nursing phenomena from direct observations (both qualitatively and quantitatively recorded) and other evidence, such as published research findings. Utilizing the results of this strategy leads directly into the larger knowledge-generating process. Thus, this strategy forms the substance of evidence-based practice. It also is employed in reviewing research literature as a preamble to a study, reaching study conclusions, and transmitting those conclusions through the educational process. If the practicing nurse, researcher, and teacher are committed to carefully grounding their work on scientific observation, then statement synthesis is not a product used, but rather a process at the heart of what each does. Statement synthesis may also be a bridge to theory synthesis (see Chapter 9 on theory synthesis). For example, Murrock and Higgins (2009) utilized statement synthesis as a step leading to development of a theory related to music and its effects on activity and health.

The strategy of statement synthesis can be helpful in graduate and undergraduate teaching aimed at helping nursing students develop skills in writing evidence-based practice statements. Often relevant data sources differ with regard to the language used to express evidence. As a result, formulating synthesized statements that capture and summarize the linkages between nursing actions or practices and care outcomes requires some tweaking of existing language. For example, findings may be expressed in terms of operational definitions (e.g., "scores on the XXX scale correlated with assessments on the YYY scale") and need to be translated into more general conceptual language.

Summary

Statement synthesis is an empirically based strategy for constructing statements that specify the manner in which two or more concepts are interrelated. The strategy encompasses a number of diverse approaches to developing statements. Specific methods range from direct observation and analysis (qualitative or quantitative) of data to use of accumulated research-based literature to construct higher-order generalizations.

Qualitative methods rely on theorists to be perceptive of processes that underlie the events confronted in the data gathering and analysis. Quantitative approaches begin with identifying numerical ways of observing reality. These are then analyzed with the aid of statistical methods to sharpen the patterns inherent in data. Literary methods aim at pulling together general statements of relationships from available research. Despite the diversity of these methods, they share in common a dependence on evidence for formulating scientific statements and a common philosophical assumption about how scientific knowledge reflects reality.

Practice Exercise

In Table 8–3, we present a continuation of the study of new mothers' beliefs and attitudes reported earlier in this chapter. The information addresses the relationship of attitudes toward the baby and attitudes toward oneself as mother as each of these relate to beliefs about the baby. The correlations between these measures were based on data collected at the end of the neonatal period. As before, the correlations are reported separately by parity and sex groups.

TABLE 8–3   Correlation Between New Mothers' Attitudes and Beliefs at the End of the Neonatal Period

Maternal Parity/Infant Sex	Correlation Among Attitudes and Beliefs[a]	
	Beliefs About Baby and Attitude Toward Baby	Beliefs About Baby and Attitude Toward Self as Mother
Primiparous/female	$-.59^b$ (28)	$-.67^b$ (28)
Primiparous/male	$-.50^b$ (43)	$-.26$ (43)
Multiparous/female	$-.39^c$ (49)	$.14$ (49)
Multiparous/male	$-.28$ (34)	$-.13$ (34)

Note: Numbers of subjects are in parentheses.

[a]The negative sign ($-.00$) on the correlations is an artifact of the opposite direction in which the attitude and belief scales are scored; for this exercise, the negative sign on the correlations may be ignored and the correlations treated essentially as positive relations among variables.

[b]$p < .001$.

[c]$p < .01$.

Look carefully at the information in Table 8–3. Formulate one or more statements about how sex and parity groups are similar or different in terms of relationships reported. Formulate an explanation for the results as you stated them.

AUTHORS' ANSWERS FOR COMPARISON

After inspecting the data, you should have noted that for all mothers, except multiparous mothers of males, beliefs about one's baby and attitude toward one's baby were significantly correlated. However, beliefs about one's baby and attitude toward oneself as mother were uncorrelated within all groups except primiparous mothers of girls.

We have earlier offered a hypothesis about the unique features of the relationship of a multiparous mother and her male infant and will not repeat those here. That hypothesis would help to explain the pattern of correlations between beliefs about the baby and attitude toward the baby. From the correlation patterns of parity and sex groups for beliefs about baby and attitude toward self as mother, we hypothesize that mothers may construct worldviews of themselves and their infants. If mothers are confident, their views of themselves will be separate from how they see their infants. Multiparous mothers are likely to view their babies separately from themselves because of their confidence in themselves as successful mothers in the past. For different reasons, such as unpredictable behavior of the male infant, primiparous mothers of males will also separate their beliefs about their infants from their attitude toward themselves as mothers. Only first-time mothers of females do not differentiate their attitude toward themselves from their beliefs about their infants. As before, your hypothesis may be as intriguing as the one offered here. What is most important, however, is that now you should be able to look at data, summarize the finding in a statement, and hypothesize about reasons behind it.

Self-Assessment Test of Introductory Statistics

For readers who wish to assess or refresh their knowledge of introductory statistics to maximally benefit from this chapter, the following self-assessment test is provided. Answers are listed at the end of the assessment.

1. Overall, the best predictor of any individual's score on a test is the
   A. variance.
   B. standard deviation.
   C. correlation.
   D. mean.
2. What effect does changing an individual's raw scores on several tests into percentages have?
   A. Splits an individual score into quartiles
   B. Locks an individual's scores into a common unit
   C. Establishes the group mean
   D. Results in the calculation of the group variance
3. The x^2 statistic is designed to analyze data that are
   A. categorical (noncontinuous).
   B. ordinal (rank ordered).
   C. interval (equal interval).
   D. ratio (true zero point).
4. A correlation coefficient reflects the
   A. average deviation from the mean.
   B. difference between two means.
   C. relationship between two variables.
   D. most frequently occurring score in a score distribution.
5. A t test and analysis of variance (ANOVA) are similar in that both
   A. apply to categorical data.
   B. test the differences between means.
   C. test the relationship between variables.
   D. may be used to compute the variance.
6. Nurse A collected information on which patients kept or broke their clinic appointments during one month. Further, Nurse A classified all these patients as "teenagers" or "non-teenagers" to determine whether teenagers had special problems in keeping appointments. To analyze Nurse A's data, which of the following is the most appropriate statistic?
   A. Measure of central tendency
   B. x^2
   C. Correlated t test
   D. Analysis of variance
7. In analyzing some other data about clinic patients, Nurse A calculated a correlation coefficient of 2.19. The size of the correlation indicates
   A. a strong relationship.
   B. a large difference.
   C. a significant finding.
   D. an error in calculation.
8. The director of the clinic told Nurse A that evidence was needed to show the effectiveness of the patient education done in the clinic. Nurse A decided to compare hypertensive patients' systolic blood pressures before and after the patient education program 1 year ago. To do this, which test statistic should Nurse A use?

A. A measure of deviation from the mean
B. x^2
C. Correlation
D. t test

ANSWERS OF SELF-ASSESSMENT TEST OF INTRODUCTORY STATISTICS

1. D; 2. B; 3. A; 4. C; 5. B; 6. B; 7. D; 8. D

References

Bennett JA. Mediator and moderator variables in nursing research: Conceptual and statistical differences. *Res Nurs Health.* 2000;23(5):415–420.

Benoliel JQ. Grounded theory and nursing knowledge. *Qual Health Res.* 1996;6:406–428.

Corbin J, Strauss AC. *Basics of Qualitative Research: Techniques and Procedures for Developing Grounded Theory.* 3rd ed. Thousand Oaks, CA: Sage Publications; 2008.

Denzin NK, Lincoln YS. *The Sage Handbook of Qualitative Research.* 4th ed. Thousand Oaks, CA: Sage Publications; 2011.

Eaves YD. A synthesis technique for grounded theory data analysis. *J Adv Nurs.* 2001;35:654–663.

Field T. Postpartum depression effects on early interactions, parenting, and safety practices: A review. *Infant Behav Dev.* 2010;33(1):1–6.

Glaser BG. *Theoretical Sensitivity.* Mill Valley, CA: Sociology Press; 1978.

Glaser BG, Strauss AL. *The Discovery of Grounded Theory: Strategies for Qualitative Research.* Chicago, IL: Aldine; 1967.

Good M, Moore SM. Clinical practice guidelines as a new source of middle-range theory: Focus on acute pain. *Nurs Outlook.* 1996;44:74–79.

Henthorn BS. Disengagement and reinforcement in the elderly. *Res Nurs Health.* 1979;2:1–8.

Hess LM, Insel KC. Chemotherapy-related change in cognitive function: A conceptual model. *Oncol Nurs Forum.* 2007;34:981–994.

Huth MM, Moore SM. Prescriptive theory of acute pain management in infants and children. *J Soc Pediatr Nurses.* 1998;3:23–32.

Kiernan M, King AC, Kraemer HC, Stefanick ML, Killen JD. Characteristics of successful and unsuccessful dieters: An application of signal detection methodology. *Ann Behav Med.* 1998;20:1–6.

Knafl KA, Grace HK, eds. *Families Across the Life Cycle.* Boston, MA: Little, Brown; 1978.

Mareno N, Annesi JJ. A statement synthesis of emotional eating and body size recognition: Advancing nursing science related to obesity research. *J Adv Nurs.* 2016;75(5):1023–1029.

Murrock CJ, Higgins PA. The theory of music, mood, and movement to improve health outcomes. *J Adv Nurs.* 2009;65:2249–2257.

Nunnally JC, Bernstein IH. *Psychometric Theory.* 3rd ed. Burr Ridge, IL: McGraw-Hill; 1994.

Osofsky JD, Danzger B. Relationships between neonatal characteristics and mother–infant interaction. *Dev Psychol.* 1974;10:124–130.

Pedhazur EJ, Schmelkin LP. *Measurement, Design, and Analysis: An Integrated Approach.* New York, NY: Psychology Press; 2013.

Polit DF. *Data Analysis and Statistics for Nursing Research.* 2nd ed. Boston, MA: Pearson; 2010.

Polit DF, Beck CT. *Nursing Research: Generating and Assessing Evidence for Nursing Practice.* 9th ed. Philadelphia, PA: Lippincott Williams & Wilkins; 2012.

Quint JC. The case for theories generated from empirical data. *Nurs Res.* 1967a;16:109–114.

Quint JC. *The Nurse and the Dying Patient.* New York, NY: Macmillan; 1967b.

Reynolds PD. *A Primer in Theory Construction.* Indianapolis, IN: Bobbs-Merrill; 1971.

Rudner R. *Philosophy of Social Science.* Englewood Cliffs, NJ: Prentice Hall; 1966.

Ruland CM, Moore SM. Theory construction based on standards of care: A proposed theory of the peaceful end of life. *Nurs Outlook.* 1998;46:169–175.

Schatzman L, Strauss AL. *Field Research: Strategies for a Natural Sociology.* Englewood Cliffs, NJ: Prentice Hall; 1973.

Schreiber RS, Stern PN. *Using Grounded Theory in Nursing.* New York, NY: Springer; 2001.

Smith GT. On construct validity: Issues of method and measurement. *Psychol Assess.* 2005;17:396–408.

Stern PN. Grounded theory methodology: Its uses and processes. *Image.* 1980;12:20–23.

Tabachnick BG, Fidell LS. *Using Multivariate Statistics.* 6th ed. Boston, MA: Pearson; 2013.

Urbina S. *Essentials of Psychological Testing.* Hoboken, NJ: Wiley; 2004.

Waltz CF, Strickland OL, Lenz ER. *Measurement in Nursing and Health Research.* 4th ed. New York, NY: Springer; 2010.

Additional Readings

READINGS IN STATISTICS

Readers who want more information on statistics may find some of the texts below of interest.

Hebel JR, McCarter RJ. *A Study Guide to Epidemiology and Biostatistics.* 7th ed. Gaithersburg, MD: Aspen; 2012.

Meyers LS, Gamst G, Guarino AJ. *Applied Multivariate Research: Design and Interpretation.* 2nd ed. Thousand Oaks, CA: Sage Publications; 2013.

Munro BH. *Statistical Methods for Health Care Research.* 5th ed. Philadelphia, PA: Lippincott; 2005.

Polit DF. *Data Analysis and Statistics for Nursing Research.* 2nd ed. Boston, MA: Pearson; 2010.

Tabachnick BG, Fidell LS. *Using Multivariate Statistics.* 6th ed. Boston, MA: Pearson; 2013.

Warner RM. *Applied Statistics: From Bivariate to Multivariate Techniques.* 2nd ed. Los Angeles, CA: Sage Publications; 2013.

READINGS IN STATEMENT CONSTRUCTION

Readers who want more information on statement construction may find some of the classic texts below of interest.

Dubin R. *Theory Building.* New York, NY: Free Press; 1978.

Hage J. *Techniques and Problems of Theory Construction in Sociology.* New York, NY: Wiley; 1972.

Mullins NC. *The Art of Theory: Construction and Use.* New York, NY: Harper & Row; 1971.

Olson S. *Ideas and Data: The Process and Practice of Social Research.* Homewood, IL: Dorsey; 1976.

Pillemer DB, Light RJ. Synthesizing outcomes: How to use research evidence from many studies. *Harvard Educ Rev.* 1980;50:176–195.

Reynolds PD. *A Primer in Theory Construction.* Indianapolis, IN: Bobbs-Merrill; 1971.

Zetterberg HL. *On Theory and Verification in Sociology.* Totowa, NJ: Bedminster Press; 1965.

9

■ ■ ■

Theory Synthesis

Questions to consider before you get started reading this chapter:

▶ Are you seeking a means to organize existing knowledge into a framework about a research problem or clinical practice area?

▶ Do you have access to databases that can aid you in identifying and retrieving existing studies for the theory or framework you are hoping to construct?

Introductory Note: If you have answered "yes" to the above two questions, then theory synthesis may be a strategy to achieve your goal. The strategy of theory synthesis exemplifies the process of transforming practice-related research about phenomena of interest into an integrated whole. Such an integrated whole allows the theorist to bring bits and pieces of knowledge together in a more useful and coherent form. This strategy is a means for making sense of a jumble of facts, or bringing order to the process of a specific nursing intervention. Because theory synthesis is intricately involved in organization of concepts and statements, readers using this strategy are urged to also read Chapters 7 and 8 on concept and statement synthesis, respectively. Readers may also find Chapter 11 on statement analysis a helpful resource in formulating statements during the process of theory synthesis.

DEFINITION AND DESCRIPTION

The aim of theory synthesis is construction of a theory—an interrelated system of ideas developed through use of evidence. In this strategy, a theorist pulls together available information about a phenomenon. Concepts and statements are organized into a network or whole, a synthesized theory. Theory synthesis involves three steps or phases:

1. Specifying focal concepts to serve as anchors for the synthesized theory.
2. Reviewing the literature to identify factors related to the focal concepts and to specify the nature of relationships.
3. Organizing concepts and statements into an integrated and efficient representation of the phenomena of interest.

Theory synthesis results in a more complex and integrative representation of phenomena than concept or statement synthesis. This is true for several reasons. In

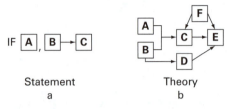

Statement
a

Theory
b

FIGURE 9–1   Example of complexity of linkages in (a) statement versus (b) theory.

contrast to concepts, which serve to highlight phenomena of interest, theories demonstrate the connections among concepts. Further, theories simultaneously embrace more aspects of phenomena and integrate them more thoroughly than statements. A statement may link only two or three concepts together (Figure 9–1a). (See Chapter 8 for a number of examples of synthesized theory statements.) By contrast, a theory may connect a number of concepts to each other and also specify complex direct and indirect linkages among concepts (Figure 9–1b). Theories offer benefits beyond linking together several concepts. A theory that is well designed moves beyond existing knowledge by pointing the way to new and surprising discoveries (Causey, 1969; Hempel, 1966, pp. 70–84). Thus, theory synthesis is not an end, but a means to new insights for use in research and practice.

Theories that are synthesized may be presented in more than one way. When the relationships within and among statements are depicted in graphic form, this constitutes a model of the phenomenon (see Chapter 3 for a fuller discussion of concepts, statements, theories, and models). In this chapter, we will use the terms *theory* and *theoretical model* interchangeably because it is often quite useful to represent beginning theories in both graphic (model) and linguistic (theory) forms. Theorists often move back and forth between expressing theories in written sentences and visual devices, such as diagrams, during theory construction. In the final stages of theory building and refinement, theories may also be expressed in mathematical form (Blalock, 1969). Here, given that this is an introductory book on theory construction, we will limit ourselves to linguistic and graphic expressions of theory.

Like other synthesis strategies, theory synthesis builds on a base of empirical evidence. In theory synthesis, a theorist may combine information from various sources during theory building: qualitative and quantitative observations, available data banks, and published research findings. In utilizing qualitative and statistical information in theory synthesis, it is helpful to first translate them into relational statements (see Chapter 8 on statement synthesis).

Because a theorist can use a variety of sources of data in theory synthesis, we will not present distinct methods for each source. Rather, we will attend to each source of data within an overall strategy for theory synthesis. A theorist may utilize evidence from each of these sources in the construction of a particular model. In theory synthesis, the source of data is less important than the salience of the evidence to the phenomenon represented by the model. Nonetheless, for some topics theorists may choose to use one source of data because of the nature and focus of the theory development project. For example, Halldorsdottir (2008) drew heavily on qualitative phenomenological studies to develop a synthesized theory of the nurse–patient relationship. In contrast, Hill (2002) focused on over 50 quantitative studies in a theory synthesis project that concentrated on feeding efficiency among preterm infants. They each used data pertinent to their purposes.

Readers also should keep in mind that a synthesized theory is limited in its generalizability or external validity by the extent and quality of evidence upon which it is based. Theoretical models drawn from a limited number of sources normally will be more restricted in focus and less generalizable than ones based on multiple and diverse sources. Synthesis strategies are more grounded in reality, however, than other strategies such as derivation because they are based on evidence. Synthesized theories, like synthesized statements, require testing or cross-validating to reaffirm their empirical validity.

A working knowledge of statistical concepts can be a valuable tool in a theory synthesis where theorists directly draw on quantitative data. Such knowledge may enable a theorist to directly utilize statistical information in theory construction. In addition, theorists who are conversant in statistics are better able to critically evaluate statements and conclusions in others' reports of statistical findings. Nevertheless, because our focus in this chapter is on the process of theory synthesis, we will keep our use of statistical information to a minimum.

EXAMPLE OF THE USE OF THEORY SYNTHESIS PROCESS

Because it is probably easiest to get a grasp on how theory synthesis works by demonstrating the process, we provide the following illustration. We draw on a literature review and qualitative study done by Ward (2002) on the topic of transformational leadership, a visionary style of leadership characterized by qualities such as power sharing that are conducive to organizational development. Our illustration is not intended as a comprehensive presentation on this topic. Readers who find the topic of particular interest are referred to Ward's original article for more complete details. (*Note:* We have identified factors related to transformational leadership by assigning an alphabetical letter [*A, B,* etc.] to it. These letters are also included in the model constructed from Ward's literature review [Figure 9–2] so that readers may trace the translation made from linguistic to graphic representation of the findings.)

From Ward's article we extracted the following antecedents of transformational leadership. Included among these antecedents are having a personal support system (*A*), having certain personal characteristics such as self-confidence (*B*), and pursuit of a

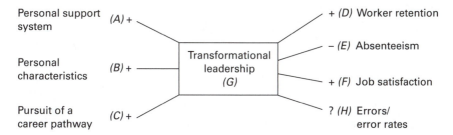

FIGURE 9–2   Model of transformational leadership. (For more complete information, see Ward [2002].)

career pathway (*C*). Studies also indicated that increased worker retention (*D*), decreased absenteeism (*E*), and increased job satisfaction (*F*) are among organizational outcomes of transformational leadership (*G*). Because Ward does not mention if errors (*H*) are reduced by transformational leadership, we cannot make a conclusion about relationships to this important organizational outcome. Having identified a series of relationships pertinent to transformational leadership, we then constructed a diagram, Figure 9–2, to represent the relationships as an interrelated network of ideas. The symbols +, −, and ? were used to designate, respectively, factors with positive, negative, and unknown relationships to transformational leadership. For simplicity, we treated the relationships as unidirectional and causal in our illustration. (See Chapter 11 on statement analysis for further discussion of the concepts of directionality and causality.)

Our example of a model of transformational leadership was based in most cases on reported research findings. Had we access to a data bank on transformational leadership, we might have generated further information pertinent to the model. Suppose we had done this and found that transformational leadership was correlated (*r* = .50) with positive lifestyle changes in employees, such as smoking reduction. We then would have added changes in lifestyle to the model as an outcome of transformational leadership. Statistical information translated into a statement of relationship may be entered into a theoretical model in the same way as relationships gleaned from the literature. Similarly, findings from qualitative research also may be added to the model.

PURPOSE AND USES

Based on the preceding illustration, it should be clear that the purpose of theory synthesis is to represent a phenomenon through an interrelated set of concepts and statements. Three specific aims for theory synthesis are listed in Table 9–1. The first of these aims targets the events that may precede a phenomenon of interest in nursing and is related to predicting or understanding factors that lead up to the phenomenon. The second aim is concerned with what are outcomes of some health-related event, such as receiving a specific diagnosis or a nursing intervention. The second is also helpful in raising awareness of effects that are undesired consequences of a clinical phenomenon, such as

TABLE 9–1   Specific Aims of Theory Synthesis and Related Examples

Aim of Theory Synthesis	Example
To represent the factors that precede or influence a particular health concern	Factors that lead women to be screened for osteoporosis, or to leave abusive relationships
To represent outcomes or effects that occur after some health-related event or intervention	Functional outcomes that are improved and follow from nursing interventions with rural older adults
To put disparate, but related, scientific information into a more theoretically organized form	Modeling the factors that lead immigrant groups to adopt acculturated dietary practices

postpartum depression. The third aim involves organizing relational statements into a system. It may entail collapsing related factors or variables into larger summary concepts. Conducting theory synthesis for this third aim is concerned with depicting relationships about a phenomenon and improving the overall form and quality with which a theory is expressed. The varied aims of theory synthesis are equally valid. The specific aim for which a theorist engages in theory synthesis will depend on the interests of the theorist and the use envisioned for the synthesized theory.

The type and amount of available evidence influences which of the three specific aims of theory synthesis will be most feasible in any given situation. For example, if only minimal information is available about the effects of some phenomenon, but a great deal is known about its antecedents or determinants, a theorist's efforts may be more profitably spent on theory synthesis related to antecedents. Generally, there must be research evidence available about relationships among at least three factors for theory synthesis to be possible. If this is not the case, the theorist should consider another strategy, for example, statement synthesis or theory derivation. The richer the pool of research information available to the theorist, the greater the complexity and precision possible in a synthesized theory.

Theory synthesis may be used in a wide variety of scientific and practical situations. It may be used to produce a compact graphic representation of research findings on a topic of interest. Literature reviews about multiple and complex relationships may be made less tedious and more informative through theory synthesis. Particularly where a graphic display of a synthesized theory is made, complex relations may be communicated more effectively than through traditional written reviews. This particular use of theory synthesis is relevant in teaching complex content about a clinical topic, applying research to the design of clinical interventions, and developing a theoretical framework for a research project.

Theory synthesis requires that a theorist systematically assess relationships among factors pertinent to a topic of interest. The process aids in highlighting areas in need of further research as the theorist methodically identifies relationships among variables; notes the directionality of the relationships; specifies whether the relationship is positive, negative, neutral, or unknown; and notes the quality and amount of evidence in support of the relationship. This information can be helpful in locating specific questions in need of further investigation.

PROCEDURES FOR THEORY SYNTHESIS

A common set of procedures comprises theory synthesis regardless of purpose. Although we outline the procedures as a set of steps or phases, their order is not absolute, nor will a theorist necessarily devote comparable time to each.

Specify Focal Concepts

A theorist begins theory synthesis by marking off a topic of interest. The theorist may do this by specifying (a) *one focal concept* or variable, such as transformational leadership, or (b) a *framework* of several focal concepts. In the former case, the theorist moves out from the focal concept, for example, transformational leadership, to other concepts or variables related to it. In the latter case, the theorist is concerned with a framework of focal concepts and how they may be interrelated. For example, the relationship of various teacher attitudes and behaviors to various nursing student attitudes and behaviors constitutes a framework of focal concepts for beginning theory synthesis. Finally, if the focal concept(s) is expressed by several terms at more than one level of abstraction, a higher-order concept(s) should be selected to capture those equivalent terms. (See Chapter 8 on statement synthesis.)

Identify Related Factors and Relationships

Guided by a single focal concept or a framework of concepts, a careful search and review of the literature is done next. During the review, note is taken of variables related to the focal concept or framework of concepts. Relationships identified are systematically recorded, and, where possible, indications are made of whether they are bi- or unidirectional; positive, neutral, negative, or unknown; and weak, ambiguous, or strong in supporting evidence. For example, double- or single-headed arrows; plus (+) or minus (−) signs; and varying number of asterisks, respectively, can be used to indicate these properties of relational statements.

   Locating relationships in research may be facilitated by finding comprehensive and thorough review articles already written. If recent reviews on the focal concepts are not available, a thorough search of the research literature is in order. Relationship statements are not located in one uniform place in research articles and reports. They may occur in the abstract, literature review, hypotheses, results, or discussion of a study. In a structured abstract, however, key relationships will be stated as conclusions. If the results of a study are not summarized in statement form, a theorist may have to trace a statement from the hypothesis section through the results section in order to determine whether it was supported by actual findings of the study.

   Identification of relationships can also be expanded to include other than literary sources of statements and concepts; for example, qualitative or quantitative observations made by the theorist may be translated into relational statements and then treated as any other statement in theory synthesis. Readers may find Chapter 8 on statement synthesis helpful in clarifying and combining statements. (Readers seeking software to facilitate theory synthesis may find the arcs© program, demonstrated in an article by Kim, Pressler, Jones, and Graves [2008], of interest.)[*]

Construct an Integrated Representation

Finally, when a theorist has collected a fairly representative listing of relational statements pertinent to one or more focal concepts, these may then be organized in terms of the overall pattern of relationships among variables. Theory developers may choose to express the synthesis work in expository form. Alternatively, diagrams may be employed to holistically depict interrelationships among concepts. Readers will recall that in our illustration variables were organized into those that appeared to be

---

[*] Information about the software program arcs© is available from Dr. Marceline Harris, RN, PHD, University of Michigan; e-mail: mrhrrs@med.umich.edu

antecedents of transformational leadership and those that appeared to be outcomes of it (see Figure 9–2). For each topic of interest, a theorist must determine a reasonable basis for organizing statements.

Several mechanisms can facilitate organizing concepts into suitable networks of ideas. One such mechanism is to collapse several highly similar variables into a more comprehensive summary concept for use in the theory. For example, kissing, cuddling, and smiling at a baby might all be amalgamated into a summary concept of *parental attachment behavior.* Similarly, return to work, normal blood sugar, and adherence to a prescribed diet may be collapsed under the concept of *adaptation to chronic disease.* Collapsing discrete variables into summary variables can make a theory more easily understood by reducing needless complexity. A more parsimonious theory will also be achieved by this method. Readers may find Chapter 7 on concept synthesis helpful in constructing summary concepts.

Another mechanism is organizing statements into what Zetterberg (1965) called an "inventory of determinants" or an "inventory of results." These refer, respectively, to the cataloging of antecedents and effects of a focal concept or variable. Structurally, these two types of inventories are quite similar. They differ only in whether the focal concept is viewed as an outcome of certain variables or a determinant of them (Figure 9–3). Organizing statements into inventories of determinants and results is often helpful where a theorist is dealing with only one focal concept or variable. This was the mechanism that we used for transformational leadership.

Yet another mechanism is Blalock's (1969) notion of theoretical "blocks." With this approach, variables that are more proximally related are organized together into a block and their interrelationships specified. Each block of variables is then related to more distally related variables in other blocks (Figure 9–4). Organizing variables and relationships into theoretical blocks is especially relevant if a theorist is constructing a "megamodel" comprising several "minimodels." Schwirian's (1981) classic synthesis of factors affecting nurses' performance in practice is a classic example of organizing diverse relationships about a phenomenon into theoretical blocks.

The mechanisms cited above are only suggestions and primarily are intended to stimulate thinking on how to depict a developing theory. The phenomena of interest to nurses are too diverse and complex to be reduced to just a few possibilities. A theorist must follow the evolving understanding that comes from carefully considering the existing evidence and their own creative processes in deciding how best to depict the phenomena of interest. For an example showing theory developers' use of their own

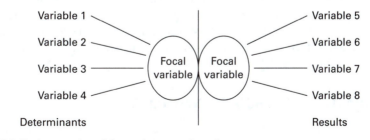

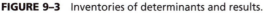

FIGURE 9–3 Inventories of determinants and results.

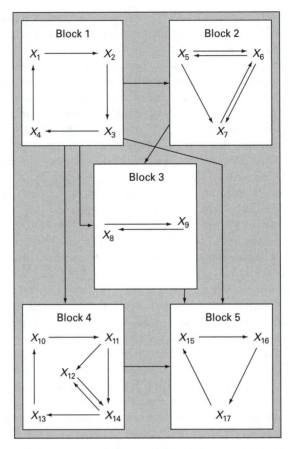

FIGURE 9–4 Variables and statements organized into theoretical blocks.
Source: BLALOCK JR, THEORY CONSTRUCTION FROM VERBAL TO MATHEMATICAL FORMULATIONS, 1st Ed., ©1969. Reprinted and Electronically reproduced by permission of Pearson Education, Inc., New York, NY.

representation of relationships, see Murrock and Higgins's (2009) diagrammatic rendering of their theory of music and its effects on physical activity and health.

To reiterate our point at the beginning of this section, the three steps or phases of theory synthesis may be varied or expanded as needed. For example, conducting the literature review first may be necessary to help theorists clarify the focal concepts of greatest interest to them. In turn, organizing the concepts into an integrated network may be embellished by organizing concepts and relational statements in diagrams and then further coding them as to the extent of research support (e.g., "***" for high support, "*" low support, and "?" conflicting support).

ILLUSTRATIONS OF THEORY SYNTHESIS

A classic and exemplary illustration of the process of theory synthesis is the model of adherence among hypertensive patients presented by Caplan, Robinson, French,

Caldwell, and Shinn (1976). Caplan et al. began model construction by specifying their focal concepts as the dependent variables of interest: adherence and the lowering of blood pressure. They then worked backward to identify predictors or determinants of these focal variables. In constructing the model, they expressed the hope that it would "serve as a heuristic aid in thinking about determinants of adherence" (p. 22). Below are key statements, largely paraphrased for brevity, that culminated in the Caplan et al. model.

Evidence supports relationships between maintaining blood pressure in normal limits and the goal of longevity, if not a long satisfying life (relationship *A*). Adherence to medical regimens that involve taking medications is an effective means of controlling high blood pressure (relationship *B*). In attaining adherence, setting specific subgoals is important in goal attainment, and "rewards need to be anticipated, or explicitly identified in advance before the person begins to strive toward the goal" (Caplan et al., 1976, p. 26), to meet the desired level of adherence (relationship *D*). Further, patients' actual adherent behaviors "serve as a feedback mechanism helping them set new goals based on past accomplishments" (relationship *D*; p. 30). Accomplishment enhances patients' perceived competence to adhere (relationship *E*). Perceived competence to adhere leads to further adherence behavior (relationship *C*).

Caplan et al. (1976) represented these relational statements in the graphic form shown in Figure 9–5. In this figure, letters are used to connect relational statements in linguistic form with their translation into graphic form. Of note in the model presented by Caplan et al. is the bidirectional relationship between adherent behavior and goal setting and attainment (*D*). Two subsequent expansions of this model were made by Caplan et al. (1976), but for brevity we have not included those here.

A number of theorists have published the results of their theory synthesis work in nursing. Several of these are shown in Table 9–2. For example, Good and Moore (1996) drew their evidence base from practice guidelines on pain management for their theory synthesis. They used the strategy of statement synthesis to transform practice guidelines into statements suitable for theory synthesis. Three statements were synthesized from the guidelines. These were then organized in the resultant

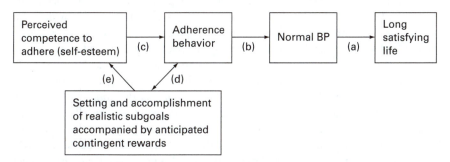

FIGURE 9–5 Model of major hypothesized predictors of adherence and their effects on blood pressure. Arrows between boxes indicate causal relationships. The letters on each arrow are used for reference in the text. *Source*: Permission granted by the Institute for Social Research of the University of Michigan to reproduce Figure 2–1 from Caplan et al. (1976). Copyright 1976 by the University of Michigan.

TABLE 9–2   Examples of Theory Syntheses

Author	Topic of Synthesized Theory
Good and Moore (1996)	Balance between analgesia and side effects in adults
Ruland and Moore (1998)	Peaceful end of life
Huth and Moore (1998)	Acute pain management in infants and children
Easton (1999)	Poststroke recovery
DeMarco (2002)	Nurses' communication patterns in the workplace
Hill (2002)	Feeding efficiency of preterm infants
Whittemore and Roy (2002)	Adaptation to the chronic disease of diabetes
Milberg and Strang (2007)	Palliative home care staff from the perspective of the family
Halldorsdottir (2008)	Nurse–patient relationship
Yao and Algase (2008)	Wandering behavior in persons with dementia
Murrock and Higgins (2009)	Theory of music and its effects on physical activity and health
Siaki, Loescher, and Trego (2013)	Culturally sensitive risk perception theory
Zeng, Sun, Gary, Li, and Liu (2014)	Model of diabetes self-management on U.S. Chinese immigrants
Zandi, Vanaki, Shiva, Mohammadi, and Bacheri-Lankarani (2016)	Caring model for women becoming mothers by surrogacy

middle-range theory of balance of analgesia and side effects. They then stated assumptions and limits of the theory. The benefits of the integrated theory were a parsimonious presentation of diverse information related to the phenomena of pain management. The work of Hill (2002) related to feeding among preterm infants also provides a further detailed illustration of the theory synthesis process. Hill's work also served to integrate extensive research related to feeding behaviors of preterm infants.

In a further example, interest in developing a theoretical basis for caring for women becoming mothers by surrogacy led Zandi et al. (2016) to use theory synthesis to construct the model, *security giving in surrogacy motherhood*. The focal concept in the model, *security giving in surrogacy motherhood*, was based on an earlier qualitative study. Building from this focal concept, they employed literature searches and identified statements related to illuminate the "caring role of nurses and what caring actions are needed to provide security" (p. 333) to women becoming mothers through surrogacy. Concepts and statements were synthesized in a theoretical model expressed in a rich description as well as diagrammatic form. This model provided a means of understanding the nurses' role and better caring for women becoming mothers by surrogacy.

ADVANTAGES AND LIMITATIONS

The strength of theory synthesis as a strategy is the resultant integration of large amounts of discrete information about a topic. By using both linguistic and graphic modalities, synthesized theories can integrate and efficiently present multiple and complex relationships. Theory synthesis is a useful strategy for summarizing research findings relevant to educational, research, and practice spheres.

Theorists may need to increase their fluency with statistical concepts in order to make accurate discriminations about structural relationships between and among concepts in their evidence base. These discriminations include clarifying causal pathways among sets of variables.

Theory synthesis is built on the premise that theory development is an incremental and cumulative process. Although this may be true at certain levels of scientific development, this may not characterize those major advances in scientific thought that have occurred by making radical reorganizations of or departures from accumulated knowledge (Kuhn, 1962).

UTILIZING THE RESULTS OF THEORY SYNTHESIS

In the context of research, theory synthesis results lay bare the conceptual structure and linkages of extant knowledge about a phenomenon. This structural knowledge may then be used to ensure operational adequacy (Fawcett, 1999) of indicators and research procedures in empirically testing synthesized theory. Consequently, even a well-designed theoretical model needs to be empirically validated. Model or theory testing is needed to provide the sound empirical base desired of theories in a scientific discipline and profession. Testing may show that a model needs to be modified. If parts of a model repeatedly do not perform under rigorous tests (e.g., do not show expected relationships), then theorists have several alternatives. They may delete nonperforming variables, introduce new variables, or rethink the whole model. For example, if the model of transformational leadership were tested, it might need to be reworked. Perhaps gender-specific concepts (Eisler & Hersen, 2000) could be added to create separate models for men and women. As before, testing is needed to determine the merit of any changes in a model.

Development of synthesized theories may be useful in teaching complex content involving multiple concepts and their interrelationships. Often when such material is presented graphically as well as linguistically, it is easier both to teach and to learn. Students may also find it easier to retain complex relationships if they are given the opportunity to sketch out relationships embedded in text format.

Synthesized theories may help nurses in practice to examine the antecedents and consequences of a clinical phenomenon, or to plan patient services based on a coherent program theory. Designing preventive interventions may be facilitated by looking at the antecedents of a clinical problem. Tracing the way that each potential antecedent might be modified in an attempt to prevent undesired clinical problems, such as hospital readmissions after surgery, can suggest how present practice might be improved. In turn, elaborating the consequences of an intervention is useful in identifying outcomes for assessing the effectiveness of an intervention. Theory synthesis is applicable to clinical problems within the hospital context, as well as in home care and community agency settings. Theory synthesis can be used to identify anteced- ents of a clinical phenomenon for use in development of risk assessment tools. In this vein, Gephart, Effken, McGrath, and Reed (2013) used theory synthesis as the foundation for development of a risk index for necrotizing enterocolitis in preterm infants.

THEORY SYNTHESIS AND INTEGRATIVE MODELS AND THEORIES

As knowledge from various disciplines converges around a phenomenon, it is tempting to build integrative models that incorporate multiple levels of analysis. For example, the UNICEF multilevel conceptual framework of the causes of child malnutrition (Figure 9–6) is recognized worldwide (https://www.unicef.org/nutrition/training/2.5/4.html).

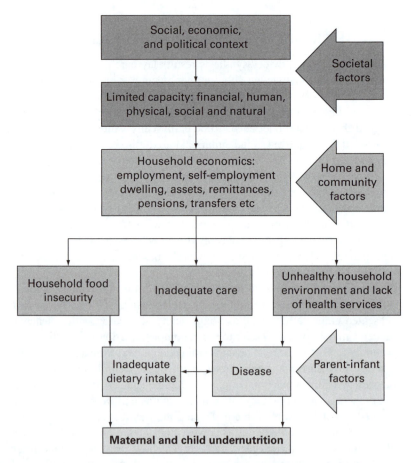

FIGURE 9–6 UNICEF conceptual framework. *Source*: Adapted from UNICEF.org. Black et al. (2008). Accessed at https://www.unicef.org/nutrition/training/2.5/4.html

In this framework, the causes of child malnutrition and mortality are depicted as starting at the societal level with regard to basic resources, then progressing to causes at the household level, and finally reaching the level of the individual child where disease conditioned by insufficient food reciprocally leads to poor food intake and further disease and finally malnutrition. Such models make major contributions to our understanding of nationally and globally significant health problems, but care is needed to appropriately construct such models. Sobal (1991), among others, has written eloquently about the issues in linking levels of analysis. While it is not our purpose to explicate these issues here, it is important to point them out. For example, concepts from one level of analysis may not be translatable to another level. To overcome this issue, Sobal has proposed creating suitable mediating processes that link otherwise incompatible terminology across levels of analysis (e.g., from the societal level across to the physiological level).

A second issue that sometimes occurs when attempting to integrate existing theories is the indiscriminate plucking of a term from one theoretical context and embedding it into another. Hempel (1966) argued that terms in theories derive their meaning from their "systemic import" within a web of theoretical relationships (p. 98). Thus, wresting a term from one theory and embedding it into another without regard for these theoretical relationships is not sound theory integration. As carefully as the spider weaves its web, so must the theorist integrate competing or parallel theories.

On the other hand, combining theories can often strengthen approaches to understanding and improving clinical care. To this end, Fassler and Naleppa (2011) adapted the theory synthesis strategy to combine practice models in the field of social work.

Summary

Because theory synthesis is based on evidence, it enables a theorist to organize and integrate a wide variety of research information on a topic of interest. In theory synthesis, sets of concepts and discrete statements are organized into an interrelated system of statements with accompanying graphic representations. Theory synthesis may incorporate information from published research literature, direct statistical information, and qualitative research. Because theory synthesis may be used for several related purposes, deciding on the specific purpose depends on the balance among the theorist's interests, the use planned for the synthesized theory, and the amount and type of information available on a topic.

Three steps or phases are involved in theory synthesis: (1) specifying focal concepts for the synthesized theory, (2) reviewing the literature to identify factors related to the focal concepts and the relationships among these, and (3) organizing concepts and statements into an integrated and efficient representation of the phenomena of interest.

Theory synthesis allows a large amount of information to be efficiently organized. If quantitative data are involved, the use of the strategy requires some statistical sophistication of the part of the theorist. The strategy assumes an incremental approach to scientific progress.

Practice Exercises

EXERCISE 1

Obesity researchers, such as Hill and Peters (1998), have argued that modern life is at odds with our evolved human regulatory systems for taking in, storing, and expending energy. Specifically, factors such as the widespread availability of energy-dense foods and growing use of energy-sparing modern conveniences have led to the rapid onset of a national obesity epidemic in the United States (Mokdad et al., 2001; Mokdad et al., 1999). One consequence of this has been growth in the number of people who are obese. Obesity, in turn, is predicted to lead to increased rates of many of its sequelae, such as cardiovascular disease, diabetes mellitus, gastric reflux syndrome, orthopedic problems, and certain cancers.

For this exercise, develop several statements regarding the antecedents and consequences of the obesity epidemic. Based on your statements, make a diagram synthesizing these statements into a model of the "epidemic of obesity."

When you have completed this exercise, compare your theoretical model with Figure 9–7. Although your model may not look exactly like ours, there should be some structural similarity to it.

EXERCISE 2

Select one of the articles in Table 9–2. After reading a copy of that article, try to answer the following questions:

- Are the source and type of evidence that were used in the synthesis process clear? Describe what those evidence sources were.
- How clearly did the authors describe their theory synthesis process (in comparison to the steps presented in this chapter)?
- How did the authors present their final theory synthesis: in text only, as a diagram, or both?
- How would you rate the quality of the synthesized theory in relation to clarity and usefulness for the authors' expressed purposes?

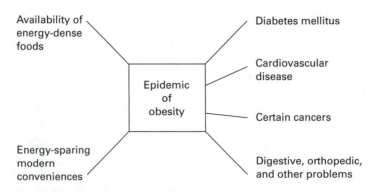

FIGURE 9–7 Model of the epidemic of obesity.

References

Black RE, Allen AH, Bhutta ZA, Caulfield LE, de Onis M, Ezzati M, et al. Maternal and child undernutrition: Global and regional exposures and health consequences. *Lancet.* 2008;371(9608):243–260.

Blalock HM. *Theory Construction: From Verbal to Mathematical Formulations.* Englewood Cliffs, NJ: Prentice Hall; 1969.

Caplan RD, Robinson EAR, French JRP, Caldwell JR, Shinn M. *Adhering to Medical Regimens: Pilot Experiments in Patient Education and Social Support.* Ann Arbor, MI: Institute for Social Research, University of Michigan; 1976.

Causey R. Scientific progress. *Tex Eng Sci Mag.* 1969;6(1):22–29.

DeMarco R. Two theories/a sharper lens: The staff nurse voice in the workplace. *J Adv Nurs.* 2002;38:549–556.

Easton KL. The poststroke journey: From agonizing to owning. *Geriatr Nurs.* 1999;20:70–76.

Eisler RM, Hersen M, eds. *Handbook of Gender, Culture, and Health.* Mahwah, NJ: Erlbaum; 2000.

Fassler A, Naleppa MJ. An innovative integrated research method: Estimating fidelity using technology for model integration and development. *Br J Soc Work.* 2011;41:761–777.

Fawcett J. *The Relationship of Theory and Research.* 3rd ed. Philadelphia, PA: Davis; 1999.

Gephart SM, Effken JA, McGrath JM, Reed PG. Expert consensus building using e-Delphi for necrotizing enterocolitis risk assessment. *J Obstet Gynecol Neonatal Nurs.* 2013;42(3):332–347.

Good M, Moore SM. Clinical practice guidelines as a new source of middle-range theory: Focus on acute pain. *Nurs Outlook.* 1996;44:74–79.

Halldorsdottir S. The dynamics of the nurse–patient relationship: Introduction of a synthesized theory from the patient's perspective. *Scand J Caring Sci.* 2008;22:643–652.

Hempel CG. *Philosophy of Natural Science.* Englewood Cliffs, NJ: Prentice Hall; 1966.

Hill AS. Toward a theory of feeding efficiency for bottle-fed preterm infants. *J Theory Constr Test.* 2002;6(1):75–81.

Hill JO, Peters JC. Environmental contributions to the obesity epidemic. *Science.* 1998;280:1371–1374.

Huth MM, Moore SM. Prescriptive theory of acute pain management in infants and children. *J Soc Pediatr Nurses.* 1998;3:23–32.

Kim J, Pressler SJ, Jones J, Graves JR. Generating scientific models of knowledge using arcs©. *Clin Nurse Spec.* 2008;22:286–292.

Kuhn TS. *The Structure of Scientific Revolutions.* Chicago, IL: University of Chicago Press; 1962.

Milberg A, Strang P. What to do when "there is nothing more to do"? A study within a salutogenic framework of family members' experience of palliative home care staff. *Psycho-Oncology.* 2007;16:741–751.

Mokdad AH, Bowman BA, Ford ES, Vinicor F, Marks JS, Koplan JP. The continuing epidemics of obesity and diabetes in the United States. *JAMA.* 2001;286:1195–1200.

Mokdad AH, Serdula MK, Dietz WH, Bowman BA, Marks JS, Koplan JP. The spread of the obesity epidemic in the United States, 1991–1998. *JAMA.* 1999;282:1519–1522.

Murrock CJ, Higgins PA. The theory of music, mood, and movement to improve health outcomes. *J Adv Nurs.* 2009;65:2249–2257.

Ruland CM, Moore SM. Theory construction based on standards of care: A proposed theory of the peaceful end of life. *Nurs Outlook.* 1998;46:169–175.

Schwirian PM. Toward an explanatory model of nursing performance. *Nurs Res.* 1981;30:247–253.

Siaki LA, Loescher LJ, Trego LL. Synthesis strategy: Building a culturally sensitive mid-range theory of risk perception using literary, quantitative, and qualitative methods. *J Adv Nurs.* 2013;69(3):726–737.

Sobal J. Obesity and socioeconomic status: A framework for examining relationships between physical and social variables. *Med Anthropol.* 1991;12:231–247.

Ward K. A vision for tomorrow: Transformational nursing leaders. *Nurs Outlook.* 2002;50:121–126.

Whittemore R, Roy C. Adapting to diabetes mellitus: A theory synthesis. *Nurs Sci Q.* 2002;15:311–317.

Yao L, Algase D. Emotional intervention strategies for dementia-related behavior: A theory synthesis. *J Neurosci Nurs.* 2008;40:106–115.

Zandi M, Vanaki Z, Shiva M, Mohammadi E, Bagheri-Lankarani N. Security giving in surrogacy motherhood process as a caring model for commissioning mothers: A theory synthesis. *Jpn J Nurs Sci.* 2016;13(3):331–344.

Zeng B, Sun W, Gary RA, Li C, Liu T. Towards a conceptual model of diabetes self-management among Chinese immigrants in the United States. *Int J Environ Res Public Health.* 2014;11(7):6727–6742.

Zetterberg HL. *On Theory and Verification in Sociology.* Totowa, NJ: Bedminster Press; 1965.

Additional Readings

Cumbie SA, Conley VM, Burman ME. Advanced practice nursing model for comprehensive care with chronic illness—Model for promoting process engagement. *Adv Nurs Sci.* 2004;27:70–80.

Dubin R. *Theory Building.* New York, NY: Free Press; 1978.

Hage J. *Techniques and Problems of Theory Construction in Sociology.* New York, NY: Wiley; 1972.

Hall JM. Alcoholism recovery in lesbian women: A theory in development. *Sch Inq Nurs Pract.* 1990;4:109–122.

Lancaster W, Lancaster J. Models and model building in nursing. *Adv Nurs Sci.* 1981;3(3):31–42.

Mullins NC. *The Art of Theory: Construction and Use.* New York, NY: Harper & Row; 1971.

Reynolds PD. *A Primer in Theory Construction.* Indianapolis, IN: Bobbs-Merrill; 1971.

Stember ML. Model building as a strategy for theory development. In: Chinn PL, ed. *Nursing Research Methodology.* Rockville, MD: Aspen; 1986.

Suppe F, Jacox AK. Philosophy of science and the development of nursing theory. In: Werley HH, Fitzpatrick JJ, eds. *Annual Review of Nursing Research.* Boston, MA: Springer; 1985, pp. 241–267.

Zetterberg HL. *On Theory and Verification in Sociology.* Totowa, NJ: Bedminster Press; 1965.

Analysis Strategies

If you have ever watched a small child take apart a toy and put it back together again in an effort to see how it works, that experience is a model case of analysis. This part introduces the strategies of concept, statement, and theory analysis. Analysis is useful when concepts, statements, or theories are already present in the literature but the theorist wishes to understand them better by taking them apart, examining the parts, and putting them all back together again. Such an analysis allows the theorist to determine the strengths or weaknesses of the concept, statement, or theory. The strategies we discuss in the next three chapters will help you to understand how to analyze theoretical structures in a systematic and logical way. Analysis, as indeed all the strategies we discuss here, is always done for a purpose. It is a rigorous process and should not be taken lightly. In most instances, the analyst chooses one of these strategies because he or she plans to use the concept, statement, or theory in a piece of his or her own work and wants to be sure it is appropriate and feasible to do so. The analyst is going to be most interested in the structure and/or function of the concept, statement, or theory as it relates to the focal concept of interest to him or her.

Chapter 10 describes the process of concept analysis. Concept analysis is a means for clarifying the meaning of concepts for various purposes. Since concepts are the basic building blocks of theory, it is critical to have the concepts sound and strong. So concept analysis is a rather good way to begin to understand how one thinks logically related to terms and their definitions and uses in theory development. As this is one of the chapters that seems to be used a lot, we have attempted to make the reasons for using this method as clear as possible. We have included a rather large table of concept analyses using the method we suggest here in an effort to provide examples of how the finished product should look.

Chapter 11 is probably the most important chapter in this section, since statement analysis is a critical part of any good theory analysis. Understanding the structure and function of relational statements contributes significantly to understanding how theories are built and how they work. Deconstructing statements to see the direction, valence, and type of relationships helps to clarify the statements. It also allows the analyst to see where there might be gaps in logic.

Chapter 12 describes the full process of theory analysis. Building on statement analysis, this chapter helps the analyst deconstruct the full theory to determine strengths, weaknesses, missing pieces, and gaps in logic. A good theory analysis can be extremely helpful if the analyst is preparing to use the theory to guide research or is considering its use for practice.

10

■ ■ ■

Concept Analysis

Questions to consider before you get started reading this chapter:

▶ Are you interested in a particular concept to use in your work but are unclear about how to measure it?

▶ Are you confronted with having to distinguish between two or more overlapping concepts?

▶ Are you interested in developing a concept as a new nursing diagnosis or intervention? Or in refining one?

▶ Are you interested in learning how to think logically about the meaning of words you are using in your research?

Introductory Note: If the answer to any of these questions is yes, then concept analysis may help you accomplish your goal. Concept analysis is a way to deconstruct a term in order to understand it better and to develop a sound definition that allows for measurement of the concept.

There has been a lot of concept analysis work since the last edition of this book. It is encouraging to note that nurse scholars and clinicians are taking nursing vocabularies seriously and making the effort to clearly define the concepts of interest to them. The only way we will be able to demonstrate the evidence base for our practice is to be able to first describe the phenomena in measurable or at least communicable ways. Concept analysis allows the theorist, researcher, or clinician to come to grips with the various possibilities within the concept of interest—to "get inside" the concept and see how it works. It is a challenging activity but provides an enormous insight into the phenomenon of interest.

DEFINITION AND DESCRIPTION

Concepts are the basic building blocks in theory construction. This may especially be true in nursing, where some concepts arise from practice experiences that then lead to further theoretical work. Thus, we want the concepts to be solid and strong to uphold the structure of the theory. For a concept to be solid and strong, it must clearly name the thing to which it refers, it must be clearly defined (structure), and its uses in the theory should be clear (function) so that anyone who sees the concept and its definition within the theory can understand exactly what is being described, explained, or predicted. Mulcahy's (2016) analysis of parental concern is a good example of a concept arising from practice.

Examining the structure and function of a concept is the purpose of concept analysis (see Chapter 3). Concepts contain within themselves the attributes or characteristics that make them unique from other concepts. Thus, we speak of concepts as containing defining characteristics or attributes that permit us to decide which phenomena match the concept and which do not. Concepts are mental constructions; they are our attempts to order our environmental stimuli in a meaningful way. Concepts, therefore, represent categories of information that contain the defining attributes. Concept analysis is a formal, linguistic exercise to determine those defining attributes. The analysis itself must be rigorous and precise, but the end product is always tentative. The reasons for this tentativeness stem from the fact that two people will often come up with somewhat different attributes for the same concept in their analyses and from the fact that scientific and general knowledge changes so quickly that what is true today is not true tomorrow.

Contributing to the tentativeness of concepts is that they also change over time—often slowly, but occasionally very quickly. Cultural, contextual, and societal factors contribute to those changes. Therefore, anyone undertaking concept analysis should be aware of the dynamic quality of ideas and the words that express those ideas. Concepts are not carved in stone. And the analyst changes over time as well. Therefore, the understanding of the concept may also change over time. This is one reason why concept analyses should never be viewed as a finished product. The best one can hope for from a concept analysis is to capture the critical elements of it at the current moment in time. However, this is not to imply that trying to determine the defining attributes of a concept of interest is futile—far from it.

Concept analysis encourages communication. If we are precise about carefully defining the attributes of the concepts we use in theory development and in research, we will make it far easier to promote understanding among our colleagues about the phenomena being discussed. And it will facilitate finding ways to recognize and/or measure those concepts in our work.

PURPOSE AND USES

Concept analysis is a process of examining the basic elements of a concept. If we know "what counts" when we describe a concept, it helps us to distinguish that concept from ones that are similar to, but not the same as, that concept. It allows us to distinguish the likeness and unlikeness between concepts. By breaking a concept into its simpler elements, it is easier to determine its internal structure. Because we have already said in Chapter 3 that a concept is expressed by a word or a term in language (Reynolds, 1971), an analysis of a concept must, perforce, be an analysis of the descriptive word and its use. Concept analysis is ultimately only a careful examination and description of a word or term and its uses in the language coupled with an explanation of how it is "like" and "not like" other related words or terms. We are concerned with both actual and possible uses of words that convey concept meanings.

Concept analysis can be useful in refining ambiguous concepts in a theory. It also helps clarify those overused or vague concepts that are prevalent in nursing practice so that everyone who subsequently uses the term will be speaking of the same thing. Concept analysis results in a precise definition that by its very nature increases the validity of the construct; that is, it will accurately reflect its theoretical base. The results of concept analysis yield to the theorist or investigator a basic understanding of the underlying attributes of the concepts. This helps to clearly define the concept and to allow the investigator or theorist to construct statements or hypotheses that accurately reflect the relationships between the concepts. The results of concept analysis are also very useful in constructing research instruments or interview guides prior to doing research.

In a classic textbook, Nunnally (1978) spoke to the need for careful conceptual development for research instruments. The results of concept analysis—the definition, list of defining attributes, and antecedents—can provide the scientist with an excellent beginning for a new tool or an excellent way to evaluate an old one. To begin a new tool, items could be constructed, using the empirical referents, to reflect each of the defining attributes. Questions could be constructed to determine whether proposed antecedents occurred. With careful psychometric testing, the new tool could be useful for continuing research by interested scientists. The results of concept analysis are also useful in evaluating existing instruments. The instruments to be used in a research project could be examined in light of the results of the concept analysis to determine whether the instruments accurately reflect the defining attributes of the relevant concepts. Developing standardized language to describe nursing practice is another primary use of concept analysis. In many cases, the terms to describe nursing diagnoses, interventions, and outcomes have been developed consensually or in practice settings without thoroughly considering the theoretical issues relating to assigning names to clients' problems/life situations, to the interventions nurses provide, or to the outcomes we can reasonably expect (Carlson-Catalano et al., 1998; Gamel, Grypdonck, Hengeveld, & Davis, 2001; Whitley, 1995). Conducting a thorough concept analysis for any potential diagnosis, intervention, or outcome would greatly facilitate taxonomic work and would thoroughly ground nursing language in the pertinent theoretical and research literature, thus providing a strong evidence base. Each nursing diagnosis, intervention, and outcome should be treated as a separate concept and be analyzed independently. For instance, most nursing diagnoses are written with three components—the health problem, the contributing factors, and the defining signs and symptoms (Gordon, 1982). These three components closely parallel the results of concept analysis—antecedents (etiology), defining characteristics (defining signs and symptoms), and definition (health problem). It seems reasonable to suggest that using the two processes iteratively would improve our taxonomies and contribute to theory development simultaneously.

The method we describe below is only one of several methods available for concept analysis. Although there has been increasing criticism of most of the concept analysis methods (we will speak to these criticisms later in this chapter), we continue to believe that this method is the easiest to understand and master, especially for beginners.

A few words of explanation might be useful before beginning. We will discuss these issues more extensively later in the chapter, but a couple of them deserve discussion here as well. First, as you begin to get really involved in this process, you are likely to feel completely overwhelmed by the task. This is normal, and the feeling will dissipate over time as you get more familiar with how the process works. Second, you are likely to feel protective of your work and be reluctant to subject it to criticism. Try to avoid this at all costs. This kind of intellectual exercise is best accomplished with feedback from peers. The product of the analysis will be far better if more than one mind is involved. Third, remember that this *is* a process, not a linear activity. You will be moving back and forth among the steps frequently, revising as you go. Circling back through some steps more than once is common. This movement, too, is normal and expected.

PROCEDURES FOR CONCEPT ANALYSIS

We have modified and simplified Wilson's (1963) classic concept analysis procedure, so there are only eight instead of eleven steps. We believe that the eight steps are sufficient to capture the essence of the process. However, should you wish to examine Wilson's entire process, you may find the citation to his seminal work in the "References" section of this chapter.

The steps are as follows:

1. Select a concept.
2. Determine the aims or purposes of analysis.
3. Identify all uses of the concept that you can discover.
4. Determine the defining attributes.
5. Identify a model case.
6. Identify borderline, related, contrary, invented, and illegitimate cases.
7. Identify antecedents and consequences.
8. Define empirical referents.

Although we will discuss the steps in concept analysis as if they were sequential, in fact they are iterative. The mental activities of a concept analysis often require that some revision be made in an earlier step because of information or ideas arising from a later one. This is to be expected. The iterative nature of the process results in a much cleaner, more precise analysis.

Select a Concept

Concept selection should be done with care. It is best to choose a concept in which you are already interested, one that is associated with your work, or one that has always bothered you. This first step is often the hardest because you may have several concepts that interest you. How do you choose just one? Generally, concept selection should reflect the topic or area of greatest interest to you. Our advice is to choose the one that is most critical to your needs. Is there one concept on which everything else depends? Is there a concept that is critical to doing the next step in your research? If so, this is the concept you should choose first. Wilson (1963) describes this process as isolating the concept—that is, examining the significance of the concept in its various contexts, boundaries, and relevance to your own work.

Choose a concept that is manageable, especially if this is your first concept analysis. It is important to avoid primitive terms that can be defined only by giving examples. It is equally important to avoid umbrella terms that are so broad that they may encompass several meanings and confuse the analysis. If the concept name is used as both a noun and a verb, it is more fruitful to choose the noun form.

Unexplored concepts can be either fruitful avenues of exploration or linguistic traps. Unexplored concepts can be found in nursing practice, can be generated from nursing research studies, or can be drawn from a theory that is as yet incomplete or that has concepts that are unclear. Analysis of one of these can be very helpful in expanding your thinking. However, by their nature (unexplored) they may lead you down a path that you do not want to tread or that takes you in the wrong direction. If this is so, you may want to consider abandoning the analysis and choosing a more relevant concept.

The bottom line is that you should choose a concept that is important and useful to your research program or to further theoretical developments in your area of interest. Choosing a trivial concept or one that does not contribute significantly to knowledge development about your phenomenon of concern is an exercise in futility and a waste of your valuable time.

Determine the Aims of Analysis

To determine the aims or purposes of the analysis is the next step. This second step helps focus attention on exactly what use you intend to make of the results of your effort. It essentially answers the question: "Why am I doing this analysis?" It is not uncommon to see articles presenting excellent concept analyses that end precipitously with no implications for "next steps." Concept analysis is not an end in itself but should be a bridge to further related work in nursing practice theory, or research.

It is very important to decide for yourself, in advance, why you are interested in conducting a concept analysis. Write it down and keep it handy during the analysis. This definition of purpose is useful if, as you begin to determine the defining attributes, you discover several dissimilar uses of the concept. The selection you make regarding which specific use of the concept you will choose should reflect the aims of the analysis.

Distinguishing between the normal, ordinary language usage of the concept and the scientific usage of the same concept might be the aim of your analysis. Others might be to clarify the meaning of an existing concept, develop an operational definition, develop a research instrument, or add to existing theory. There are other possible purposes. Whatever the purpose is for your analysis, keep it clearly in mind as you work.

Before you begin, be sure to examine the literature to see whether the concept has already been analyzed by someone else. If it has been, read the analysis carefully to see whether the analysis fits your needs. If it does, use it. Concept analysis is rigorous and time consuming. It is a waste of time and energy to repeat an analysis if one already exists that meets your needs.

In our analysis of attachment at the end of this chapter, you will see that because we were interested in the concept of attachment as it applied to mothers and babies, we had to distinguish between animate and inanimate instances of attachment. If our aim had not been related to animate attachment, we might have made different decisions about how to proceed when we realized there would be differences.

Identify Uses of the Concept

Using dictionaries, thesauruses, available literature, and even friends and colleagues, identify as many uses of the concept as you can find. At this initial stage, do not limit yourself to only one aspect of the concept. You must consider all uses of the term. Do not limit your search to just nursing or medical literature as this may bias your understanding of the true nature of the concept. Ignoring the physical aspects of a concept and focusing only on the psychosocial aspects, for instance, may deprive you of a great deal of valuable information. Remember to include both implicit and explicit uses of the concept. Extensive reading in as many different sources as possible is invaluable. Even slang expressions can be helpful.

This review of literature helps you support or validate your ultimate choices of the defining attributes and provides the evidence base for your analysis. For instance, if you were examining the concept of "coping," you would discover that not only are there psychological uses for the term but there are also copings on buildings, coping saws, a method of trimming a falcon's beak called coping, and a coping that is an ecclesiastical garment similar to a cloak. All of these uses of the term must be included in your final analysis.

Failing to identify or, worse, ignoring some uses of a concept may result in an analysis that severely limits the usefulness of the outcome. A few years ago, one of our students was analyzing the concept "presence" as it relates to the care of hospitalized children. In the initial phase, the student reported many positive uses of the concept but none that were negative. When other students mentioned things such as "evil presence" or "presence of a hostile army on the border," the student was reluctant to consider those aspects of presence. Yet, in the final analysis, one critical attribute of the nurse's presence with a hospitalized child turned out to be the potential for threat engendered in the presence of the nurse. If the concept of presence is of interest to you, Smith's (2001) excellent article is recommended, along with the commentary by Chase (2001) for a thorough and interesting review of the concept of presence.

Once you have identified all the usages of the concept, both ordinary and scientific, you may have to decide whether to continue to consider all aspects of the concept or only those pertinent to the scientific use. We generally feel that when possible you should continue to consider all aspects of the concept usage because that is likely to yield richer meanings. However, at times that will clearly be impractical or unhelpful. In these cases, use the aims of your analysis to guide your decision making.

Often your literature review will be extensive and you may feel overwhelmed. First, remember you are only looking for the definitions and uses of the term. You do not have to read all of every source. Although you may want to, sometimes it is not practical or feasible. We often suggest that our students write brief summaries of each source and keep them with the source materials or to make a database or an Excel chart to manage their literature. For an excellent example of how this can be done, you may want to read the concept analysis of healing done by the staff of the Samueli Institute (Firth et al., 2015).

During your review of the literature and in the process of collecting instances of concept use, you will find other instances that are similar or related to the concept being analyzed but are not quite the real thing. Keep a list of these instances. They will be helpful to you when you begin to define borderline or related cases.

Determine the Defining Attributes

Determining the defining attributes of a concept is the heart of concept analysis. The effort is to try to show the cluster of attributes that are the most frequently associated with the concept and that allow the analyst the broadest insight into the concept. As you examine as many of the different instances of a concept as you can find, make notes of the characteristics of the concept that appear over and over again. This list of characteristics, called defining characteristics or defining attributes, functions very much like the criteria for making differential diagnoses in medicine. That is, they help you and others name the occurrence of a specific phenomenon as differentiated from another similar or related one. In the case of defining attributes, more is not necessarily better. In fact, the best analyses refine the defining attributes to the fewest number that will still differentiate the concept of interest from surrounding concepts. If the analysis is done well, the defining characteristics, standing alone, should immediately call the concept to mind. For good examples of this, see Trendall's (2000) analysis of chronic fatigue and Mulder's (2006) analysis of effective breastfeeding.

The defining attributes are not immutable. They may change as your understanding of the concept improves. They will certainly change during the analysis as you use the cases to help you understand what counts as the core meaning of the concept. They may change slightly over time if the concept changes. Or they may change when used in a different context than the one under study.

If, when you have gathered all the instances of a concept, there are a large number of possible meanings, then a decision is clearly necessary regarding which will be the most useful and which will provide you the greatest help in relation to the aims of your analysis. You may decide to choose more than one meaning and continue analyzing using several meanings. For example, in the analysis of the concept of "attachment" at the end of this chapter we found that attachment can occur in both animate and inanimate forms. We chose to examine which attributes were common to both kinds and then to continue our analysis further to include the specific defining attributes for animate attachment because our area of interest was in mother–infant attachment (Avant, 1979). Consideration of the social or nursing care context in which the concept is to be used may be important in your decision as it was to us in the example. The final decision is up to you.

The three characteristics that seemed to be most obvious among all those divergent uses of the term *coping* that we listed earlier for instance were (1) the attribute of covering something—an action, a cape, a window, or a beak; (2) the attribute of protection—one's psyche, the garment under the cape, or the flowers under the window; and (3) the attribute of adjusting or rebalancing. We decided that the idea of the *coping saw* was not relevant to the general concept because it does not reflect any of the three attributes that occur in all the other instances we found. We will use this, in fact, as the example of an "illegitimate" case later in the analysis—one in which the term is used incorrectly in relation to its generally accepted meaning.

Bennett, Wang, Moore, and Nagle (2017) provide an excellent example of defining attributes in their analysis of the concept of "care partner." The three attributes were the care provider, the person needing care but participating in the care, and a relationship between the two. In Ellis-Stoll and Popkess-Vawter's (1998) study, the defining attributes of empowerment were identified as mutual participation, active listening, and individualized knowledge acquisition. The model case presented regarded James, a postcoronary bypass patient in rehabilitation. In the model case, the defining attributes were clearly observable. Another excellent example is Xyrichis and Ream's (2008) analysis of teamwork. The three defining attributes of exercising concerted effort, employing interdependent collaboration, and utilizing shared decision making are clearly there in the model case. This demonstration of the defining characteristics is one of the principal reasons for the model case. The model case helps you to be sure that you have the defining characteristics correct.

Identify Model Case(s)

A model case is an example of the use of the concept that demonstrates all the defining attributes of the concept. That is, the model case should be a pure case of the concept, a paradigmatic example, or a pure exemplar. Basically, the model case is one that we are absolutely sure is an instance of the concept. Wilson (1963) suggests that the model case is one in which the analyst can say, "Well, if that isn't an example of it, then nothing is." The model case can come first in your analysis, may be developed simultaneously with the attributes, or may emerge after the attributes are tentatively determined.

Model cases may be actual examples from real life, found in the literature, or even constructed by you. The model case may be a nursing example or not. That depends on you. Sometimes using a nursing model case helps you understand the concept, but sometimes it obscures your ability to be objective about the concept meanings. You must find the examples and set them up in such a way as to be useful to your analysis. Some concepts lend themselves more easily than others to this effort.

When a concept is familiar to you, the model case often comes first in your analysis. Because you are familiar with it, you know about instances of it. Thus, you can compare your experience to the defining attributes you have found for the concept. Do they match? If not, why not? What things are different, missing, or additional in either the defining attributes or the model case that makes them inconsistent? The answers to these questions can help you refine the defining attributes. Wilson (1963) calls this back-and-forth examination of cases and defining attributes an internal dialogue. It is a kind of constant comparative reflection that takes place while you are actively working on the analysis. It helps you come to grips with the internal structure of the concept and hence to clarify its meaning and context.

However, the internal dialogue can take you only so far. At some point, you will want to think aloud about your analysis. It is often helpful and sometimes necessary to seek out a thoughtful colleague or two who can listen with a fresh ear as you talk through your examples. If there are flaws or errors you haven't seen, it is likely that someone else can spot them for you. Moody (1990) suggests that this is a "test of necessity." At times, the best you will be able to do may be a little fuzzy at the edges, especially if the concept has several synonyms or related concepts that overlap the concept of interest. Don't despair. The effort here is to try to keep the case as paradigmatic as possible.

In our coping example, for instance, the model case was stated as follows:

A young woman is walking along a street wearing high heels and a silk dress. On her briefcase is a pouch with an umbrella in it. As she walks, it begins to rain heavily. She takes out her umbrella and raises it. She begins to run, but stumbles. She stops, removes her shoes quickly, and resumes running to the nearest shelter.

This model case includes all three of the critical attributes, covering, protection, and rebalancing. There are several other examples, or cases, of coping that could have been used instead. We tried to use one that was simple and commonplace for demonstration.

Identify Additional Cases

Examining other cases is another part of the internal dialogue. Teasing out the defining attributes that most closely represent the concept of interest may be difficult because they may overlap with some related concepts. Examining cases that are not exactly the same as the concept of interest but are similar to it or contrary to it in some ways will help you make better judgments about which defining attributes or characteristics have the best fit. We will discuss several types of cases that have proved useful in the past. The basic purpose for these cases is to help you decide what counts as a defining attribute for the concept of interest and what doesn't count. The cases we suggest here are borderline, related, invented, and contrary ones. Again, these cases may be real-life examples, may come from the literature, or may be constructed by you as exemplars.

Borderline cases are those examples or instances that contain most of the defining attributes of the concept being examined but not all of them. They may contain most or even all of the defining characteristics but differ substantially in one of them, such as length of time or intensity of occurrence. These cases are inconsistent in some way from the concept under consideration, and, as such, they help us see why the model case is not inconsistent. In this way, we help clarify our thinking about the defining attributes of the concept of interest. Again using the coping example, a borderline case might be that of a college student who was facing a big exam. He had not studied until the evening before the test, then he "crammed all night." He finished the examination, but failed the test because he kept falling asleep during the exam. This meets the attributes of covering and protection. However, the example breaks down when it comes to rebalancing. Even though he took the test and may even have known the answers, his continual falling asleep caused him to fail the test. If he were completely rebalanced, thus staying awake, he would probably have passed the test.

Consider the two concepts of anxiety and fear as borderline cases of each other. These two concepts are very closely related to one another and yet are not exactly the same. What makes them different? According to Bay and Algase (1999, p. 107), anxiety is a "heightened sense of uneasiness to a potential threat, which is inconsistent with the expected event and results when there is a mismatch between the next likely event and the actual event." Fear, on the other hand, is a "sufficiently potent, biologically driven, motivated state wherein a single salient threat guides behavior. Fear is a defensive response to perceived threat or the result of exposure to a single cue presented in an environment reminiscent of the original fear experience" (p. 107). Here is a real-life model case of anxiety: A woman is walking in the jungle. She worries that there might be wild animals somewhere around but she doesn't see any or hear any. The model case for fear might be as follows: A woman is walking in the jungle. She worries that there are wild animals around and she hears a lion roaring somewhere. She turns a corner and there is a lion in her path facing her. The primary difference between the two concepts is that fear has a real source of threat to survival, whereas anxiety has an unspecified source of threat. This example shows how distinguishing between the concept under analysis and a concept that is very much like it is crucial to concept development.

Another example of a borderline case may make things even clearer. Because concepts help us classify things, we gave students an exercise in class. We asked them to categorize the contents of their closet. One student classified her clothes as "things I wear above my waist" and "things I wear below my waist." She was puzzled as to how to classify the belts because they were worn *at* the waist. This is a classic, indeed a concrete, example of a borderline case because the belt may fit into either category and yet belongs to neither. Her dilemma was to decide whether the belt fits one of the categories and why or to decide that she needed a third category, thus a third defining characteristic. Eventually, she decided that the belt fits the category of "below the waist" since she only wore it with her jeans, which were "below the waist."

Related cases are instances of concepts that are related to the concept being studied but that do not contain all the defining attributes. They are similar to the concept being studied; they are in some way connected to the main concept. The related cases help us understand how the concept being studied fits into the network of concepts surrounding it. Concepts that could be developed into related cases in our coping example, for instance, might be stress, conflict, achievement, and adaptation.

Related cases are those cases that demonstrate ideas that are very similar to the main concept but that differ from them when examined closely. It is the close examination that helps you clarify what counts as the defining attributes of the concept under analysis and what doesn't count. Related cases have names of their own and should be identified with their names in the analysis. This will help readers see how you made the decisions that you made. It will also help readers determine what the constellation of surrounding concepts looks like.

Haas's (1999a, 1999b) study of quality of life is an excellent example of using related cases to help clarify the defining attributes of the concept. Haas reviewed the literature and found several concepts that were often used interchangeably with quality of life: functional status, satisfaction with life, well-being, and health status. Her careful analysis of how each concept differed from quality of life substantially aided her in identifying the most robust defining attributes for quality of life. Manojlovich and Sidani (2008) give an excellent example of the difference between the concept of "dose" and the related case of "strength." Their analysis of "nurse dose" is a striking and clear example of how using more than one strategy (analysis and derivation) results in a stronger theoretical concept.

In Prufeta and Spano-Szekely's (2016) analysis of emotional intelligence, they used Goleman's 2004 defining attributes of self-awareness, self-regulation, motivation, empathy, and social skill. The related case they used was personality traits such as introversion or extroversion. These traits are closely related to emotional intelligence but are not the same.

Contrary cases are clear examples of "not the concept." Again, Wilson (1963) suggests that it can be said of the contrary case, "Well, whatever the concept is, that is certainly not an instance of it." In our coping example, for instance, the contrary case might describe a host who is preparing dinner for a group of people. The roast burns on one end. The host becomes upset, throws out the whole roast, and sends the guests home unfed. We can see from this example the host's behavior is not an example of coping. It meets none of the three critical attributes we have said must pertain to an instance of coping—covering, protection, and rebalancing.

Kissinger's (1998) analysis of the concept of overconfidence has a wonderful example of a contrary case. In the contrary case, a nurse finds her patient short of breath, rushes out to another nurse, and says, "What should I do? I've seen her like this before, but I am just so unsure. Please help!" (p. 24). It is clear that whatever overconfidence is, this is not an example of it.

Henson's (1997) study of mutuality is a good example of how negative or contrary cases can help determine the final set of defining attributes. Henson used cases describing paternalism, intrusiveness, and autonomy to help clarify what mutuality was and was not. Henson determined that mutuality actually resided between paternalism and autonomy. It is the middle ground of shared decision making between the obtrusiveness of paternalism on the part of health professionals and the fierce independence of absolute autonomy of the client. Agrimson and Taft's (2008) analysis of spiritual crisis also has a nice example of a contrary case as does Mathes' (2016) analysis of mindfulness. Moody (1990) suggests that a "test of sufficiency" is useful related to contrary cases. If one can construct a contrary case in which all the attributes of the model case are included, then an essential defining attribute has been omitted. This is a good example of why one uses the cases iteratively to refine the analysis.

Contrary cases are often very helpful to the analyst because it is often easier to say what something is *not* than what it is. Discovering what a concept is not helps us see in what ways the concept being analyzed is different from the contrary case. This, in turn, gives us information about what the concept should have as defining attributes if the ones from the contrary case are clearly excluded.

Invented cases are cases that contain ideas outside our own experience. They often read like science fiction. Invented cases are useful when you are examining a very familiar concept such as "man," or "love," or one that is so commonplace as to be taken for granted, such as "air." Often to get a true picture of the critical defining attributes, you must take the concept out of its ordinary context and put it into an invented one. Not all concept analyses need invented cases. If the concept is clear and the model case and other cases help you complete the analysis without difficulty or ambiguity, then you probably don't need to use an invented case. They are fun to do, though!

Here is an example using our coping concept. Suppose that a being from another planet visited Earth. Her physiology is such that when she becomes upset or frightened in our atmosphere, she floats straight up into the air, often bumping her head sharply on ceilings. She begins carrying a cement block in her backpack to keep her on the ground. In addition, she pads her helmet and wears it constantly. This is an example of coping in an invented case.

The last type of case is also not always included in a concept analysis. It is the **illegitimate** case. These cases give an example of the concept term used improperly or out of context. In the case of the coping saw, the use of the term *coping* demonstrates neither the attribute of "covering" nor the one of "protection" and so is illegitimately used. These cases are helpful when you come across one meaning for a term that is completely different from all the others. It may have one or two of the critical attributes, but most of the attributes will not apply at all. In the "attachment" analysis at the end of this chapter, the term *attachment* as used to mean those pieces that fit onto a sewing machine contains only the attribute of "touch" and none of the other four.

Once the cases have been put together, they must be compared to the defining attributes one more time to ensure that all the defining attributes have been discovered. Sometimes, once the model case is in place and compared with the other cases and the proposed defining attributes, some areas of overlap, vagueness, or contradiction will become apparent. It is at this point that further refinement becomes necessary. An analysis is not complete until there are no overlapping attributes and no contradictions between the defining attributes and the model case. Remember, the cases may be developed before or during your analysis. They are put together to help you refine the defining attributes as you work.

Identify Antecedents and Consequences

Identifying antecedents and consequences are the next steps in a concept analysis. Although these two steps are often ignored or dealt with lightly, they may shed considerable light on the social contexts in which the concept is generally used. They are also helpful in further refining the defining attributes. A defining attribute cannot be either an antecedent or a consequence. **Antecedents** are those events or incidents that must occur or be in place prior to the occurrence of the concept. Thus, an antecedent cannot also be a defining attribute for the same concept. For example, Ward (1986) gives a clear example of antecedents of role strain, identifying as the antecedents role conflict, role accumulation, rigidity of time and place, which role demands must be met, and the amount of activity prescribed by some roles. Clearly these antecedents are not the same as role strain itself but must be present for role strain to happen. Another good example is Cookman's (2005) analysis of attachment in older adulthood (see Box 10–1).

Consequences, on the other hand, are those events or incidents that occur as a result of the occurrence of the concept—in other words, the outcomes of the

BOX 10–1   Cookman's Analysis of Attachment

Cookman's analysis of attachment in older adulthood identifies fear-provoking situations, challenging situations, and conflictual interactions as antecedents. Compare these to the antecedents we propose for maternal attachment in the "Practice Exercise" section at the end of this chapter. How are they different? How are they similar? Why?

concept. For example, Meraviglia (1999) examined the concept of spirituality and found 12 outcomes resulting from the concept of spirituality. The outcomes were, for example, meaning in life, hope, self-transcendence, trust, creativity, religiousness, and health. Cookman (2005), in the analysis above, found environmental interaction and resource mobilization to be consequences of attachment in older adulthood. Compare his consequences to the ones related to mother–infant attachment found at the end of this chapter.

In our coping example, one antecedent was an intensely stressful stimulus (the burned roast); the consequence was the regaining of balance. Another clear example presents itself: If we examine the concept of "pregnancy," one of the antecedents is clearly ovulation, whereas a consequence is some kind of delivery experience whether or not the pregnancy goes to term or produces a viable baby.

In a classic book, Zetterberg (1965) has spoken of constructing theoretical models of determinants and results around a focal variable or construct. (See Chapter 9 for a more thorough discussion of his ideas.) His notion of determinants and results is very close to the notion of antecedents and consequences in concept analysis. Thus, determining antecedents and consequences can be extremely useful theoretically. Antecedents are particularly useful in helping the theorist identify underlying assumptions about the concept being studied. In our attachment example at the end of this chapter, you will see that one of the antecedents is the ability to distinguish between internal and external stimuli. This implies that an assumption of living, sentient beings has been made. Consequences are useful in determining often-neglected ideas, variables, or relationships that may yield fruitful new research directions.

Define Empirical Referents

Determining the empirical referents for the defining attributes is the final step in a concept analysis. When a concept analysis is nearing completion, the question arises, "If we are to measure this concept or determine its existence in the real world, how do we do so?" **Empirical referents** are classes or categories of actual phenomena that by their existence or presence demonstrate the occurrence of the concept itself. As an example, *kissing* might be used as an empirical referent for the concept of "affection." In our coping example, an empirical referent might be "ability to successfully solve a problem in a stressful situation." In many cases, the defining attributes and the empirical referents will be identical. However, there are times when the concept being analyzed is highly abstract and so are its defining attributes. When that happens, empirical referents are necessary. Empirical referents are not tools to measure the concept. They

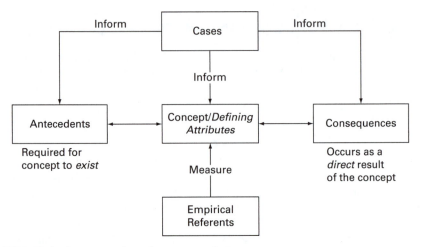

FIGURE 10–1   Representation of concept analysis process.

are the means by which you can recognize or measure the defining characteristics or attributes. Thus, the empirical referents relate directly to the defining attributes, not the entire concept itself.

Empirical referents, once identified, are extremely useful in instrument development because they are clearly linked to the theoretical base of the concept, thus contributing to both the content and construct validity of any new instrument. They are also very useful in practice because they provide the clinician with clear, observable phenomena by which to determine the existence of the concept in particular clients. Corbett and Quinn Griffin's (2016) analysis of triage nurse expertise has a nice example of empirical referents. The Boyd (1985), Bu and Jezewski (2006), Manojlovich and Sidani (2008), Meize-Grochowski (1984), Rew (1986), and Ward (1986) articles listed in the "References" section of this chapter also have good examples of empirical referents.

Figure 10–1 is a graphic representation of the concept analysis process. It depicts the relationships among the various steps.

ADVANTAGES AND LIMITATIONS

Concept analysis clarifies the symbols (words or terms) used in communication. The main advantage of concept analysis is that it renders very precise theoretical as well as operational definitions based on the empirical referents for use in theory and research. Another advantage is that concept analysis can help clarify those terms in nursing that have become catchphrases and hence have lost their meanings. A third advantage is its utility for tool development and nursing language development. Additionally, the rigorousness of this intellectual exercise is extremely good practice in thinking.

There are few firm rules for concept analysis. Table 10–1 provides several examples of concept analyses using the method delineated here. There are other methods that are similar but have slightly different foci or steps. The analyst must choose

TABLE 10–1 Examples of Concept Analyses Using Methods by Walker and Avant

Concept(s)	Author(s)	Journal/Book	Year
Abuse of aging caregivers	Ayres and Woodtli	*J Adv Nurs*	2001
Autonomy	Keenan	*J Adv Nurs*	1999
Attachment in older adulthood	Cookman	*J Adv Nurs*	2005
Bioterrorism preparedness	Rebmann	*J Adv Nurs*	2006
Care partner	Bennett et al.	*Nurs Outlook*	2017
Caregiver abuse	Ayres and Woodtli	*J Adv Nurs*	2001
Chronic fatigue	Trendall	*J Adv Nurs*	2000
Contamination	Green and Polk	*Int J Nurs Terminol Classif*	2009
Decisional conflict	Ervin and Pierangeli	*Worldviews Evid Based Nurs*	2005
Developmental care in the NICU	Aita and Snider	*J Adv Nurs*	2003
Emotional intelligence	Prufeta and Spano-Szekely	In *Nursing Concept Analysis: Application to Research and Practice*	2016
Empowerment	Ellis-Stoll and Popkess-Vawter	*Adv Nurs Sci*	1998
Effective breastfeeding	Mulder	*JOGNN*	2006
Fear and anxiety	Bay and Algase	*Nurs Diagn*	1999
Fear	Whitley	*Nurs Diagn*	1992
Healing	Firth et al.	*Glob Adv Health Med*	2015
Health literacy	Speros	*J Adv Nurs*	2005
Health-related quality of life in young people	Taylor, Gibson, and Franck	*J Clin Nurs*	2008
Hopelessness	Dunn	*J Nurs Scholarsh*	2005
Hot flash experience in men	Engstrom	*Oncol Nurs Forum*	2005
Infant feeding responsiveness	Mentro, Steward, and Garvin	*J Adv Nurs*	2002
Interactive teaching	Ridley	*J Nurs Educ*	2007
Intuition	Rew	*Adv Nurs Sci*	1986
Impaired memory and chronic confusion	Alfradique de Souza, Santana, and Cassiano	*J Nurs UFPE Online*	2015
Maternal attachment	Avant	*Adv Nurs Sci*	1979

TABLE 10–1 Continued

Concept(s)	Author(s)	Journal/Book	Year
Mother–daughter identification	Boyd	*Adv Nurs Sci*	1985
Mutuality	Henson	*Image*	1997
Nurse dose	Manojlovich and Sidoni	*Res Nurs Health*	2008
Nursing productivity	Holcomb, Hoffart, and Fox	*J Adv Nurs*	2002
Overconfidence	Kissinger	*Nurs Forum*	1998
Pain management	Davis	*Adv Nurs Sci*	1992
Patient advocacy	Bu and Jezewski	*J Adv Nurs*	2006
Parental concern	Mulcahy	In *Nursing Concept Analysis: Application to Research and Practice*	2016
Peer support	Dennis	*Int J Nurs Stud*	2003
Preceptorship	Billay and Yonge	*Nurs Educ Today*	2004
Presence	Smith	*Sch Inq Nurs Pract*	2001
Postoperative recovery	Allvin, Berg, Idvall, and Nilsson	*J Adv Nurs*	2007
Postpartum weight self-management	Ohlendorf	*Res Theory Nurs Pract*	2013
Psychological acculturation	Al-Omari and Pallikkathayil	*J Transcult Nurs*	2008
Psychological distress	Ridner	*J Adv Nurs*	2004
Quality of life	Haas	*West J Nurs Res*	1999a
Resilience	Gillespie, Chaboyer, and Wallis	*Contemp Nurs*	2007
Role strain	Ward	*Adv Nurs Sci*	1986
Self-mutilation	Hicks and Hinck	*J Adv Nurs*	2008
Spirituality	Meraviglia	*J Holist Nurs*	1999
Spiritual crisis	Agrimson and Taft	*J Adv Nurs*	2008
Symptom management	Fu, LeMone, and McDaniel	*Oncol Nurs Forum*	2004
Teamwork	Xyrichis and Ream	*J Adv Nurs*	2008
Triage nurse expertise	Corbett and Quinn-Griffin	In *Nursing Concept Analysis: Application to Research and Practice*	2016
Trust	Meize- Grochowski	*J Adv Nurs*	1984

his or her own preferred method. In the long run, whatever method or set of rules one uses, the goal is to obtain the clearest and cleanest definition possible. In every case, however, the theorist must work painstakingly and is likely to encounter pitfalls that will hinder the analysis. These pitfalls, which tend to obscure the meanings you want to convey (Wilson, 1963), include the following:

1. *The tendency to moralize when the concept being analyzed has some value implications.* Many concepts hold some implicit, if not explicit, value to us. As we begin a concept analysis, it is important to recognize that just choosing the concept demonstrates a bias on our part. We must be doubly careful, then, to treat the concept objectively as subject matter rather than subjectively as a persuasive weapon.

2. *The feeling of being absolutely in over your head.* Because there are no firm rules in concept analysis, this may make you very anxious. There is no way we can say to you, "First do this, then do that, and when you have done so, all will be wonderful." We have attempted to give you guidelines, but the actual intellectual work must be yours. Once you have begun, the anxiety subsides and the fun begins.

3. *The feeling that concept analysis is too easy.* Some people initially grow impatient with the process and tend to throw up their hands with the comment, "Well, everybody knows that term means so-and-so. Why do we need to keep on with this?" The point is that not everybody knows what it means. Concept analysis is not easy; it is a vigorous intellectual exercise, but it is fruitful and useful and even enjoyable.

4. *The compulsion to analyze everything, or the "how-do-you-turn-it-off syndrome,"* as one of our students calls it. This occurs fairly often in students. The process of analysis somehow gets their creative juices flowing, and they get very excited. The result is that often they don't want to stop. There are some concepts more worthy of analysis than others, but all analyses must finally come to an end. In addition, analysis is only one strategy in theory development. Some energy should be saved for the rest!

5. *The need to protect oneself from others' criticism or debate* during the process of analysis. Good concept analysis cannot occur in a vacuum. Only the insights and criticisms of others can fully expand the analyst's ideas. The willingness to look foolish is one of the criteria for creativity. If you restrain yourself in discussions or fail to seek criticism because you may look silly or dumb, you are cutting yourself off from successful concept development. In dealing with concept analysis, it is vital to say something and then trust that it will lead somewhere.

6. *The feeling that verbal facility equals thinking.* There is sometimes a tendency to engage in superficial fluency instead of productive dialogue. Most of us know people who can talk or write easily but have little of real substance to say. There are times in concept analysis when the analyst must struggle with difficult and substantive problems. It is often tempting to go for the hasty solution or to beg the question by substituting verbiage for substance. But the results of hasty analysis are meager and unproductive. It is far more helpful to hang in there with the difficulties until you solve them in a way that provides the best results, not the easiest.

7. *The attempt to add superfluous defining attributes.* Doing so can confound the results of the analysis because many of the added attributes are not critical to the concept and may even overlap the antecedents and consequences. A rule of thumb is to quit when you're done with the original analysis. In this case, more is not always better.

Although any or all of these pitfalls may potentially hinder analysis, a sense of proportion, a little risk taking, a sense of humor, and a low anxiety level are all helpful in the process of analysis. This is a new way of thinking for many people and as such requires a little getting used to in the beginning. It is a very important aspect to theory construction. Because concepts are the bricks of theory development, it is critical that they be structurally sound. If a theory contains careful concept analyses, all who read the theory or use it in practice will be able to clearly understand what is meant by the concepts within it and their relationships to each other.

Even beautifully analyzed concepts can contribute merely the basics of theory. Only when concepts are studied for relationships among them and relational statements are constructed can real forward progress be made in theory construction.

UTILIZING THE RESULTS OF CONCEPT ANALYSIS

Several uses of the results of concept analysis have been discussed. These are refining ambiguous terms in theory, education, research, and practice; providing operational definitions with a clear theoretical base; providing an understanding of the underlying attributes of a concept; facilitating instrument development in research; and providing assistance in the development of nursing language.

Once a concept has been analyzed, what is the next step for the theorist? This depends in part on the aims of the analysis. If one of the aims, for instance, is to develop an instrument, then the next step would be to construct items that would reflect the defining attributes of the concept, based on the empirical referents. If the aim is to propose a nursing diagnosis, intervention, or outcome name, then the next step would be to clinically validate the defining attributes (Alfradique de Souza, 2016). Using the empirical referents for the defining attributes and assessing clients for the presence or absence of the attributes would help substantiate the potential diagnosis, intervention activities, or outcome criteria. If the aim is to construct an operational definition, the next step would be to attempt to find a research instrument that accurately reflects the defining attributes of the concept.

Concept analysis alone will not provide useful theories for nursing education, research, or practice. Only when the concepts are linked to each other will useful theories result (see Chapter 3). In the meantime, scientists, educators, and clinicians should continue to examine concepts critically in an effort to refine nursing knowledge and to discover what those linkages are.

RESPONSE TO CRITICISM OF THIS METHOD

This and other methods of concept analysis have recently come under criticism for not delineating the philosophical or ontological underpinnings of the various methods proposed (Beckwith, Dickinson, & Kendall, 2008; Bergdahl & Bertero, 2016; Draper, 2014; Duncan, Cloutier, & Bailey, 2007; Hupcey, Morse, Lenz, & Tasón, 1996; Risjord, 2008; Weaver & Mitcham, 2008). The methods are also criticized as being too realistic or too simplistic or somehow do not allow the analyst to ground the concept within its context or within a particular theory.

Some of the criticism concerns the published analyses in the literature. In fact, we too have commented about this issue (Walker & Avant, 2005). Not all concept analyses are suitable for publishing. Conducting a concept analysis may be a worthy student learning experience; deciding to publish a concept analysis requires that the analytic paper advance understanding of the concept to enhance its application in practice and research. Although manuscripts reporting concept analysis may be well written, reviewers and editors need to ensure that authors make the relevant connections to future research and practice. If authors are unable to do so in a compelling way, then the contribution of the analysis is likely to be insufficient to merit publication. Thus, we argue for strengthening the process for reviewing concept analysis manuscripts.

One of the critics (Draper, 2014) also commented that concept analysis does not contribute to the body of knowledge. On this issue, we beg to differ. Many concept analyses have been the springboard for research programs or are conducted within the research program to clarify ambiguous or unclear issues within the program. Although it is not within the scope of this chapter to provide a comprehensive list of these contributions, in the following paragraphs we will document three examples of concept analyses that are contributing to nursing knowledge.

One good example is the work of Ohlendorf (2012). She began by investigating the information needs related to postpartum weight self-management and stages of change in the trajectory of postpartum weight self-management (2012). Subsequently, she conducted a concept analysis of postpartum weight self-management (2013) to clarify the meaning. Subsequently, she used the analysis for further research into predictors of engagement in postpartum weight management (Ohlendorf, Weiss, & Oswald, 2015) in which she proposed a mid-range theory for use in practice.

A second example is similar. The Samueli Institute, a research nonprofit organization dedicated to exploring the science of healing, well-being, and resilience, developed a conceptual framework on optimal healing environments (Sakallaris, MacAllister, Voss, Smith, & Jonas, 2015) to guide its work. However, the staff decided they needed to clearly understand and agree about the meanings of the concepts in the framework. Firth et al. (2015) chose healing as the first concept to be analyzed. Subsequently, they analyzed all of the concepts in the framework and developed definitions for each one. Sakallaris et al. (2015) report that the framework has been used to evaluate healing environments and to change philosophies and practices at several hospitals.

The third example comes from the nursing diagnosis literature. The NANDA International organization has been using concept analysis as one criterion for the submission of new diagnoses for many years. Every new diagnosis is evaluated based on the defining attributes of the concept analysis. Great care is taken to clarify the diagnoses for use in practice. One such program of research is that of Alfradique de Souza et al. (2015). They conducted a small study to differentiate the two similar concepts of impaired memory and chronic confusion but were unable to fully distinguish them. During her doctoral work, Alfradique de Souza repeated the study with a large sample and was able to differentiate the two concepts (2016).

Other criticism of the method we propose here has implied that the strategy of concept analysis is positivistic, reductionistic, and rigid and requires a correspondence theory of truth (Gift, 1995; Hupcey, Morse, Lenz, & Tasón, 1996; Penrod & Hupcey, 2005; Rodgers, 1989). It has never been our intent to subscribe to these tenets. Indeed, it is not the intent of most current philosophers of science to subscribe to such outmoded views (Schumacher & Gortner, 1992). We have never suggested that our method or Wilson's is the only method of concept analysis. However, concept analysis, using whatever technique, is a reasonable and logical method that has served the development of science over time.

Finally, some of the above-mentioned critiques have actually misinterpreted some portions of the method we and others proposed or make assumptions about the purposes of the method that are not entirely justified. Some of the criticisms are put forward as a means for justifying a different concept analysis method (All & Huycke, 2007). All of the criticisms contain some merit. These authors make good points, and it is a pleasure to see the discussions arising about these issues. They are certainly worthy endeavors and are to be encouraged for the betterment of the discipline and our science.

We must point out, however, that this level of sophisticated discourse was never the intent or within the scope of this book, especially in its first edition in 1983. The intent of this book has always been for the introduction of theoretical methods to the novice who is often filled with anxiety about the whole idea of actually developing theory. As we have said from the beginning, this is intended to be a kind of primer in theory development and was never intended to be used alone or in the absence of other material related to philosophy of science and knowledge development. We continue to believe that this simplified method, if taught and used correctly, is sufficient to introduce students to thinking carefully about language and its uses and to understanding how carefully defined concepts contribute to the building of theory. Helping students achieve a more sophisticated philosophical understanding is the responsibility of the professor and the students in dialogue with one another and the literature.

Summary

The process of concept analysis has been the focus of this chapter. This strategy employs the processes of analysis to extract the defining attributes of a concept. There are no rules for accomplishing the analysis. Selection of the concept and the theorist's familiarity with the literature will have some impact on where the theorist begins. The steps in concept analysis include selecting the concept, determining the aims of analysis, identifying all uses of the concept, determining the defining attributes of the concept, identifying model cases, examining additional cases, identifying antecedents and consequences, and determining empirical referents.

Concept analysis increases the richness of our vocabulary and provides precise and rigorously constructed theoretical and operational definitions for use in theory and research. However, concept analysis is limited by the level of theory that can be attained using only concepts. In the next chapters, we will describe some strategies for going beyond concepts to develop statements about how concepts are related to each other.

Nursing science will be judged by whether it solves "significant disciplinary problems" (DeGroot, 1988), "offers defensible interpretations of multiple realities of interest to nurses" (Coward, 1990), or provides practitioners with an adequate and holistic knowledge base from which to practice (Avant, 1991). It is our belief that concept analysis, using the method proposed here, will be a useful tool in fulfilling these criteria. We leave it up to the reader to make the final judgment as to the usefulness and validity of the method.

An Additional Example and Practice Exercise

To aid you with the subsequent practice exercise, we present below a brief summary of a concept analysis of "attachment." This is by no means a complete, formal analysis. It is presented merely to show how one looks as it is developed.

Concept: Attachment.
Aim of Analysis: Develop operational definition of theoretical concept.
Defining Attributes: In all cases of attachment, each of the following attributes is present.

1. Visual contact must have been made between the person and the object of attachment.
2. The person must have touched the object of attachment at some time during the process of attachment.
3. There must be some positive affect associated with the object of attachment.
   Cases of animate attachment have the following attributes in addition to the ones above:
4. There must be reciprocal interaction between the two parties in attachment.
5. Vocalization by at least one of the two parties is supportive of attachment process.

MODEL CASES

Person-to-Object Attachment

A woman explains to her friend that she simply can't throw out her old bathrobe because she has had it since she married and is just too "attached to it."

Person-to-Person Attachment

An 8-month-old boy is playing in the room where his mother is working on her laptop. As he plays, he occasionally looks around at her, or comes over and touches her. When she leaves the room, he cries and begins to search for her. When she returns, he climbs into her lap. She hugs him close and talks to him until he is ready to continue playing.

Contrary Case: Nonattachment

A 22-year-old woman delivers a baby under general anesthesia and cesarean section as a result of abruptio placenta. The infant is about 26 weeks' gestation and weighs 2 pounds. He is immediately transferred to the regional perinatal center 200 miles away. When the mother wakes from anesthesia, she is told she has a 2-pound baby boy and also about his transfer. She is told the baby will stay in the hospital until he weighs about 5 pounds. Due to postpartum complications, the mother is not released from the hospital for 3 weeks. Even though her husband brings reports of the baby, she says, "Do I really have a baby?"

Borderline Case: At-Risk Attachment

Jeffrey is being seen at the health clinic for possible child abuse. Jeffrey is blind due to retrolental fibroplasia. He also has spastic cerebral palsy. Jeffrey's mother says she gets angry because he won't look at her or cuddle when she picks him up. When he cries too long, she hits him. This is borderline attachment because two defining characteristics, touch and vocalization, are met. Visual contact, positive affect, and reciprocal interaction are absent or severely diminished. Attachment may still occur, but it will be difficult.

Related Cases

Love	Deprivation
Separation	Dependency
Detachment	Symbiosis

Illegitimate Case

A salesperson demonstrating a new sewing machine makes a point of explaining "the most useful attachment—the buttonholer."

Antecedents

1. Ability to distinguish between internal and external stimuli.
2. Ability to receive and respond to cues of the persons involved in attachment process.

Consequences

1. Proximity-maintaining behavior
2. Separation anxiety

Empirical Referents—Examples

1. Eye-to-eye contact
2. Patting, stroking, holding hands, and so on
3. Speaking positively about the person
4. Speaking, singing, and reading to the person

Practice Exercise

Analyze the concept of "play" using the foregoing analysis as a guide. Some of your defining attributes probably were similar to the ones below.

1. Movement or activity
2. One animate entity
3. Voluntariness or choice
4. Expectation of diversion or pleasure
5. Novelty or unpredictability
6. Creativity

Did you remember to include the ideas "play on words," "play in the steering wheel," "play" as in a drama, and so forth?

Using the defining attributes above, develop a model case that includes all of them.

What are some related concepts? How about "games," "work," "exercise," "performance," "imitate," and "sport"?

Try developing a contrary case using "work" as "not play." Use the concept "exercise" as a borderline case.

Complete the analysis using the outline given.

References

Agrimson LB, Taft LB. Spiritual crisis: A concept analysis. *J Adv Nurs.* 2008;65(2):456–461.

Aita M, Snider L. The art of developmental care in the NICU: A concept analysis. *J Adv Nurs.* 2003;41(3):223–232.

Alfradique de Souza P. Concept clarification of nursing diagnoses of impaired memory and chronic confusion: A preliminary study. Paper presented at the NNN International Conference on Nursing Knowledge, NNN Network/Portugal, Porto, Portugal, 2016.

Alfradique de Souza P, Santana RF, Cassiano KM. Differential validation of nursing diagnoses of impaired memory and chronic confusion. *J Nurs UFPE Online.* 2015;9(7):9078–9085.

All AC, Huycke LI. Serial concept maps: Tools for concept analysis. *J Nurs Educ.* 2007;46(5):217–224.

Allvin R, Berg K, Idvall E, Nilsson U. Postoperative recovery: A concept analysis. *J Adv Nurs.* 2007;57(5):552–558.

Al-Omari H, Pallikkathayil L. Psychological acculturation: A concept analysis with implications for nursing practice. *J Transcult Nurs.* 2008;19(2):126–133.

Avant K. Nursing diagnosis: Maternal attachment. *Adv Nurs Sci.* 1979;2(1):45–56.

Avant KC. The theory-research dialectic: A different approach. *Nurs Sci Q.* 1991;4(1):2.

Ayres MM, Woodtli A. Concept analysis: Abuse of ageing caregivers by elderly care recipients. *J Adv Nurs.* 2001;35(3):326–334.

Bay EJ, Algase DL. Fear and anxiety: A simultaneous concept analysis. *Nurs Diagn.* 1999;10(3):103–111.

Beckwith S, Dickinson A, Kendall S. The "con" of concept analysis. A discussion paper which explores and critiques the ontological focus, reliability and antecedents of concept analysis frameworks. *Int J Nurs Stud.* 2008;45:1831–1841.

Bennett PN, Wang W, Moore M, Nagle C. Care partner: A concept analysis. *Nurs Outlook.* 2017;65(2):184–194.

Bergdahl E, Bertero CM. Concept analysis and the building blocks of theory: Misconceptions regarding theory development. *J Adv Nurs.* 2016;130(2):1–9.

Billay DB, Yonge O. Contributing to the development of preceptorship. *Nurs Educ Today.* 2004;24:566–574.

Boyd C. Toward an understanding of mother–daughter identification using concept analysis. *Adv Nurs Sci.* 1985;7(3):78–86.

Bu X, Jezewski MA. Developing a mid-range theory of patient advocacy through concept analysis. *J Adv Nurs.* 2006;57(1):101–110.

Carlson-Catalano J, Lunney M, Paradiso C, Bruno J, Luise BK, Martin T, et al. Clinical validation of ineffective breathing pattern, ineffective airway clearance, and impaired gas exchange. *Image.* 1998;30(3):243–248.

Chase S. Response to "The concept of nursing presence: State of the science." *Sch Inq Nurs Pract.* 2001;15(4):323–325.

Cookman C. Attachment in older adulthood: Concept clarification. *J Adv Nurs.* 2005;50(5):528–535.

Corbett A, Quinn Griffin MT. Triage nurse expertise. In: Fitzpatrick J, McCarth G, eds. *Nursing Concept Analysis: Application to Research and Practice.* New York, NY: Springer Publishing Co.; 2016, pp. 249–255.

Coward DD. Critical multiplism: A research strategy for nursing science. *Image.* 1990;22 (3):163–166.

Davis G. The meaning of pain management: A concept analysis. *Adv Nurs Sci.* 1992;15 (1):77–86.

DeGroot HA. Scientific inquiry in nursing: A model for a new age. *Adv Nurs Sci.* 1988;10 (3):1–21.

Dennis CL. Peer support within a health care context: A concept analysis. *Int J Nurs Stud.* 2003;40:321–332.

Draper P. A critique of concept analysis. *J Adv Nurs.* 2014;70(6):1207–1208.

Duncan C, Cloutier JD, Bailey PH. Concept analysis: The importance of differentiating the ontological focus. *J Adv Nurs.* 2007;58(3):293–300.

Dunn SL. Hopelessness as a response to physical illness. *J Nurs Scholarsh.* 2005;37 (2):148–154.

Ellis-Stoll CC, Popkess-Vawter S. A concept analysis on the process of empowerment. *Adv Nurs Sci.* 1998;21(2):62–68.

Engstrom C. Hot flash experience in men with prostate cancer: A concept analysis. *Oncol Nurs Forum.* 2005;32(5):1043–1048.

Ervin NE, Pierangeli LT. The concept of decisional control: Building the base for evidence-based nursing practice. *Worldviews Evid Based Nurs.* 2005;2(1):16–24.

Firth K, Smith K, Sakallaris B, Bellanti DM, Crawford C, Avant K. Healing: A concept analysis. *Glob Adv Health Med.* 2015;4(6):44–50.

Fu MR, LeMone P, McDaniel RW. An integrated approach to an analysis of symptom management in patients with cancer. *Oncol Nurs Forum.* 2004;31(1):65–70.

Gamel C, Grypdonck M, Hengeveld M, Davis B. A method to develop a nursing intervention: The contribution of qualitative studies to the process. *J Adv Nurs.* 2001;33 (6):806–819.

Gift AG, ed. Concept development in nursing. *Sch Inq Nurs Pract.* 1995;10(3, special issue).

Gillespie BM, Chaboyer W, Wallis M. Development of a theoretically derived model of resilience through concept analysis. *Contemp Nurse.* 2007;25:124–133.

Goleman D. What makes a leader? *Harv Bus Rev.* 2004;82(1):82–91.

Gordon M. *Nursing Diagnosis: Process and Application.* New York, NY: McGraw-Hill; 1982.

Green PM, Polk LV. Contamination: Concept analysis and nursing implications. *Int J Nurs Terminol Classif.* 2009;20(4):189–197.

Haas BK. A multidisciplinary concept analysis of quality of life. *West J Nurs Res.* 1999a;21 (6):728–742.

Haas BK. Classification and integration of similar quality of life concepts. *J Nurs Scholarsh.* 1999b;31(3):215–220.

Henson RH. Analysis of the concept of mutuality. *Image.* 1997;29(1):77–81.

Hicks MH, Hinck SM. Concept analysis of self-mutilation. *J Adv Nurs.* 2008;64(4):408–413.

Holcomb BR, Hoffart N, Fox MH. Defining and measuring nursing productivity: A concept analysis and pilot study. *J Adv Nurs.* 2002;38(4):378–386.

Hupcey JE, Morse JM, Lenz ER, Tasón M. Wilsonian methods of concept analysis: A critique. *Sch Inq Nurs Pract.* 1996;10(3):185–210.

Keenan J. A concept analysis of autonomy. *J Adv Nurs.* 1999;29(3):556–562.

Kissinger JA. Overconfidence: A concept analysis. *Nurs Forum.* 1998;33(2):18–26.

Manojlovich M, Sidani S. Nurse dose: What's in a concept? *Res Nurs Health.* 2008;31:310–319.

Mathes J. Mindfulness. In: Fitzpatrick J, McCarth G, eds. *Nursing Concept Analysis: Application to Research and Practice.* New York, NY: Springer Publishing Co.; 2016, pp. 209–214.

Meize-Grochowski R. An analysis of the concept of trust. *J Adv Nurs.* 1984;9:563–572.

Mentro AM, Steward DK, Garvin BJ. Infant feeding responsiveness: A conceptual analysis. *J Adv Nurs.* 2002;37(2):208–216.

Meraviglia MG. Critical analysis of spirituality and its empirical indicators: Prayer and meaning in life. *J Holist Nurs.* 1999;17(1):18–33.

Moody LE. *Advancing Nursing Science Through Research.* London, UK: Sage Publications; 1990.

Mulcahy H. Parental concern. In: Fitzpatrick J, McCarth G, eds. *Nursing Concept Analysis: Application to Research and Practice.* New York, NY: Springer Publishing Co.; 2016, pp. 83–91.

Mulder PJ. A concept analysis of effective breastfeeding. *JOGNN.* 2006;35(3):332–339.

Nunnally J. *Psychometric Theory.* New York, NY: McGraw-Hill; 1978.

Ohlendorf J. Postpartum weight self-management: A concept analysis. *Res Theory Nurs Pract.* 2013;27(1):35–52.

Ohlendorf JM. Stages of change in the trajectory of postpartum weight self-management. *J Obstet Gynecol Neonatal Nurs.* 2012;41(1):57–70.

Ohlendorf JM, Weiss ME, Oswald D. Predictors of engagement in postpartum weight self-management behaviours in the first 12 weeks after birth. *J Adv Nurs.* 2015;71(8):1833–1846.

Ohlendorf JM, Weiss ME, Ryan P. Weight-management information needs of postpartum women. *MCN Am J Matern Child Nurs.* 2012;37(1):56–63.

Penrod J, Hupcey JE. Enhancing methodological clarity: Principle-based concept analysis. *J Adv Nurs.* 2005;50(4):403–409.

Prufeta P, Spano-Szekely L. Emotional intelligence. In: Fitzpatrick J, McCarth G, eds. *Nursing Concept Analysis: Application to Research and Practice.* New York, NY: Springer Publishing Co.; 2016, pp. 187–194.

Rebmann T. Defining bioterrorism preparedness for nurses: Concept analysis. *J Adv Nurs.* 2006;54(5):623–632.

Rew L. Intuition: Concept analysis of a group phenomenon. *Adv Nurs Sci.* 1986;8(2):21–28.

Reynolds PD. *A Primer in Theory Construction.* Indianapolis, IN: Bobbs-Merrill; 1971.

Ridley RT. Interactive teaching: A concept analysis. *J Nurs Educ.* 2007;46(5):203–209.

Ridner SH. Psychological distress: Concept analysis. *J Adv Nurs.* 2004;45(5):536–545.

Risjord M. Rethinking concept analysis. *J Adv Nurs.* 2008;65(3):684–691.

Rodgers BL. Concepts, analysis and the development of nursing knowledge: The evolutionary cycle. *J Adv Nurs.* 1989;14:330–335.

Sakallaris B, MacAllister L, Voss M, Smith K, Jonas W. Optimal health environments. *Glob Adv Health Med.* 2015;4(3):40–45.

Schumacher KL, Gortner SR. (Mis)conceptions and reconceptions about traditional science. *Adv Nurs Sci.* 1992;14(4):1–11.

Smith TD. The concept of nursing presence: State of the science. *Sch Inq Nurs Pract.* 2001;15(4):299–322.

Speros C. Health literacy: Concept analysis. *J Adv Nurs.* 2005;50(6):633–640.

Taylor RM, Gibson F, Franck LS. A concept analysis of health-related quality of life in young people with chronic illness. *J Clin Nurs.* 2008;17:1823–1833.

Trendall J. Concept analysis: Chronic fatigue. *J Adv Nurs.* 2000;32(5):1126–1131.

Walker L, Avant K. Letters to the editor. Discourse on concept analysis. *J Holist Nurs.* 2005;23(1):11–12.

Ward C. The meaning of role strain. *Adv Nurs Sci.* 1986;8(2):39–49.

Weaver K, Mitcham C. Nursing concept analysis in North America: State of the art. *Nurs Philos.* 2008;9:180–194.

Whitley GG. Concept analysis of fear. *Nurs Diagn.* 1992;3(4):155–161.

Whitley GG. Concept analysis as foundational to nursing diagnosis research. *Nurs Diagn.* 1995;6(2):91–92.

Wilson J. *Thinking with Concepts.* New York, NY: Cambridge University Press; 1963.

Xyrichis A, Ream E. Teamwork: A concept analysis. *J Adv Nurs.* 2008;61(2):232–241.

Zetterberg HL. *On Theory and Verification in Sociology.* Totowa, NJ: Bedminster Press; 1965.

Additional Readings

Arakelian M. An assessment and nursing application of the concept of locus of control. *Adv Nurs Sci.* 1980;3(1):25–42.

Brown AJ. A concept analysis of respect: Applying the hybrid model in cross-cultural settings. *West J Nurs Res.* 1997;19(6):762–780.

Carnevali D. Conceptualizing, a nursing skill. In: Mitchell PH, ed. *Concepts Basic to Nursing.* 2nd ed. New York, NY: McGraw-Hill; 1977.

Carper B. Fundamental patterns of knowing in nursing. *Adv Nurs Sci.* 1978;1(1):13–23.

Chinn PL, Jacobs K. A model for theory development in nursing. *Adv Nurs Sci.* 1978;1(1):1–12.

Deatrick JA, Knafl KA, Murphy-Moore C. Clarifying the concept of normalization. *Image.* 1999;31(3):209–214.

Doona ME, Haggerty LA, Chase SK. Nursing presence: An existential exploration of the concept. *Sch Inq Nurs Pract.* 1997;11(1):3–20.

Englemann S. *Conceptual Learning.* San Rafael, CA: Dimensions; 1969.

Goulet C, Bell L, Tribble DS, Paul D, Lang A. A concept analysis of parent–infant attachment. *J Adv Nurs.* 1998;28(5):1071–1081.

Hempel CG. *Fundamentals of Concept Formation in Empirical Science.* Chicago, IL: University of Chicago Press; 1952.

Hupcey JE, Penrod J, Morse JM, Mitcham C. An exploration and advancement of the concept of trust. *J Adv Nurs.* 2001;36(2):282–293.

Hutchfield K. Family-centred care: A concept analysis. *J Adv Nurs.* 1999;29(5):1178–1187.

Jacelon CS, Connelly TW, Brown R, Proulx K, Vo T. A concept analysis of dignity for older adults. *J Adv Nurs.* 2004;48(1):76–83.

Jenner CA. The art of nursing: A concept analysis. *Nurs Forum.* 1997;32(4):5–11.

Klausmeier HJ, Ripple RE. *Learning and Human Abilities.* New York, NY: Harper & Row; 1971.

Kunyk D, Olson JK. Clarification of conceptualizations of empathy. *J Adv Nurs.* 2001; 35(3):317–325.

Lyth GM. Clinical supervision: A concept analysis. *J Adv Nurs.* 2000;31(3):722–729.

Maijala H, Munnukka T, Nikkonen M. Feeling of "lacking" as the core of envy: A conceptual analysis of envy. *J Adv Nurs.* 2000;31(6):1342–1350.

Marck P. Therapeutic reciprocity: A caring phenomenon. *Adv Nurs Sci.* 1990;13(1):49–59.

Matthews C, Gaul A. Nursing diagnosis from the perspective of concept attainment and critical thinking. *Adv Nurs Sci.* 1979;2(1):17–26.

Meeberg GA. Quality of life: A concept analysis. *J Adv Nurs.* 1993;18:32–38.

Montes-Sandoval L. An analysis of the concept of pain. *J Adv Nurs.* 1999;29(4):935–941.

Norris CM. Restlessness: A nursing phenomenon in search of meaning. *Nurs Outlook.* 1975; 23:103–107.

Paley J. Positivism and qualitative nursing research. *Sch Inq Nurs Pract.* 2001;15(4):371–387.

Penrod J. Refinement of the concept of uncertainty. *J Adv Nurs.* 2001;34(2):238–245.

Popper KR. *Conjectures and Refutations.* 4th ed. London, England: Routledge & Kegan Paul; 1972.

Rawnsley M. The concept of privacy. *Adv Nurs Sci.* 1980;2(2):25–32.

Richmond JP, McKenna H. Homophobia: An evolutionary analysis of the concept as applied to nursing. *J Adv Nurs.* 1998;28(2):362–369.

Roberts KT, Whall A. Serenity as a goal for nursing practice. *Image.* 1996;28(4):359–364.

Robinson DS, McKenna HP. Loss: An analysis of a concept of particular interest to nursing. *J Adv Nurs.* 1998;27:779–784.

Rodgers BL, Kanfl KA. *Concept Development in Nursing: Foundations, Techniques, and Applications.* 2nd ed. Philadelphia, PA: W.B. Saunders; 1999.

Ryles SM. A concept analysis of empowerment: Its relationship to mental health nursing. *J Adv Nurs.* 1999;29(3):600–607.

Schoenfelder DP, Crowell CM, the NDEC Team. From risk for trauma to unintentional injury risk: Falls—A concept analysis. *Nurs Diagn.* 1999;10(4):149–157.

Schroetter SA, Wendler MC. Capstone experience: Analysis of an educational concept for nursing. *J Prof Nurs.* 2008;24(2):71–79.

Simpson SM. Near death experience: A concept analysis as applied to nursing. *J Adv Nurs.* 2001;36(4):520–526.

Smith J. The idea of health: A philosophical inquiry. *Adv Nurs Sci.* 1981;3(3):43–50.

Stern PN. Grounded theory methodology: Its uses and processes. *Image.* 1980;12(2):20–23.

Suppe F. Response to "positivism and qualitative nursing research." *Sch Inq Nurs Pract.* 2001;15(4):389–397.

Swanson EA, Hensen DP, Specht J, Johnson ML, Maas M. Caregiving: Concept analysis and outcomes. *Sch Inq Nurs Pract.* 1997;11(1):65–79.

Teasdale K. The concept of reassurance in nursing. *J Adv Nurs.* 1989;14:444–450.

Wade GH. A concept analysis of personal transformation. *J Adv Nurs.* 1998;28(4):713–719.

Wall LM. Exercise: A unitary concept. *Nurs Sci Q.* 1999;12(1):68–72.

11

■ ■ ■

Statement Analysis

Questions to consider before you get started reading this chapter:

▶ Are you interested in testing a hypothesis or statement of relationships that you think will forward your research program but don't know how sound the statement is or whether it is worth spending time and resources examining?

▶ Have you read a research article and found it confusing or highly complex and difficult to understand?

Introductory Note: If either of these situations occurs, then statement analysis may be the best method to help you clear up the situation. Statement analysis may be used alone to examine hypotheses in a study or propositions in a theory. It allows the analyst to carefully examine a single statement to determine its accuracy, completeness, and testability. In addition, it provides a set of skills essential to theory analysis. Much of the examination of the logic of a theory is a result of a good solid analysis of each statement in the theory. So, even though you may not see many formal articles about analyses of statements, it is a method you need to be very familiar with in order to do the work of science. Use the practice exercises in this chapter to help you grasp the differences among the types of statements.

DEFINITION AND DESCRIPTION

Examining relational statements to determine in what form they are presented and what relationship the concepts within those statements have to one another is the basic process of statement analysis. Statement analysis focuses on each concept within a statement, the relationships among the concepts, and the role that the statement plays as a whole.

In Chapter 3, we listed two types of nonrelational statements used in theory. The first was what Reynolds (1971) called an *existence* statement that simply identifies a concept or an object and claims its existence. For example, we might say, "the phenomenon of a person's subjective feelings is termed the *affect*." The name of the concept "affect" is claimed to exist and is identified by a brief summary statement. Existence statements occur in theories to provide background and explanation prior to positing relationships.

A *definition* is the second type of nonrelational statement in a theory. A definition describes the characteristics of a concept. It may be a *theoretical* definition—one that is abstract and useful to the theory, but with no empirical referents named—or it may be an *operational* definition, in which the method of measurement is clearly spelled out. Leaving rods and cones out of it for now, let us assume that the concept of "color blindness" has a theoretical definition that implies visual inability to distinguish accurately between colors. The operational definition of color blindness, then, might include criteria such as which colors would be included in testing, how many times the test must be run, and how many wrong answers constitute failure before color blindness can be said to be present. Definitions are useful in theory because they provide the basis for clear communication between the theorist and the reader or user.

Relational statements are a bit more complex than either existence statements or definitions. Relational statements form the skeleton of a theory. Each statement describes some type of relationship among or between the concepts within it. When they occur singly, they form the basis for research or at least further reflection on the phenomenon in question. When they occur in groups and are not interrelated, they provide the stimulus for thinking and exploring their possible linkages. If they occur in groups and are interrelated, they are called "theory" and form the basis for research programs.

Relational statements come in several forms or types. Suffice it to say that relational statements may be causal, probabilistic, concurrent, conditional, time ordered, necessary, or sufficient (Hardy, 1974; Reynolds, 1971). Each of these forms will be discussed further later in this chapter.

PURPOSE AND USES

Statement analysis is a rigorous exercise. The purposes of statement analysis are (1) to classify statements as to form and (2) to examine the relationships among the concepts. The exercise provides a means of examining statements in an orderly way to determine whether the statements are useful, informative, and logically correct. It is an essential first step in theory analysis as you will see in Chapter 12.

Statement analysis provides a way of looking at and formalizing theoretical constructions that are already available in the literature or through research. Statement analysis is suited to situations in which one or more statements about a phenomenon exist but have not yet been organized into a theoretical system. The strategy is also useful in providing the theorist with information about the structure and function of the statements being considered. It is particularly useful because once the statement has been analyzed, any obvious deficiencies in it may be corrected or modified.

When a theorist is building a new theory, carefully examining the proposed relational statements using statement analysis will help the theorist clean up any problems before subjecting the new theory to criticism and scrutiny from the scholarly community.

STEPS IN STATEMENT ANALYSIS

There are seven steps in statement analysis. Each of the steps will be discussed individually for clarity and understanding. But as in all of the strategies discussed in this book, the steps in statement analysis are not linear but iterative. The analyst will go back and forth through the various steps to be sure that things have been interpreted correctly. The more iterations achieved, the more likely a reasonable analysis will ensue. The steps in statement analysis are as follows: (1) select the statement(s) to be analyzed; (2) simplify the statement; (3) classify the statement; (4) examine concepts within the statement for definition and validity; (5) specify relationships among concepts by type, sign, and symmetry; (6) examine the logic; and (7) determine testability.

Select the Statement

Selecting a statement to be analyzed involves some commitment to the idea behind the statement. Anyone attempting statement analysis should have clearly in mind what reason he or she has for doing so. Perhaps some doubt exists about the statement, or perhaps the idea is exciting, provoking examination of the content or structure for soundness before refuting or acting upon it in some way. In any case, the theorist should have the rationale for analysis clearly in mind before beginning.

One difficulty in selecting a statement is that some verbal or written theories suffer from a woeful lack of specificity in their relational statements. Theories, especially in the social and behavioral sciences, may be elaborately verbal (Blalock, 1969). On close inspection, however, it may prove quite difficult to isolate one single relational statement. It then becomes the task of the analyst to extract or construct simple relational statements from all the verbiage. This exercise requires very careful reading to accurately reflect the meaning the original theorist intended. Checking with colleagues or even the original theorist is often a big help when confronted by such a problem.

Finally, a statement selected for analysis must be relevant. That is, it is far better to select a prominent or major statement in a theory than to select an insignificant one. To tell the difference in major and minor statements, examine the statement's breadth. A major statement will yield more information to the analyst than a minor one will. In addition, if the major statement has validity, the likelihood increases that the minor one does too.

Simplify the Statement If Necessary

Simplifying a statement is needed only if one of two things occurs. The first is the problem of the elaborate verbal model that must be reduced to manageable statements. The second problem is complexity, which may occur in theories where one concept may be linked to several others simultaneously. When this happens, it simplifies analysis to break the concept linkages into several shorter, more manageable statements. Assume a statement could be diagrammed as the one in Figure 11–1. It is clear that the analyst might find the job much easier to handle if the formulation looked more like the one in Figure 11–2. The analyst now has four simple discrete relationships to examine instead of one set of complex relationships. It is also clear, however, that

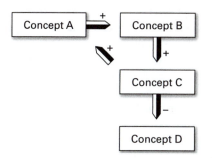

FIGURE 11–1 A complicated statement. See Figure 11–2 for simplification.

great care must be exercised when simplifying statements or relationships may be overlooked or misconstrued.

Cooley's (1999) excellent analysis of Corbin and Strauss's (1991) trajectory theory of chronic illness management gives some nice examples of how to simplify complex propositions into manageable and analyzable statements. Corbin and Strauss's Proposition 1 stated, "Yet courses can be extended, kept stable, and their symptoms controlled through proper management" (p. 162). Cooley restated it to read: "Trajectory management can control symptoms, keep stable or extend the trajectory" (p. 81). She used the placeholders *TM* for trajectory management and *T* for trajectory. She then diagrammed the statement as

$$TM \xrightarrow{+} T.$$

Classify the Statement

As discussed, there are three basic classifications of statements: (1) existence statements, (2) definitions, and (3) relational statements.

Existence statements claim existence for concepts (Reynolds, 1971). The statement "That object is called a refrigerator" is an existence statement. Existence statements are

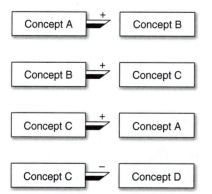

FIGURE 11–2 The statement in Figure 11–1 broken down into several shorter, more manageable statements.

not definitions and thus do not describe characteristics of the concept. They simply assert that something is so. Existence statements can be accurate or inaccurate. If the object in our example is really a dishwasher, then the statement is inaccurate. If the object in the statement corresponds to reality (it *is* a refrigerator), then the existence statement is accurate. Determining whether a refrigerator corresponds to reality is not hard as the refrigerator is a concrete object. A statement that claims the existence of an abstract concept, on the other hand, may present the analyst with some difficulty in deciding whether the concept is accurate. As we discussed in the previous chapter, concepts may not be given the correct name or the characteristics of the concept may change over time. The analyst may have to take the statement as accurate until proven otherwise.

Definitions have three subforms—descriptive, stipulative, and operational (Hempel, 1966). A **descriptive** definition explains the accepted meaning for a term already in use. It explicates the term in other words that are already understood by the reader. It generally can be considered accurate. For example, a descriptive definition of *kitten* might read: "A kitten is the biological offspring of an adult female cat."

If the definition describes the term in such a way that it has a distinctive use assigned by the author and that may depart from the widely accepted use, then it is a **stipulative** definition. These definitions cannot be considered either accurate or inaccurate because they are specifically formulated only for use in the way the author of the theory has decreed. A stipulative definition of *kitten* might read: "For the purpose of this study, a kitten shall be defined as any healthy female offspring of a healthy female cat that is less than 8 weeks old." A stipulative definition is not the same as an operational definition.

An **operational** definition includes the specific means for measuring or testing each scientific term within it. An operational definition must be so precise that different scientists can use it repetitively and still obtain objective results. In our definition of *kitten*, for instance, the operational definition might be: "For the purposes of this study, a kitten shall be any healthy offspring of a healthy female cat weighing between 4 and 12 ounces and no less than 3 days or more than 8 days old." Operational definitions may also include the measurement instrument to be used. For instance, if researchers wanted to test the relationship between stress and coping in adolescents, they would specify a particular set of questionnaires (X's stress scale and Y's coping scale) to be used in the study.

Relational statements specify relationships between concepts. Some relational statements may be so well supported empirically and logically that they function as laws or axioms within the theory. Others may be less well supported by data or logic and serve as propositions or empirical generalizations. Relational statements may also be hypotheses that are as yet unsupported by data even if they may appear reasonable and logical. Identifying the relational statements is very important when reaching step 5 in the statement analysis. It is that step in which the analyst specifies which type of relationship the statement exemplifies.

Examine the Concepts Within the Statement

Perhaps the easiest part of statement analysis is identifying the concepts within the statement to be analyzed. Scan the statement for the major ideas expressed within it. The names, or terms, for these ideas are the pertinent concepts.

There are three actions involved in examining the concepts once they are identified. The first is to determine the definitions of the terms that reflect the concepts. The definition should reflect all the defining attributes of the concept so that everyone who reads the theory will know precisely how the theorist intends the term to be used. (For a discussion of determining defining attributes for a concept, see Chapter 10.) If the concept is not adequately defined, can its meaning be determined from the context of the theoretical formulation? If so, the analyst should use this material to help formulate additions to the definition that will aid the analysis and even, perhaps, help refine the theory. If not, then the analyst must simply state that the concepts are inadequately defined for the purpose of analysis.

Determining whether the concepts as they are defined are theoretically valid is the second step in the examination of concepts in a statement. The analyst attempts to determine whether the concepts, as they are defined, accurately reflect the general semantic usage for that concept. This process involves a brief review of the relevant literature concerning the concept being considered. If the concept is being used in the same ways as it has previously been used in the literature and the definition reflects it, the concept may be considered valid. When the theorist has conducted a careful concept analysis, the concept is considered valid even if it does not reflect the relevant literature but goes beyond traditional usage. In fact, the validity of the concept may be more certain after analysis than a concept defined by tradition alone.

Finally, determine whether the concepts, as they are defined, are used consistently throughout the discussions related to the formation of the statement. Occasionally, an author will subtly change the meaning of a concept in an attempt to make the meaning clear or will define the concept clearly and then change it slightly to reflect the measuring instrument's definition. The analyst should be aware of this possibility and make a note of any changes that may occur. This conceptual drift can seriously undermine both the clarity and validity of the statement or theory in which it occurs.

Specify Relationships by Type, Sign, and Symmetry

Assessment of a relational statement for type, sign, and symmetry is done to determine its function within the theory. In the interest of clarity and simplicity, we assume that all relational statements are linear until proven otherwise. (Statement analysis can often provide the clue to curvilinear relationships. If you can't classify a statement or determine its sign, it may express a nonlinear relationship.)

TYPE   Several types of relational statements may occur. These are causal, probabilistic, concurrent, conditional, time ordered, necessary, and sufficient (Hardy, 1974). We will consider each type briefly giving examples of each. It is possible for a statement to be more than one type at the same time. For instance, a statement may be both probabilistic and conditional. We give examples of some types that often occur together later in practice exercises.

A **causal** statement is one in which the first concept is said to be the "cause" of the other. Causal statements are often deduced from laws. Therefore, there are very few causal statements in the social and behavioral sciences primarily because they encompass so many intervening variables that may influence causation. Causality is easier to demonstrate in the physical sciences. For example, the statement "Raising the temperature of a gas held under constant pressure will increase its volume" is a causal statement. It asserts that some event (raising the temperature of a gas under constant pressure) causes another event (increased gas volume). This is the simplest form of causal statement, although there are more complex ones involving several causal factors for one phenomenon. Causal statements are difficult to find in health and social sciences, especially in beginning attempts at theory construction, because the caused outcome must always happen if the causal event or events occur.

It is often helpful to use symbols, or placeholders, for the concepts in statements to avoid becoming confused by the content of the concepts during analysis. Using the symbols G_p for gas under pressure, T for temperature, and GV for gas volume, the analyst could diagram the previous causal statement; thus

$$\text{If } \uparrow T \rightarrow G_p, \text{ then always } \uparrow GV.$$

If the event (GV) always occurs, it can be labeled a causal statement.

A statement is called **probabilistic** if the event occurs some of the time or most of the time, but not *all* of the time. Probabilistic statements are usually derived from statistical data. They assert that if one event occurs, the second event probably will also occur. An excellent example of a probabilistic statement is that cigarette smoking (CS) is highly likely to lead to lung cancer (LC). There is no direct causality in this statement because everyone who smokes does not develop lung cancer. But the probability of developing lung cancer is increased significantly in the presence of cigarette smoking. This probabilistic relationship, if diagrammed, might look like this:

$$\text{If } CS \rightarrow \text{ then probably } LC.$$

When a statement asserts that if event A occurs, event B also occurs, it is asserting that the relationship between the concepts is **concurrent**. There may or may not be any causation between the two events—they simply exist together. An example of this kind of statement might be: "A low level of educational preparation and a low income often occur together." The statement does not infer that lack of education *causes* poverty. Another example of concurrence can be found in Muhlenkamp and Parsons's (1972) classic study of nurses and is confirmed in Kaiser and Bickle's (1980) study. These authors found that nurses have personality characteristics that are highly feminine rather than masculine, that is, higher in personality characteristics such as nurturance versus dominance. This is a good example of a concurrent statement. It simply asserts that nurses (N) and feminine personality (FP) characteristics occur together. It makes no other claim. A diagram of this statement would be

$$\text{If } N, \text{ also } FP.$$

Sometimes a relationship between two concepts occurs only in the presence of a third concept. This type of statement is a **conditional** statement. A good example of a conditional statement is one found in a series of studies by Acton, Irvin, Jensen, Hopkins, and Miller (1997) on the mediating effects of self-care resources. In their studies, they found that the relationship between high levels of stress (HS) and diminished well-being (*DMB*) was improved when subjects had higher levels of social support (*SS*), self-worth (*SW*), and hope (*H*). This can be simplistically diagrammed as

If *HS*, then *DMB*, but not in the presence of *SS*, *SW*, and *H*.

Time-ordered statements are those that indicate that some amount of time intervenes between the first concept or event and the second one. An example of a time-ordered statement is the classic one indicating that when a person experiences numerous stressful life events (*SLE*) within a year, the likelihood of that person becoming ill (*I*) is quite high (Erickson, Tomlin, & Swain, 1990; Holmes & Rahe, 1968; Rahe, 1972). This relationship is time ordered because time passes between the first episodes of stress and the resultant illness. This statement can be diagrammed like this:

If *SLE*, then later *I*.

A statement that indicates that one and only one concept or event can lead to the second concept or event reflects a **necessary** relationship. Necessary relationships function very much as differential diagnoses do in medicine. That is, a patient can be positively said to have cancer, for instance, if and only if there is a pathologist's report of malignant cells on biopsy. In the same way, relationships among concepts may occur only under certain conditions. An example from nursing might be a statement relating to stress and adaptation. Roy's (1976), Neuman's (1980), and Erickson et al.'s (1990) models of nursing have all stated that adaptation (*A*) occurs as a response to stressors (*S*). Stressors then become necessary before adaptation can occur. The diagram would look like this:

If and only if *S*, then *A*.

Statements in which the first concept or event and the second concept or event are related, regardless of anything else, demonstrate **sufficient** relationships. Using the stressor–adaptation idea above, we can see that if stressors occur, then adaptation will begin in the person whether or not she or he wills it and whether or not someone intervenes. In other words, the presence of the first concept guarantees the presence of the second concept. A sufficient relationship could be diagrammed this way:

If *S*, then *A*, regardless of anything else.

When first introduced to statement analysis, some students mistakenly believe that a statement can be only one type at a time. This is clearly not the case. For instance, most relational statements are probabilistic in addition to being conditional or concurrent or time ordered and so on.

SIGN Signs generally fall into one of three categories: positive, negative, or unknown (Mullins, 1971; Reynolds, 1971). The rule of thumb is that if the concepts vary in the same direction, that is, as one increases or decreases so does the other, then the relationship is positive. If one concept increases while the other decreases, the relationship is said to be negative. If you have no information about the way the concepts vary, the relationship is unknown. Below are three probabilistic statements and one statement inferred from the first three with their relationships drawn to help you see how this is done:

When members of a group become anxious (*A*), hostility (*H*) increases.

$$A \overset{+}{\rightarrow} H$$

Hostility is related to a decrease in group cohesiveness (*GC*).

$$H \overset{-}{\rightarrow} GC$$

Creativity (*C*) decreases as anxiety increases in groups.

$$A \overset{-}{\rightarrow} C$$

Inferred: Anxiety has a negative impact on group cohesiveness.

$$A \overset{-}{\rightarrow} GC$$

This inferred statement was derived logically from the first two statements. Because both *A* and *GC* are related to *H*, they are therefore related to each other.

What we cannot tell from these four statements is what effect creativity and group cohesiveness have on each other. So that might look like this:

$$C \overset{?}{\rightarrow} GC.$$

SYMMETRY   So far, all our examples have been asymmetrical, that is, one-direction relationships. In asymmetrical statements, the relationship goes from only one concept to the next but is never reciprocated. There are many examples of asymmetrical relationships in our discussions. One example is the statement above that anxiety is negatively related to group cohesiveness. But, relationships can be symmetrical as well (Blalock, 1969) where each concept affects the other. An example of a symmetrical statement might be one from research done by one of us on maternal attachment behaviors (Avant, 1981). High attachment scores (*At*) were associated with low anxiety (*Ax*) scores and high anxiety scores were associated with low attachment scores in primiparous women. This relationship can be diagrammed like this:

$$At \overset{-}{\leftrightarrow} Ax.$$

Examine the Logic

Origin, reasonableness, and adequacy are the criteria for examining the logic of relationships. When examining the origin of a statement, ask yourself whether the statement is constructed deductively, that is from a more general law, or inductively, from observation or available data. If the statement is deductive in origin, its logic should be adequate because a conclusion in a valid deductive argument cannot be false if the premises are true. If the statement is inductive, its logic cannot be judged except by the amount of empirical support it has and by comparison to existing knowledge (Hempel, 1966). If it has strong support both in empirical testing and in agreement with existing literature, its logic is probably adequate. The logic can also be determined by examining the relationships of the concepts to each other. If the relationship cannot be classified by type, sign, or symmetry, there may be a logical flaw.

Determining the reasonableness of a statement also uses comparison to existing knowledge. Simply ask whether this statement seems reasonable given what you already know on the subject. If it makes sense in light of existing knowledge, it is reasonable.

Determining adequacy of a single statement is more difficult than determining adequacy of a theory because we cannot construct matrices or models to demonstrate where logical gaps may occur. It is possible, however, to draw a simple diagram as we have done in the previous section labeling the concepts by letters or numbers and determining types and signs that are relevant. If you are unable to do any one of the three, there is some flaw in the statement.

Determine Testability

In this final step of the analysis, determine whether or not there are operational measures that can be used in the real world to obtain data that will support or refute the statement being analyzed. It is at this point that the analyst will run up against the situation Hempel calls "testability-in-principle." Basically, this is a statement that could be tested empirically if the tools were available to measure the concepts; but they are not available (Hempel, 1966). He considers these statements just as useful in theory construction as the empirically testable statements. We feel that the criterion of testability can be met if a statement is either testable in principle or actually testable because so many concepts in nursing may lack the instruments to measure them. This is not to imply, however, that all statements are therefore testable.

In order for a statement to meet the criterion of testability, it must render some test implications. That is, you should be able to say: "If I tested this under the specified conditions, then the outcome hypothesized should actually happen." A relatively new statement might render fewer testable ideas than one that has more age and support, but if it is testable at all, it meets the criterion. Any statement that cannot produce one testable idea or that is constructed in such a way that the concepts have vague meanings cannot meet the criterion of testability until modified.

ADVANTAGES AND LIMITATIONS

The primary advantage of statement analysis is that it provides a systematic way of examining the relationships among concepts. In addition, it assists the theorist in examining the structure and function of statements. Statement analysis is also a fundamental skill necessary for theory analysis. But perhaps the most important function of statement analysis occurs when the theorist is thinking carefully and systematically about the linkages between concepts. He or she may discover other linkages or relationships that are important to the final theoretical formulations during that thinking time. In just such analysis situations, many scientists have happened on to significant theoretical ideas. Analyzing just one statement may be a limitation of statement analysis, especially if it is part of a theoretical whole. Removing the statement from its context can often result in loss of valuable information, and the analysis is hindered.

In addition, determining the logic of a statement is often more difficult when it is removed from the theory. The final limitation of the statement analysis process is that it does take a little time and it is rigorous. This is a limitation only as it applies to the theorist, however; this very intense and time-consuming effort ultimately proves very valuable in assessing statements.

UTILIZING THE RESULTS OF STATEMENT ANALYSIS

Statement analysis results in formalized statements with their underlying structures and functions made explicit. But what does a theorist do with the resulting information? It can be used in a variety of ways in education, practice, research, and theory development.

Analyzed statements can be used as springboards for discussion in the classroom. Discussions may include ideas about which concepts were clear, which ones were related to each other, and how, or what, inconsistencies were discovered. The amount of empirical evidence for or against the statement can provide the basis for designing classroom activities such as proposals for research studies to produce either more evidence in support of the statement or more evidence to falsify it. The amount of empirical evidence could also be used to launch a discussion about the efficacy of the statement to guide clinical practice.

Another possible use for statement analysis in education would be having a faculty interest group discuss the issues raised from analyzing several similar statements or several statements about the same selected topic. This discussion could lead to curriculum changes or to faculty research projects. A series of faculty discussions and analyses had just such a result in the development of the theory of unpleasant symptoms (Lenz, Pugh, Milligan, Gift, & Suppe, 1997; Lenz, Suppe, Gift, Pugh, & Milligan, 1995).

Statement analysis can guide clinicians in the judicious use of research findings. Knowing whether or not a statement is associational, causal, or time ordered can inform decisions about when to use the statement and under what conditions. Certain nursing diagnoses may be considered or certain nursing interventions or outcomes chosen as a result of a statement analysis not previously available to the nurse. In addition, faced with the choice of two potential interventions, the nurse using results from a statement analysis would know which one has the most empirical support, thus leading to a more educated decision.

Statement analysis allows the researcher or theorist to identify the problems in a statement and to take the appropriate next step. Concepts may need clarifying. Inconsistencies, unclear definitions, and gaps in knowledge can become apparent. Together, these clarifications provide direction for planning concept analyses, reformulating ideas, or proposing new hypotheses to test (Bu & Jezeweskio, 2006). Connell, Shaw, Holmes, and Foster's (2001) article on family participation in Alzheimer's research offers an excellent example of how statement analysis can be useful in research and practice.

If the analysis has demonstrated that the statement is sound, the theorist can begin to look for other concepts and linkages to add to what is already known. This is how theories are built—one step at a time.

Summary

Statement analysis is a process of systematically examining the relationships among concepts. There are seven steps involved: selecting the statement; simplifying it if necessary; classifying it; examining the concepts for definition and validity; specifying relationships by type, sign, and symmetry; examining the logic; and determining the testability.

Once a statement has been analyzed, any deficiencies in the statement are clear and may be corrected. Furthermore, the process of thinking aloud, discussions, and written assessments often generate additional ideas and statements, either by deduction or by serendipity, that are valuable additions to future theoretical formulations.

Practice Exercises

Below are several statements paraphrased from a study of faculty attitudes (Ruiz, 1981).

A. Classify each statement as one of the following:
   a. Relational statement
   b. Descriptive definition
   c. Stipulative definition
   d. Operational definition

   1. Ethnocentrism means ethnic narrow-mindedness.
   2. Dogmatism shall be defined as close-mindedness.
   3. Intolerance of ambiguity and dogmatism are the two factors underlying ethnocentrism for this study.
   4. Faculty who are highly dogmatic view patients with different ethnocultural backgrounds as annoying and superstitious.
   5. Faculty who have high ethnocentrism scores have negative attitudes toward culturally different patients.

B. Using statement 4, simplify it into two statements and diagram them.

C. Using statements 4 and 5, examine the concepts and specify the relationships by type, sign, and symmetry. Determine the logic and testability of each.

ANSWERS

A. 1. b; 2. c; 3. d; 4. a; 5. a

B. 1. Dogmatic faculty (*DF*) view patients with differing ethnocultural (*DEB*) backgrounds as annoying (*A*):

$$\text{If } DF, \text{ then } A, \text{ but only if } DEB.$$

   2. Dogmatic faculty (*DF*) view patients with differing ethnocultural backgrounds (*DEB*) as superstitious (*S*):

$$\text{If } DF, \text{ then } S, \text{ but only if } DEB.$$

C. Statement 4 can be diagrammed as $DF \xrightarrow{-} A$ and *S*, but only if *DEB*.

Statement 5 can be diagrammed as ethnocentric faculty $(EF) \xrightarrow{-}$ attitudes toward culturally different patients (*ACDP*) or $EF \xrightarrow{-} ACDP$.

Both statements 4 and 5 are probabilistic because they are drawn from statistical data. Statement 4, as it is diagrammed in Practice Exercise B, is conditional as well. Both statements are asymmetrical. The signs are negative because less dogmatic faculty had more positive views of ethnocentric patients.

Some of the concepts from statements 4 and 5, such as "patient," "faculty," "ethnocultural background," "annoying," and "superstitious," are undefined. If these concepts were intended to be used in their common language meanings, the author should state that clearly. Otherwise, each should be defined. The two concepts that were defined, "ethnocentrism" and "dogmatism," are given only in vague, equally undefined terms in this exercise. (They were operationally defined in the actual study.) The concept of "intolerance of ambiguity" is not defined but is used as part of an operational definition. This is clearly to be avoided. None of the concept definitions are unambiguous.

The statements are logical. They are testable only if better concept definitions are constructed so that operational measures can be found for them. It can be said that the concepts are measurable or the statement testable only when there are careful operational definitions that reflect the theoretical definitions.

Since we gave you the answers to the exercise above, you may want to try the same exercise without having the answers available. Below are two statements from a study of the effects of emotional autonomy, self-care behaviors, and depression on health adaptation in adolescents (Chen et al., 2017). Perform a statement analysis like the one above on these statements.

1. "Emotional autonomy directly and negatively affected self-care behavior and life satisfaction quality of life but directly and positively affected depressive symptoms." (p. 73)
2. "Depressive symptoms directly and negatively influenced self-care behaviors and life satisfaction quality of life, but did not significantly influence HbA1c levels." (p. 73)

References

Acton GJ, Irvin BL, Jensen BA, Hopkins BA, Miller EW. Explicating middle-range theory through methodological diversity. *Adv Nurs Sci.* 1997;19(3):78–85.

Avant K. Anxiety as a potential factor affecting maternal attachment. *J Obstet Gynecol Neonatal Nurs.* 1981;10(6):416–420.

Blalock H Jr. *Theory Construction: From Verbal to Mathematical Formulations.* Englewood Cliffs, NJ: Prentice Hall; 1969.

Bu X, Jezeweskio MA. Developing a mid-range theory of patient advocacy through concept analysis. *J Adv Nurs.* 2006;57(1):101–110.

Chen C-Y, Lo F-S, Chen B-H, Lu M-H, Hsin Y-M, Wang R-H. Pathways of emotional autonomy, self-care behaviors, and depressive symptoms on health adaptation in adolescents with type 1 diabetes. *Nurs Outlook.* 2017;65(1):68–76.

Connell CM, Shaw BA, Holmes SB, Foster NL. Caregiver's attitudes toward their family members' participation in Alzheimer disease research: Implications for recruitment and retention. *Alzheimer Dis Assoc Disord.* 2001;15(3):137–145.

Cooley ME. Analysis and evaluation of the trajectory of chronic illness management. *Sch Inq Nurs Pract.* 1999;13(2):75–95.

Corbin JM, Strauss A. A nursing model for chronic illness management based upon the trajectory framework. *Sch Inq Nurs Pract.* 1991;5:155–174.

Erickson HC, Tomlin E, Swain MA. *Modeling and Role-Modeling: A Theory and Paradigm for Nursing.* Lexington, SC: Pine Press; 1990.

Hardy M. Theories: Components, development, and evaluation. *Nurs Res.* 1974;23:100–107.

Hempel C. *Philosophy of Natural Science.* Englewood Cliffs, NJ: Prentice Hall; 1966.

Holmes R, Rahe R. The social readjustment rating scale. *J Psychosom Res.* 1968;11:213–218.

Kaiser J, Bickle I. Attitude change as a motivational factor in producing behavior change related to implementing primary nursing. *Nurs Res.* 1980;19(5):290–300.

Lenz ER, Pugh LC, Milligan RA, Gift AG, Suppe F. The middle-range theory of unpleasant symptoms: An update. *Adv Nurs Sci.* 1997;19(3):14–27.

Lenz ER, Suppe F, Gift AG, Pugh LC, Milligan RA. Collaborative development of middle-range nursing theories: Toward a theory of unpleasant symptoms. *Adv Nurs Sci.* 1995;17(3):1–13.

Muhlenkamp A, Parsons J. Characteristics of nurses: An overview of recent research published in a nursing research periodical. *J Vocat Behav.* 1972;2:261–273.

Mullins N. *The Art of Theory: Construction and Use.* New York, NY: Harper & Row; 1971.

Neuman B. The Betty Neuman health-care systems model. In: Riehl JP, Roy C, eds. *Conceptual Models for Nursing Practice.* 2nd ed. New York, NY: Appleton-Century-Crofts; 1980.

Rahe R. Subject's recent life changes and their near future illness susceptibility. *Adv Psychosom Med.* 1972;8:2–19.

Reynolds P. *A Primer in Theory Construction.* Indianapolis, IN: Bobbs-Merrill; 1971.

Roy C. *Introduction to Nursing: An Adaptation Model.* Englewood Cliffs, NJ: Prentice Hall; 1976.

Ruiz M. Open-closed mindedness, intolerance of ambiguity and nursing faculty attitudes toward culturally different patients. *Nurs Res.* 1981;30(3):177–181.

Additional Readings

Greenwood D. *The Nature of Science and Other Essays.* New York, NY: Philosophical Library; 1959.

Hage J. *Techniques and Problems of Theory Construction in Sociology.* New York, NY: Wiley; 1972.

Lerner D, ed. *Parts and Wholes.* New York, NY: Free Press of Glencoe; 1963.

Zetterberg HL. *On Theory and Verification in Sociology.* 3rd ed. New York, NY: Bedminster Press; 1965.

12

■ ■ ■

Theory Analysis

Questions to consider before you get started reading this chapter:

▶ Are you interested in a particular theory that might be useful in your research or practice but not sure how valid it is?

▶ Are you planning to use a theory in your work but need to know where its strengths and weaknesses lie?

▶ Are you interested in a theory but parts of it do not seem to contribute to your understanding?

Introductory Note: If any of these issues are confronting you, theory analysis is likely the best strategy to use for resolving them. Theory analysis is a formal way to break the theory into its component parts and examine them for consistency, logic, and usability.

We have been delightedly surprised at how many theories are undergoing analysis and revision over the last several years. This is a very encouraging trend. It reveals the rapid nature of the development of the science of nursing. There are also many more middle-range theories under development. They provide the discipline with a rich source of potential knowledge about how nursing works and how effective and efficient nursing care is. We encourage researchers, advanced practice nurses, staff nurses, and students to examine any theory they intend to teach or to use in practice to be sure that it is a valid theory and is reliable in its description, explanation, prediction, and prescription or control.

DEFINITION AND DESCRIPTION

Theory is usually constructed to express a unique, unifying idea about a phenomenon that answers previously unanswered questions and provides new insights into the nature of the phenomenon. A theory should provide a parsimonious, precise example, or model, of the real world or the world as it is experienced. Thus, theory is defined as a set of interrelated relational statements about a phenomenon that is useful for description, explanation, prediction, and prescription or control (Chinn & Jacobs, 1987; Dickoff, James, & Wiedenbach, 1968a, 1968b; Hardy, 1974; Hempel, 1965; Reynolds, 1971).

A theory purporting to describe, explain, or predict something should provide the reader with a clear idea of what the phenomenon is and does, what events affect it, and how it affects other phenomena. Therefore, theory analysis is the systematic examination of the theory for meaning, logical adequacy, usefulness, generality, parsimony, and testability.

In theory analysis, as in all analysis strategies, the theory is broken down into parts. Each is examined individually as it relates to every other. In addition, the theoretical structure as a whole is examined to determine such things as validity and approximation to the real world.

PURPOSE AND USES

Theory analysis allows you to examine both the strengths and the weaknesses of a theory. In addition, a theory analysis may determine the need for additional development or refinement of the original theory.

Theory analysis provides a systematic, objective way of examining a theory that may lead to insights and formulations previously undiscovered. This then adds to the body of knowledge in the nursing discipline. As Popper (1965) pointed out in a classic work, science is interested in novel ideas and interesting theories because their very novelty or interest prompts the scientist to put them to empirical test. Theory analysis offers one way of determining what needs to be put to the test and often suggests how it can be done.

A formal theory analysis is relevant only if the theory has the possibility of being useful in an educational, clinical practice, or research setting. If the theory demonstrates no potential for usefulness, then the analysis becomes a futile exercise. It has been our experience that the primary purpose for conducting a theory analysis prior to using that theory in education or clinical practice is to discover the strong points the theory offers to guide practice. One wants to be sure the theory is well supported and effective if one is to use it in practice.

However, a theory analysis for the purposes of research usually focuses on the weak points or the unsubstantiated linkages among its concepts. The reason for this distinction is that the analysis provides evidence the researcher needs to justify conducting a study concerning new or unclear relationships within the original theory.

Understanding is the main aim of **analysis**. To truly understand something, we must put aside our own values and biases and look objectively at the object of analysis. Because a theory analysis is both systematic and objective, it provides a way to examine the content and structure of a theory without being influenced by subjective evaluation. Leaving our personal values out of the analysis allows us to see the theory more clearly, and the original theorist's values will become more evident.

The main aim of **evaluation**, on the other hand, is decision and/or action. Here, our own values and biases become important to the outcome. Evaluation of theory should only be done *after* a thorough analysis is made. Then, we should feel free to evaluate the theory's potential contribution to scientific knowledge and to make judgments about its worth in establishing a basis for making decisions or taking action (Chinn & Kramer, 2014; Fawcett, 1980, 1989, 1993, 1995, 2000, 2005; Fawcett & DeSanto-Madeya, 2013).

PROCEDURES FOR THEORY ANALYSIS

The steps in theory analysis were synthesized from the works of Popper (1961, 1965), Reynolds (1971), Hardy (1974), Fawcett (1980, 1989, 2000), and Chinn and Jacobs (1987). Despite their age, these authors' works collectively formed the existing foundation of knowledge in theory development. Without their pioneering efforts, nursing theory development would be seriously behind and this book might not exist.

There are six steps in theory analysis: (1) identify the origins of the theory, (2) examine the meaning of the theory, (3) analyze the logical adequacy of the theory, (4) determine the usefulness of the theory, (5) define the degree of generalizability and the parsimony of the theory, and (6) determine the testability of the theory. Each of these steps will first be defined briefly and then discussed in detail.

The **origins** of a theory refer to its initial development. The analyst investigates what prompted its development, whether the theory is inductive or deductive in form, and whether evidence exists to support or refute the theory.

The **meaning** (Hardy, 1974) of a theory has to do with the theory's concepts and how they relate to each other. Essentially, the meaning is reflected in the language of the theory and calls for a careful examination of the specific language used by the original theorist.

The **logical adequacy** (Hardy, 1974) of a theory denotes the logical structure of the concepts and statements independent of their meaning. The analyst looks for any logical fallacies in the structure of the theory and examines the accuracy with which predictions can be made from the theory.

The **usefulness** of a theory concerns how practical and helpful the theory is to the discipline in providing a sense of understanding or predictable outcomes. A theory that provides a practitioner with realistic guides to practice so that Intervention A consistently leads to Patient Behavior B, for instance, is obviously more useful than one that does not.

Generalizability, or **transferability**, explains the extent to which generalizations can be made from the theory. The more widely the theory can be applied, the more generalizable it becomes.

Parsimony refers to how simply and briefly a theory can be stated while still being complete in its explanation of the phenomenon in question. Many mathematical theories are parsimonious, for example, because they offer an explanation in only a few equations. Social science theories are rarely parsimonious, on the other hand, because they deal with such complex human phenomena that they defy mathematical expression.

Testability has to do with whether the theory can be supported by empirical data. If a theory cannot generate hypotheses that can be subjected to empirical research, it is not testable.

We believe that all of these six steps are important to a complete theory analysis. Some authors disagree. Fawcett and DeSanto-Madeya (2013) state that the last two steps determining parsimony and testability are really related to theory evaluation. Granted, when one completes the analysis and begins to evaluate the theory, one may place heavier values on some of the steps than on others. But, if a theory has poorly defined and inconsistently used concepts, for instance, it will not be capable of test, will not have parsimony, and will not be useful. The value assigned to a theory rests primarily on what the analysis reveals, but it also reflects one's own feelings and biases to a certain extent. This is to be expected; no scientist can ever be completely objective. We will now more thoroughly discuss each of the analysis steps.

Origins

The first step is to determine what prompted the development of the theory. Sometimes the theorist will offer an explicit explanation. Otherwise, the analyst may only be able to surmise this from the context of the discussion. Understanding the origin of a theory and the purpose for which it was developed often proves very helpful to the analyst in understanding how the theory was put together and why. Begin by reading the theory carefully, identifying the major ideas or concepts, and isolating the relational statements. In addition, find out if the theory was developed deductively (from a more general law) or inductively (from data). If the theory was developed from another theory or from some other hypothesis, it can be considered deductive in origin. It can be considered inductive in origin if observations of relationships from qualitative or quantitative data, literature, or clinical practice generated the theory. Later when determining its logical adequacy, the inductive or deductive form of origin will be important. Finally, it is often helpful to identify any underlying assumptions on which the theory is built. These underlying assumptions can be important to interpretation and when considering the usefulness of the theory. Some authors will identify their assumptions explicitly. However, in many cases you may have to determine what the assumptions are from the context and description of the theory itself.

Meaning

Examining meaning and logical adequacy is the most lengthy process in a theory analysis but also the most valuable. Meaning, in theory analysis, refers to the semantics of the theory. An analyst must examine the language used in the theory by looking at the concepts and statements within it. The steps are as follows: identify the concepts, examine their definitions and use, identify the statements, and examine the relationships among concepts as demonstrated in the statements. (This is essentially statement analysis. If you feel you need to know more about how to examine the relationships, see Chapter 11.)

IDENTIFY CONCEPTS Look for the major ideas in the theory. All relevant terms that reflect those ideas should be clearly stated and defined. It is often difficult to identify the major concepts in an elaborate verbal model. Probably the best approach is to read with a pencil and paper at hand. As new terms appear, write them down with their definitions, if given. This saves time in the long run and makes it very clear where definitions are missing. If you are working electronically, either highlight the concepts and their definitions or set up a database to capture the information. In either case, be sure to note the page numbers where you found the concepts and definitions to aid your writing later.

Determine whether each concept is primitive, concrete, or abstract. As described in Chapters 3 and 10, primitive terms are those names for concepts that derive their meanings from common experience in the discipline and can only be defined by using examples (Wilson, 1969). Concrete concepts must be directly measurable and are restricted by time and space. Abstract concepts are not limited by time or space and may not be directly measurable. Classifying the concepts in this way will aid the analyst in assessing the concrete or abstract nature of the entire theory.

EXAMINE DEFINITIONS AND USE There are four possible options in regard to definitions: a theoretical definition, an operational definition, a descriptive definition, and no definition.

A **theoretical** definition uses other theoretical terms to define a concept and place it within the context of the theory but does not specify any operational rules for classifying or measuring it. A theoretical definition is usually fairly abstract and may use lower-order concepts to define higher-order ones. The most important criterion, though, is the lack of measurement specification in the definition.

A theoretical definition may provide the theorist with a way of expressing the richness of the concept within the theory and the means for classifying a phenomenon as either an example of the concept or not, but an **operational** definition provides the means for measuring the concept in question.

Operational definitions are useful in research but often artificially limit the concept. It is useful to the analyst, however, if both types of definitions are formulated for the major theoretical concepts. It is also very important to be sure that the operational definitions accurately reflect the theoretical definitions.

A **descriptive** definition, one that simply lists or describes the attributes of a concept much as in a dictionary, says nothing about the context in which the concept is used, nor does it specify operational measures. Having a descriptive definition is better than the last option, **no definitions** at all, but provides very limited data to the analyst. When only limited definitions are available, the analyst may find it difficult to make a truly objective analysis and equally difficult to use the theory for the purpose intended. When a theory contains only descriptive definitions or no definitions, it is often in a very early stage of development. It will be valuable if the analyst can make thoughtful suggestions about how further development should proceed.

The major concern in considering the way in which the concepts are used is with consistency of use, that is, whether or not the theorist uses the concepts consistently, as they are defined, throughout the theory. This is vital information for anyone who proposes to apply the theory. If a theorist defines a concept in one way and then subtly, or not so subtly, alters the meaning as the theory develops, then all the formulations using that concept become suspect until the ambiguity of the definition can be cleared up. Otherwise, the analyst may attempt to predict outcomes from an early statement in a theory only to find that a later statement contradicts those same outcomes.

Additional research work regarding a theory may cause changes to be made in concept definitions or even in whole sections of a theory. It is to be expected that some refinements should be made. However, when such changes are necessitated, then the initial studies using the original concepts may not be useful in the support of the theory. They may need to be repeated and the initial relational statements retested for validity using the new concept definitions.

IDENTIFY STATEMENTS   Once the major concepts and definitions in the theory have been identified and examined, the analyst then concentrates specifically on relational statements. Relational statements identify the ways the concepts relate to each other. This process is not always easy, especially in elaborate verbal theories. Refer to the major concepts identified in the previous step when postulating relationships among them.

Look for explicit relational statements first. If you are dealing with research reports, you may look in the results section for the major relational statements. At other times, it may be necessary to start with the hypothesis section and work forward to the data analysis in order to find the relationships. Then go back and look for any relationships that may be implied or alluded to by the author or demonstrated but not reported in the tables or data analysis section. Another place to look for relationships is in a graphic model if the author provides one. Such a model often provides a picture of the major relationships among the concepts. If such a model is provided, compare the graphic model with the verbal description of the theory. The two should be completely congruent in terms of the major concepts and relationships. If they are not congruent, the theory should be considered flawed and in need of further refinement to clear up the discrepancies.

When working from a verbal explanation written in non–research-report format, such as a descriptive article or a book chapter, it is often best to identify each concept as it appears along with any concepts that lie close to it on the page. Read carefully to see whether association between any of the concepts is mentioned. Often the last few paragraphs or the summary of the article or chapter will offer some relationships, although we have found that summaries often give only the major relationships. Therefore, using summaries alone often leaves much of the richness of the theory in obscurity and hinders the analysis. For excellent examples of identifying statements and examining their relationships, see Cooley's (1999) analysis of the trajectory theory of chronic illness management or Linder's (2010) analysis of the UCSF symptom management theory of chronic illness.

EXAMINE RELATIONSHIPS   Determining what types of relationships are specified, what boundaries are present, and whether the statements are used consistently is the first task in examining the relationships among concepts as demonstrated in the statements. In addition, the analyst must assess whether or not each statement has any valid empirical support. For the purpose of theory analysis, determining types of relationships will refer to questions of causation, association, and linearity. (For a more detailed method of statement analysis, refer to Chapter 11.)

As discussed in Chapter 11, causal relationships are those that specify that one concept always occurs as a direct result of the other concept. If any probability exists in the relationship whatsoever, it is not a true causal relationship (Hardy, 1974).

Associational relationships are those that specify that two concepts are related positively, negatively, or in no known way. This means that there is correlation between the two concepts but not causation. A positive association (+) indicates that both concepts vary together; that is, if one increases, so does the other. A negative association (−) indicates that the concepts vary inversely; that is, as one concept increases, the other concept decreases. When two concepts occur simultaneously but there is no known relationship, the statement is given a question mark (?) as designation.

Linearity is assumed until proven otherwise. It is by far the easiest relationship to determine and test. Linearity assumes that a change in one variable or concept quickly produces an arithmetic change in the other concept or variable. When the correlation coefficients are calculated, the correlation will be strong and the slope of best fit a straight line.

There are other types of relational linkages, however, that can be determined either by deduction or by using data analysis, such as curvilinearity or power curves (Hage, 1972). The most difficult one to determine by analysis is the curvilinear linkage. Curvilinearity assumes that as one concept increases, the other concept also increases until a certain point is reached; then the second concept begins to decrease. The classic example of curvilinearity is the inverted U-shaped curve discussed in Chapter 5. Curvilinearity may be deduced by examining the formal theoretical and relational statements, or it may be determined by statistical analysis of data. If there are small but significant correlation coefficients among the data, it is often useful to subject them to nonlinear analysis strategies to determine whether the relationships are nonlinear. Figure 12–1 shows models of the U, the inverted U, and the power curve.

The power curve shows an incremental relationship among concepts. That is, if one concept is shown to increase or decrease by a certain amount, the second concept changes at an accelerated rate in either a positive or a negative direction. Power curves are often called exponential curves because the changes in the second concept are often expressed mathematically in terms of exponents. Many of the system theories that use inputs and outputs also use power curves, as do some of the developmental and learning theories. Most power curves represent extensive periods (20 years or more) because they must take into account minor fluctuations and individual differences. Power curves can also be used to explain changes in interventions such as weight loss. Often weight plateaus after an initial loss but will move downward again if the level of exercise intensity, for example, increases (Chaput et al., 2007).

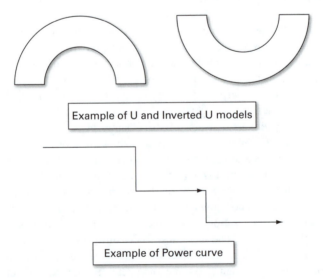

Example of U and Inverted U models

Example of Power curve

FIGURE 12–1 Models of the U, the inverted U, and the power curve.

Next, determine what boundaries are present for the theory. Boundaries have to do with the actual content of the theory. Some theories, like practice theories, for instance, have a very narrow focus and their boundaries, or limits, are clearly determined. In effect, a theory with narrow boundaries states exactly how far it can go in explaining specific phenomena and clarifying where the theory starts and stops. For example, a theory would have narrow boundaries if it addressed only a specific type of preoperative teaching for adults facing abdominal surgery in an American hospital.

A middle-range theory will have somewhat wider boundaries and will be more abstract than a narrow theory. The content may be very specific, but its application will encompass a wider group of events, or populations, than the narrow theory. An example might be a theory that speaks to several predictable effects from two preoperative teaching strategies on adult surgical patients.

A theory with wide boundaries is highly abstract, covers a large content area, and is applicable in a large number of cases. To extend our preoperative teaching example a bit further, a theory with wide boundaries might reflect the effects of any preoperative teaching strategies on any preoperative patients from any cultural background, regardless of age or diagnosis.

Next, determine whether the statements are used consistently. Look at all the statements: relational as well as existence and definitional. The theorist should use the statements in exactly the same way at all times. If this is not done, the theory loses credibility and becomes invalid for systematic use. And it is also very confusing for the reader!

Finally, assess the empirical support for the statements. Is there any? If not, the theory will have less validity than one that does. If research or empirical evidence exists to support the statements, the analyst must evaluate the strength of the evidence. Using the criteria for evaluating evidence-based practice research may help you here if you feel uncertain about evaluating strength of evidence. If the research studies are too numerous to review thoroughly, a generous sampling is permissible.

Determine from the reading how much research supports or refutes the statements in the theory. To do this, look at the hypotheses in the research studies. If they are in the null form, that is, stating that there will be no relationship among the variables and the research hypothesis is rejected, it supports the theory (Kerlinger, 1986). If the hypothesis is supported, implying no relationship, then it refutes the theory. This sounds confusing, but it is only a function of the way the logic works. Rejecting a null hypothesis is like stating a double negative in English grammar; two "nos" make a "yes." If the hypothesis is not in the null form but actually specifies a relationship, then if the hypothesis is rejected, it refutes the theory, and if it is accepted, it supports the theory.

Supporting evidence for a statement must be evaluated quantitatively as well as qualitatively. A brief series of questions is sufficient to give the analyst a general idea of the validity of the research. They are as follows (Kerlinger, 1986):

1. Do the research questions or hypotheses accurately reflect the theoretical concepts?

2. Are the sampling and sample size adequate for the method chosen?
3. Is the methodology sound and appropriate for the questions or hypotheses proposed?
4. Is the data analysis accurate and appropriate?
5. Are the results reported accurately?
6. Are the conclusions justified?
7. Is the study replicable?

If the answers to these questions are satisfactory, the support is sound. However, if one sound study is good as support for a statement, 4 or even 10 sound studies are that much better.

Logical Adequacy

Because this is basically a strategies book, we will not go as far as the linguistic philosophers in determining the logical adequacy of a theory. Linguistic philosophical analysis can get very complicated as it is based on formal logic. We will limit ourselves to only a few considerations: (1) Is there a system whereby predictions can be made from the theory independent of its content? (2) Can scientists in the discipline in which the theory is developed agree on those predictions? (3) Does the actual content make sense? (4) Are there obvious logical fallacies?

PREDICTIONS INDEPENDENT OF CONTENT   In several previous chapters, we have used letters of the alphabet and arrows with pluses or minuses over them to denote symbolically how concepts are related to each other. This is precisely the same kind of system that can be used to determine predictions from a theory that are independent of its content. That is, each of the concepts is given a meaningless label such as *A*, *B*, or *C* and then the relationships are diagrammed, as are the predictions that can be made from those relationships. This step is important when you are concerned with the logical structure of the theory. If the structure is not logical, predicted relationships may be fallacious. This is not to imply that the content itself is unimportant—only that at this time it is not considered.

Content is analyzed in the meaning steps and also in question 3 in this step. If the theory being analyzed cannot be examined in this way, it leaves much to be desired in terms of logical adequacy. This diagramming effort also points out unclear or unstudied relationships among concepts that are useful for further theory development or research. Below are several relational statements from a theory about the hearing accuracy of a barn owl (Knudsen, 1981).

1. An owl's strike accuracy deteriorates with increases in angle between sound source and head orientation.
2. An owl's ability to locate the origin of a sound is dependent on the presence of high frequencies in the sound.
3. The amount of sound amplification provided by the feathers of the facial ruff varies with the sound frequency.
4. The strike accuracy of the owl increases sharply as the number of frequencies in a sound is increased.

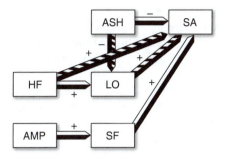

FIGURE 12–2 Diagram of statements 1 through 4 in the text.

As the original theory is stated, the outcome is strike accuracy. One should be alert to implied relationships. For example, logically the owl must be able to locate the sound source to improve strike accuracy. The statements may be restated as follows:

1. Angle of sound source and head orientation: (*ASH*) $\overset{-}{\rightarrow}$ strike accuracy (*SA*).
2. High frequencies in the sound: (*HF*) $\overset{+}{\rightarrow}$ location of origin (*LO*).
3. Amount of sound amplification: (*AMP*) $\overset{+}{\rightarrow}$ sound frequency (*SF*).
4. Number of sound frequencies: (*SF*) $\overset{+}{\rightarrow}$ strike accuracy (*SA*).

Once they are written and labels assigned, a diagram may be drawn as we have done in Figure 12–2. The relationships that have been specified in the theory are drawn with solid lines. Striped lines indicate the relationships that are implied. All other relationships are unknown.

Now look at Figure 12–3. This is similar to a correlation table, in which all the variables are listed horizontally as well as vertically and the sign of the relationship is placed in the correct box. Implied relationships are enclosed in parentheses.

As you can see, the matrix is easier to read and the implied relationships can be seen more clearly than in Figure 12–2. Either is acceptable if it helps you get the structure of the relationships clear. If neither is helpful or you feel confused, refer to Chapter 11 on statement analysis for additional help or review.

	SA	LO	AMP	ASH	HF	SF
SA	+	(+)	?	–	(+)	+
LO		+	?	(–)	+	?
AMP			+	?	?	+
ASH				+	?	?
HF					+	?
SF						+

FIGURE 12–3 Another type of matrix showing statements in Figure 12–2.

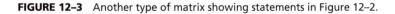

AGREEMENT OF SCIENTISTS   A theory must be sufficiently precise in its representation for scientists to agree on the predictions that can be made from it. If scientists cannot agree on the possible predictions, the theory is not useful in any scientific sense. If the theory is not scientifically useful, it cannot be added to any body of knowledge (except, of course, to the body of knowledge of things that don't work yet). For an excellent example of how to determine agreement among scientists, see Carter and Kulbok's (1995) evaluation of the Interaction Model of Client Health Behavior.

MAKING SENSE   A theory may make a great deal of sense to one scientist and no sense to another with a different background. For instance, a theory that makes sense to a maternity nurse may make little sense to one in cardiac care. If scientists with relevant and similar backgrounds all say the theory makes no sense, then it probably doesn't. For a theory to make sense, it must provide insights or understanding about a phenomenon. If it does not, perhaps the theorist needs to spend additional time simplifying or more clearly defining what the theory purports to demonstrate in order to meet the criterion of making sense.

LOGICAL FALLACIES   Look for logical fallacies. This is where the deductive or inductive origins of the theory become important. In a deductive theory, if all the premises are true and the deduction is valid, then the conclusions, or inferences, drawn from those premises are also true (Toulmin, 1958). Therefore, the analyst must determine whether or not the premises of the theory are true. This usually involves a brief review of literature and an evaluation of any supporting evidence to determine the truth of the premise. In this case, truth comes from the validity of the research on which the original premises are based. If the premises are correct, then the conclusion will also be correct.

In traditional philosophical analysis, there are three possible problems with an inductive theory: (1) the premises are correct, but the conclusion is incorrect; (2) the premises are incorrect, but the conclusion is correct; or (3) both premises and conclusion are incorrect (Toulmin, 1958). Again, the analyst must return to the literature and to evidence that supports or refutes the premises. In this case, the evidence will be logically inconclusive because the theory is inductive. The analyst will simply have to use the notion of the *preponderance of evidence* to determine the relative truth of the premises. If the evidence strongly supports the premises, one can assume truth for the purposes of analysis.

Because the truth of the premises does not guarantee the truth of the conclusion, determining the correctness of the conclusion is more difficult in an inductive theory. All the analyst can do here is examine the research that supports the conclusion for validity and determine whether the conclusion makes sense, given the stated premises and the research evidence. If the conclusion makes sense and if the research is valid and meets all the criteria for a good research study, then the analyst is justified in assuming that the conclusion is correct. If the conclusion fails to make sense or if the research is poor, no assumptions can be made at all about the conclusion. We simply will not know whether the conclusion is correct.

In more postmodern philosophy, there is less emphasis on the issue of inductive evidence of a theory's validity. Because much of grounded theory, for instance, is generated from inductive and often qualitative research, other criteria for validity are used for the research. For an in-depth discussion of this issue, Sandelowski's (1986) classic article is excellent. Other resources such as textbooks on qualitative research mentioned elsewhere in this book are also good. For the purposes of theory analysis, either set of criteria will work well to help you evaluate the soundness of the research evidence.

Inductive theory is always logically inconclusive; thus, we are always left a bit in doubt about the theory's validity. This doubt does not preclude our use of well-supported theory. It only serves to remind us that there may be a better explanation that has not been discovered yet.

Although the final four steps in theory analysis are not so rigorous or time consuming, they are an important part of a thorough analysis. There are several examples of theory analyses in the literature (Haigh, 2002; Henderson, 1995; Jacono, 1995; Jezewski, 1995; Linder, 2010).

Usefulness

If the theory provides new insights into a phenomenon, if it helps the scientist explain the phenomenon better or differently, or if it helps the scientist make better predictions, then it is a useful theory (Berthold, 1968). It adds significantly to the body of knowledge. If the theory does none of these things, it is not a useful theory. Usefulness of theory thus has to do with how helpful the theory is to the scientist in providing a sense of understanding about the phenomenon in question (Reynolds, 1971). For example, Skelly, Leeman, Carlson, Soward, and Burns (2008) examined the relevance and usefulness of the UCSF symptom management model for meeting the needs of African Americans with diabetes.

The analyst must consider three issues in determining usefulness: (1) How much research has the theory generated (Reynolds, 1971)? (2) To what clinical problem is the theory relevant (Barnum, 1998)? (3) Does the theory have the potential to influence nursing practice, education, administration, or research (Meleis, 1990)? It is at this point in the analysis that the *content* becomes important. An analyst cannot answer these three questions without considering the content of the theory. If the theory contains subject matter that is already in the scientific domain, it should shed new light on the phenomenon or should provide information that allows clarification, new predictions, or the exertion of control where none previously existed. If the theory covers subject matter that has not been in the scientific domain, it should make some significant difference in that field of science in which it was developed. The theory should generate a significant number of research studies if it is useful. It should be relevant, or at least *potentially* relevant, to a clinical practice setting. It should be capable of influencing, or potentially capable of influencing, nursing practice, education, administration, or research (Meleis, 1990). In the example above, Skelly et al. (2008) determined that the UCSF symptom management model was an innovative one for use in tailoring culturally sensitive interventions to increase diabetes self-care.

Generalizability

How widely the theory can be used in explaining or predicting phenomena reflects the criterion of generalizability or transferability (Lincoln & Guba, 1985). Generalizability can be determined by examining the boundaries of the theory and by evaluating the research that supports the theory. We have said earlier in this chapter that the boundaries of the theory are content related and have to do with how wide the focus of the content is. The wider the focus of a theory, the more generalizable it is likely to be. The more broadly it can be applied, the more generalizable it is. Feminist theorists and critical social theorists use a slightly different set of criteria to evaluate the transferability of a theory. For more detailed discussions of these theories and how they are to be evaluated, we recommend Lincoln and Guba (1985) or Hall and Stevens (1991).

The analyst must have some skills in research critique in order to determine the adequacy of theoretical support because the research evidence that supports the theory is important in determining generalizability. If the research evidence is sound, that is, valid and with adequate sample size, derived from diverse populations, and reproducible, the theory will be more generalizable than one in which there is little support or the research support is of poor quality. It is not our purpose here to provide research critique skills. Any good research textbook can be helpful to the reader who perceives a need for additional help.

Parsimony

A parsimonious theory is one that is elegant in its simplicity even though it may be broad in its content. Perhaps the best example of parsimony is from Einstein's theory of relativity, $E = MC^2$. This particular statement of the theory revolutionized physics and is very broad in its boundaries but is very simple in its expression. A parsimonious theory explains a complex phenomenon simply and briefly without sacrificing the theory's content, structure, or completeness.

Most theories, especially those in the behavioral sciences, cannot be reduced to such a mathematical model. The analyst must examine the theory to see if its formulations are as clear and as brief as they can be. The propositions or relational statements should be precise and should not overlap. If there are several statements, determine whether some of them could be reduced to one or two broader, more general, relational statements.

Many theorists provide graphics or models as a way of helping themselves and others visualize the relations of the concepts to each other. As we mentioned earlier, if such a model is provided, it should accurately reflect the verbal material in the theory. It must also actually help make the theory clearer. If it does not help clarify the verbal material, it is not a useful model and does not aid in increasing the parsimony of the theory.

Testability

We support the idea that for a theory to be truly valid, it must be testable at least in principle. This implies that hypotheses can be generated from the theory, research carried out, and the theory supported by the evidence or modified because of it. A theory that has strong empirical evidence to support it is a stronger theory than one that does not. If a theory cannot generate hypotheses, it is not useful to scientists and does not add to the body of knowledge. Thompson, Fazio, Kustra, Patrick, and Stanley (2016) conducted a scoping review and theory analysis of the use of complexity theory in health services research. Their findings demonstrated that complexity was defined in multiple ways and was operationalized very differently in the studies. Therefore, they concluded that generalizability was limited. Their conclusion was that the concepts needed clear and agreed upon definitions that could be used consistently before the theory would be very useful in health services research.

There has been some discussion over the years among philosophers of science as to whether or not the criterion of testability is crucial to theory (Hempel, 1965; Hempel, 1966; Popper, 1965; Reynolds, 1971). The debate seems to center on whether or not a theory that provides a great deal of understanding but that by its nature is untestable is a legitimate theory. We do not propose to enter this argument. It seems to us that even a theory that by its nature is untestable as a whole may yield testable hypotheses and relational statements that lend support to the total theory.

ADVANTAGES AND LIMITATIONS

The major advantage of theory analysis is the insight into relationships among the concepts and their linkages to each other that the strategy provides. In addition, the analysis strategy allows the theorist to see the strengths of the theory as well as its weaknesses. The theorist is then free to decide whether or not the theory is useful for practice or research or whether the theory needs additional testing and validation before use. Where a theory has untested linkages discovered through analysis, it is a spur to the theorist to test those linkages. This both strengthens the theory and adds to the body of knowledge. The major limitation of theory analysis is that analysis examines only parts and their relationship to the whole. It can expose only what is missing but cannot generate new information. In addition, theory analysis requires evaluation and criticism of supporting evidence. Where the analyst may be limited in the critical skills of research evaluation, important information regarding the soundness of a theory may be disregarded or misinterpreted. This results in a limited analysis and may yield unsatisfactory results.

UTILIZING THE RESULTS OF THEORY ANALYSIS

Theory analysis provides a means of systematic examination of the structure and content of theory for new insights into a phenomenon or to determine its strengths and weaknesses. But what does one do with the analysis when it is completed? The results of theory analysis can be very useful in education, practice, research, and theory development.

Theory analysis can be used very effectively in the classroom. We have used it successfully to teach students how to examine theories critically. Assigning a theory to a group of students to analyze and then having them report to the class often generates meaningful discussion and debate among the students. Another use of the results of theory analysis is in preparing conceptual frameworks for students' papers. Students have found theory analysis an excellent way to define gaps or inconsistencies in the knowledge about some phenomenon in which they are interested. Yet a third use of the results of theory analysis is in faculty development. As we proposed in the statement analysis chapter, having faculty discussions related to the results of theory analysis on a single topic of interest may generate many useful ideas to be used in curriculum design or in generating faculty research.

The results of theory analysis may provide the clinician with knowledge about the soundness of any theory being considered for adoption in practice. In addition, knowing which theoretical relationships are well supported provides guidelines for the choice of appropriate interventions and some indications of their efficacy. Given the current emphasis on evidence-based practice, the results of theory analysis will assist clinicians to determine whether or not a particular theory might be appropriate for their practice.

Theory analysis is particularly helpful in research because it provides a clear idea of the form and structure of the theory in addition to the relevance of content, and inconsistencies and gaps present. The missing links or inconsistencies are fruitful sources of new research ideas. They also point to the next hypotheses that need to be tested. In theory development, the inconsistencies, gaps, and missing links provide the stimulus to the theorist to keep on working. In addition, the results provide clues to the obvious next steps to be taken to refine the theory.

Summary

Theory analysis consists of systematically examining a theory for its origins, meaning, logical adequacy, usefulness, generalizability/parsimony, and testability. Each of these six steps stands alone in a theory analysis and yet each is related to the other. This paradoxical relationship is generated by the act of analysis itself. To do a thorough analysis, one must consider each of the steps, giving them all careful attention. Yet, the results of each of the steps are interdependent on the results of the others.

Like many of the strategies presented in this book, the steps of theory analysis are also iterative. That is, the analyst must go back and forth among the steps during the analysis in addition to moving sequentially through them.

For instance, the logical adequacy, usefulness, generalizability, parsimony, and testability of a theory will be affected if concepts are undefined and statements are only definitional in nature. If the meaning is adequately handled but the logical structure is missing or fallacious, then usefulness, generalizability, parsimony, and testability will be severely limited. If a theory is untestable and fails to generate hypotheses, it is not useful, generalizable, parsimonious, or particularly meaningful. So each step is independent and yet interdependent as well. It is this interdependence that makes the strategy so useful in theory construction. The analysis strategy provides a mechanism for determining the strengths and weaknesses of the theory prior to using it as a guide to practice or in research.

With theory analysis, linkages that have not been examined become obvious. This, in turn, should lead to additional testing, thus adding support to the theory or pointing out where modifications need to be made. The whole process is complex but the results are well worth the effort. It frequently leads to new insights about the theory being examined, thus adding to the body of knowledge.

Theory analysis, like all analysis strategies, is rigorous and takes time. It is also limited in that it does not generate new information outside the confines of the theory.

Finally, by pointing out where additional theoretical work is needed, theory analysis is a way of promoting additional theory construction. When pointing out where additional work is needed, however, it is helpful to remember that comparing anything to the ideal tends to stifle development (Zetterberg, 1965). The best approach is to compare the analyzed theory to similar theories at the same stage of development. To what extent does this theory meet the criteria as compared to others similar to it? Because most theories are generated in the context of discovery, it is more helpful to be encouraging than to be severely critical.

Practice Exercise 1

Read Younger's (1991) "A Theory of Mastery." It is a psychosocial nursing theory and is substantially middle range in focus. It is therefore suitable to use for your practice exercise.

Conduct a theory analysis. When you have completed your own analysis, compare it to the one below. Keep in mind that your analysis will probably be more comprehensive than the one we have included here. Our intention is to give you only clues as to the major strengths and weaknesses of the theory. The example we have provided is merely a sample to demonstrate each step. Remember that although one person's analysis may differ somewhat from another's, they may both be equally valid.

ORIGINS

Younger developed the theory of mastery in an effort to explain "how individuals who experience illness or other stressful health conditions and enter into a state of stress may emerge, not demoralized and vulnerable, but healthy and possibly stronger" (p. 77). In addition, she states that a second purpose was to explicate the theory base for the new instrument she is developing. The theory appears to be a deductive synthesis based on various philosophical and empirical works of others, but Younger is not explicit about whether it is a deductive system.

MEANING

1. The major concepts identified by Younger in addition to mastery are

   certainty
   change
   acceptance
   growth

   In addition to the five major concepts, Younger mentions several related concepts. These are coping, adjustment, efficacy, resilience, hardiness, and control. In each case, she attempts to identify how the related concepts are different from mastery.

   Not identified as a part of the theory or related concepts but discussed in the section on the definition of mastery are such concepts as quality of life, bonds of connectedness with others, stress, self-curing, self-caring, hypervigilance, compulsive repetition, sleep disturbance, fearfulness, passivity, and alienation. These concepts are part of the discussions about antecedents and consequences of mastery or the lack of achievement of mastery.

2. The major concepts certainty, change, acceptance, growth, and mastery are all carefully defined. Indeed, it appears from the discussion that all five have been subjected to concept analysis. As a result, these five concepts have excellent descriptive and theoretical definitions that are used consistently throughout the piece. There are no operational definitions given here. However, it appears that these may be forthcoming as one of the purposes of the article was to give a theory base for a new instrument.

3. The relational statements are harder to come by in this work than are the concepts. Each concept in the theory is described as a process that must be completed before mastery can be achieved. Below are the statements Younger makes explicitly (mainly on p. 87) about the relationships among the concepts:

   a. A critical dose of certainty is necessary for change and acceptance.
   b. Change and acceptance are necessary for growth to occur.
   c. Change, acceptance, and growth feed back to increase certainty.
   d. Change is sufficient for growth.
   e. Change and acceptance are dynamically interrelated.
   f. Acceptance, qualified, is sufficient for growth.
   g. Stress initiates the process of mastery.
   h. Mastery affects quality of life and wellness.

Each of the statements indicates a positive relationship. The boundaries are moderately wide. The theory is abstract but is sufficiently circumscribed to be considered a middle-range theory.

   The statements are all made toward the end of the article and are not used again once they are made. Therefore, no judgment can be made about the degree to which the author uses them consistently. One must look to later works to make this judgment.

   There is no empirical support given for any of the statements. There is some philosophical and historical background given as justification for them but no testing has been done as yet using this new theory.

LOGICAL ADEQUACY

1. It is possible to make predictions independent of content. The matrix shown in Figure 12–4 demonstrates where the predictions are specified and where they are implied. Some of the major concepts of the theory are included here, although there are several other relevant concepts mentioned in the narrative.

   certainty (CT), acceptance (A)
   stress (S), wellness (W)
   change (CG), growth (G)
   quality of life (QOL)

   Obviously, there are many implied, but unspecified, relationships in the theory. Some of the implied relationships are supported in other research in the field but are not indicated in Younger's article. Readers may also be interested in the analysis of the theory of mastery when it was merged with the theory of organismic integration (Fearon-Lynch & Stover, 2015).

2. We did not locate any direct tests of the theory and so agreement of scientists is probable but not confirmed by the use of the theory in others' work to date. However, the theory

	CT	CG	A	G	S	QOL	W
CT	+	+	+	+	(−)	(+)	(+)
CG		+	+	+	(−)	(−)	(−)
A			+	+	(−)	(+)	(+)
G				+	(−)	(+)	(+)
S					+	(−)	(−)
QOL						+	(+)
W							+

FIGURE 12–4   Matrix of concepts in theory of mastery.

was successfully applied to development of the Mastery of Stress instrument, which measures the theory concepts of certainty, change, acceptance, and growth (Younger, 1993). Although the theory is still untested, it is capable of test. Therefore, this criterion is met in principle but not in fact.

3. The theory makes sense as it is built on several sound philosophical and scientific traditions. It is appealing in its simplicity. However, it is a bit redundant of other similar theories. It is very close indeed to various theories of self-efficacy for instance.

4. There are no logical fallacies, although there are some logical relationships that as yet go unspecified and are only implied in the theory.

USEFULNESS

The theory has the potential to be useful. Even though it is somewhat similar to other theories of coping and self-efficacy, it is specifically focused on threats to health as a primary stressor. For this reason alone, it may prove very helpful to practitioners and researchers in nursing.

GENERALIZABILITY OR TRANSFERABILITY

The theory has relatively wide boundaries, but so far has not been tested or verified through research. Certainly it would apply to anyone experiencing stress, particularly health-related stress. Its potential for explanatory power is excellent.

PARSIMONY

The theory is relatively new and therefore is probably too parsimonious. It seems that there is a natural evolution or progression of new theories such that they often start small and parsimonious, grow substantially during the justification phases, and then are reduced to smaller and more parsimonious models over time. This theory may undergo substantial changes and revisions before it is considered to be adequately developed.

TESTABILITY

Given appropriate, reliable, and valid instruments to measure the concepts in this theory *as they are defined*, the theory is testable. The concepts are very carefully defined, so any instruments being considered for testing them should be examined carefully to be sure that they reflect the defining attributes of each of the concepts.

Practice Exercise 2

Choose a theory that interests you or is relevant to your research, preferably a mid-range theory. Perform a theory analysis.

> How well did the theory perform?
> Was the meaning clear and consistent?
> Was it logically adequate?
> Was it understandable and generalizable?
> Is it potentially useful?
>
> Did the analysis give you a different understanding of the theory?
> Are you still as interested in the theory as you were before the analysis?

References

Barnum B. *Nursing Theory: Analysis, Application, and Evaluation.* 5th ed. Philadelphia, PA: Lippincott Williams & Wilkins; 1998.

Berthold JS. Symposium on theory development in nursing. *Nurs Res.* 1968;17(3):196–197.

Carter KF, Kulbok PA. Evaluation of the Interaction Model of Client Health Behavior through the first decade of research. *Adv Nurs Sci.* 1995;18(1):62–73.

Chaput JP, Drapeau V, Hetherington M, Lemieux S, Provencher V, Tremblay A. Psychobiological effects observed in obese men experiencing body weight loss plateau. *Depress Anxiety.* 2007;24(7):518–521.

Chinn P, Jacobs M. *Theory and Nursing: A Systematic Approach.* 2nd ed. St. Louis, MO: Mosby; 1987.

Chinn P, Kramer M. *Integrated Theory and Knowledge Development in Nursing.* 8th ed. St Louis, MO: Mosby; 2014.

Cooley ME. Analysis and evaluation of the Trajectory Theory of Chronic Illness Management. *Sch Inq Nurs Pract.* 1999;13(2):75–95.

Dickoff J, James P, Wiedenbach E. Theory in a practice discipline, part I. *Nurs Res.* 1968a;17:415–435.

Dickoff J, James P, Wiedenbach E. Theory in a practice discipline, part II. *Nurs Res.* 1968b;17:545–554.

Fawcett J. A framework for analysis and evaluation of conceptual models of nursing. *Nurs Educ.* 1980;5(6):10–14.

Fawcett J. *Analysis and Evaluation of Conceptual Models of Nursing.* 2nd ed. Philadelphia, PA: Davis; 1989.

Fawcett J. *Analysis and Evaluation of Nursing Theories.* Philadelphia, PA: Davis; 1993.

Fawcett J. *Analysis and Evaluation of Conceptual Models of Nursing.* 3rd ed. Philadelphia, PA: Davis; 1995.

Fawcett J. *Analysis and Evaluation of Contemporary Nursing Knowledge: Nursing Models and Theories.* Philadelphia, PA: Davis; 2000.

Fawcett, J. *Contemporary Nursing Knowledge: Analysis And Evaluation of Nursing Models and Theories.* 2nd ed. Philadelphia, PA: F. A. Davis; 2005.

Fawcett J, DeSanto-Madeya S. *Contemporary Nursing Knowledge: Analysis and Evaluation of Nursing Models and Theories.* 3rd ed. Philadelphia, PA: Davis; 2013.

Fearon-Lynch JA, Stover CM. A middle-range theory for diabetes self-management. *Adv Nurs Sci.* 2015;38(4):330–346.

Hage J. *Techniques and Problems of Theory Construction in Sociology.* New York, NY: Wiley; 1972.

Haigh C. Using chaos theory: The implication for nursing. *J Adv Nurs.* 2002;37(5):462–469.

Hall JM, Stevens PE. Rigor in feminist research. *Adv Nurs Sci.* 1991;13(3):16–29.

Hardy M. Theories: Components, development, evaluation. *Nurs Res.* 1974;23(2):100–106.

Hempel CG. *Aspects of Scientific Explanation.* New York, NY: Free Press; 1965.

Hempel CG. *Philosophy of Natural Science.* Englewood Cliffs, NJ: Prentice Hall; 1966.

Henderson DJ. Consciousness raising in participatory research: Method and methodology for emancipatory nursing inquiry. *Adv Nurs Sci.* 1995;17(3):58–69.

Jacono BJ. A holistic exploration of barriers to theory utilization. *J Adv Nurs.* 1995;21(3):515–519.

Jezewski MA. Evolution of a grounded theory: Conflict resolution through culture brokering. *Adv Nurs Sci.* 1995;17(3):14–30.

Kerlinger F. *Foundations of Behavioral Research.* 3rd ed. New York, NY: Holt, Rinehart & Winston; 1986.

Knudsen EL. The hearing of the barn owl. *Sci Am.* 1981;245(6):113–125.

Lincoln YS, Guba EQ. *Naturalistic Inquiry.* Beverly Hills, CA: Sage Publications; 1985.

Linder L. Analysis of the UCSF symptom management theory: Implications for pediatric oncology nursing. *J Pediatr Oncol Nurs.* 2010;27(6):316–324.

Meleis A. *Theoretical Nursing: Development and Progress.* Philadelphia, PA: Lippincott; 1990.

Popper KR. *Conjectures and Refutations: The Growth of Scientific Knowledge.* New York, NY: Harper & Row; 1965.

Popper KR. *The Logic of Scientific Discovery.* New York, NY: Science Editions; 1961.

Reynolds PD. *A Primer in Theory Construction.* Indianapolis, IN: Bobbs-Merrill; 1971.

Sandelowski M. The problem of rigor in qualitative research. *Adv Nurs Sci.* 1986;8(3):27–37.

Skelly AH, Leeman J, Carlson J, Soward AC, Burns D. Conceptual model of symptom-focused diabetes care for African Americans. *J Nurs Scholarsh.* 2008;40(3):261–267.

Thompson DS, Fazio X, Kustra E, Patrick L, Stanley D. Scoping review of complexity theory in health services research. *BMC Health Serv Res.* 2016;16:87.

Toulmin S. *The Uses of Argument.* London, England: Cambridge University Press; 1958.

Wilson J. *Thinking with Concepts.* New York, NY: Cambridge University Press; 1969.

Younger JB. A theory of mastery. *Adv Nurs Sci.* 1991;14(1):76–89.

Younger JB. Development and testing of the mastery of stress instrument. *Nurs Res.* 1993;42(2):68–73.

Zetterberg HL. *On Theory and Verification in Sociology.* Totowa, NJ: Bedminster Press; 1965.

Additional Readings

Aldous J. Strategies for developing family theory. *J Marriage Fam.* 1970;32:250–257.

Blalock HM. *Theory Construction: From Verbal to Mathematical Formulations.* Englewood Cliffs, NJ: Prentice Hall; 1969.

Copi I, Cohen C, McMahon K. *Introduction to Logic.* 14th ed. New York, NY: Routledge; 2011.

Hanson NR. *Patterns of Discovery.* London, England: Cambridge University Press; 1958.

Hutchinson SA, Wilson HS. The theory of unpleasant symptoms and Alzheimer's disease. *Sch Inq Nurs Pract.* 1998;12(2):143–158.

Kaplan A. *The Conduct of Inquiry.* New York, NY: Chandler; 1964.

Lenz ER, Gift AG. Response to "The theory of unpleasant symptoms and Alzheimer's disease." *Sch Inq Nurs Pract.* 1998;12(2):159–162.

Lenz ER, Pugh LC, Milligan RA, Gift A, Suppe F. The middle-range theory of unpleasant symptoms: An update. *Adv Nurs Sci.* 1997;19(3):14–27.

Lenz ER, Suppe F, Gift F, Pugh LC, Milligan RA. Collaborative development of middle-range nursing theories: Toward a theory of unpleasant symptoms. *Adv Nurs Sci.* 1995;17(3):1–13.

Paley J. Benner's remnants: Culture, tradition and everyday understanding. *J Adv Nurs.* 2002;38(6):566–573.

Roberson MR, Kelley JH. Using Orem's theory in transcultural settings: A critique. *Nurs Forum.* 1996;31(3):22–28.

Silva MC. Response to "Analysis and evaluation of the trajectory theory of chronic illness management." *Sch Inq Nurs Pract.* 1999;13(2):96–109.

5

∎ ∎ ∎

Perspectives on Theory and Its Credibility

In this final part of the book, we broaden our view to look beyond the work of theory development to the processes of validating, testing, and refining theory. Rudner (1966) used the terms *context of discovery* and *context of justification*, respectively, to logically differentiate between the processes of developing and evaluating ideas. We, too, believe it can be useful to distinguish between the processes of theory development and processes of testing and validation, which aid in evaluating the soundness of theories. For example, theoretical ideas often are formulated without immediate knowledge of their ultimate usefulness or accuracy. Prematurely evaluating such preliminary theoretical work can lead to rejection of a promising idea and stifle the creative process. Evaluation of more mature theory, on the other hand, serves to highlight its strengths and weaknesses by examining the outcomes of theory testing and comparing the theory with other criteria, such as logical consistency. An integral part of evaluation of a theory or its related concepts and statements is validating and testing such work. Because the processes of developing, testing, revising, and further developing theoretical ideas are often ongoing, there is no final hard-and-fast line between the *context of discovery* and *context of justification* in the life of a given theoretical project.

Nonetheless, having some benchmarks for testing and validating theoretical work can be useful. Thus, in Chapter 13, we focus on testing concepts, statements, and theories. This is an important activity in the evolving theoretical basis for the nursing discipline. Theory testing involves logical operations, empirical research, and thoughtful interpretation of findings—all of which are briefly addressed in the final chapter that follows. We also present four principles to bear in mind in the process of theory testing. The aftermath of theory testing often leads to further development of the theoretical project. So the work begins anew. As Smith (2005) has noted, "[N]o theory is ever fully proved or disproved" (p. 397).

REFERENCES

Rudner R. *Philosophy of Social Science.* Englewood Cliffs, NJ: Prentice Hall; 1966.

Smith GT. On construct validity: Issues of method and measurement. *Psychol Assess.* 2005;17:396–408.

13

■ ■ ■

Assessing the Credibility and Scope of Nursing Knowledge Development: Concepts, Statements, and Theories

Questions to consider before you get started reading this chapter:

▶ Now that you have developed a concept, set of statements, or a theoretical model, are you grappling about the next step to evaluate your work?

▶ Are you confused about whether testing of nursing ideas should take place through use in practice or through structured research?

▶ Are you trying to link what you know from research classes with producing evidence that contributes to nursing knowledge and practice?

▶ Given that nursing research is entering its 7th decade, are you wondering what advances and understandings have been achieved?

Introductory Note: Shifting gears from theory development to theory testing can be both exhilarating and trying. Readers should be aware that they may experience a feeling of being at sea. Despite having taken research methods courses, the specific methods of concept, statement, and theory testing may not be easily extracted from those didactic experiences. Thus, in this chapter, we have aimed at providing a bridge between research methods and the testing of fruits from concept, statement, and theory development efforts. Because these intellectual products may vary widely, there is no one method that can be applied to all cases. As always, judgment is involved. In closing, we note that scholarly knowledge development in nursing is reaching into its 7th decade. Thus, we end this chapter with a brief commentary on the scope and central concerns of nursing as a scholarly practice discipline.

A GLANCE AT CONCEPT, STATEMENT, AND THEORY TESTING

The preceding chapters have covered the context, terminology, and strategies of theory development. In this chapter, we shift our emphasis to the vital next phase of testing that follows the initial development of concepts, statements, and theory. Although *testing* and *empirical validation* are similar terms, their usage may vary. Often validation is used in the context of efforts to substantiate concepts and their defining attributes, whereas testing is used in efforts to substantiate statements and theories. However, these characteristic uses of the two terms do not preclude permutations, such as validating concepts in the process of theory testing. Figure 13–1 presents a model of the phases in the development of nursing science. The first phase depicted in the model includes developing concepts, statements, and theories in nursing. The subsequent phases comprise testing, revision, and retesting of the theory and demonstrate the continuing nature of building the theory base for nursing.

In this chapter, we assume that the concept, statement, or theory that has been the focus of a theorist's developmental activities is of sufficient import to warrant testing. Along this line, the noted methodologist Marx (1963) observed:

> We need to recognize most explicitly that both discovery and confirmation are necessary to effective scientific work. The most ingenious theories are limited [sic] value until empirical tests are produced; the best confirmed proposition is of little value unless it deals with meaningful variables. (p. 13)

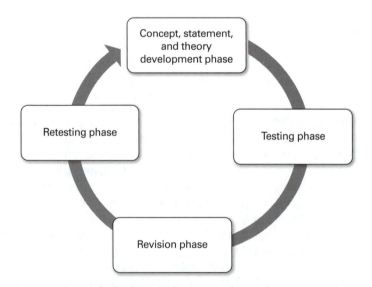

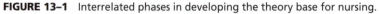

FIGURE 13–1   Interrelated phases in developing the theory base for nursing.

Furthermore, it is important to remember that the topic of concept, statement, and theory testing is embedded in diverse philosophical issues about the nature of science, scientific knowledge, and research methodologies. Some of these issues have been briefly profiled in Chapter 1. Although exposition of such issues is not possible here, interested readers may find the following classic sources useful: Coward (1990) on worldviews of scientific inquiry; Schumacher and Gortner (1992) on misconceptions in nursing about traditional science; Silva and Sorrell (1992) on alternative approaches (critical reasoning, personal experience, and application to practice) for testing nursing theories; and Weaver and Olson (2006) on pluralistic methods within a larger program of integrative approaches to nursing science.

Finally, although the topics of concept, statement, and theory testing are presented in separate sections below to permit us to highlight the focal concerns for each type of testing, there is much overlap between these activities. Consequently, Table 13–1 presents four broad principles that pertain to concept, statement, and theory testing. Several principles address the interrelatedness of concept, statement, and theory testing. For example, according to Principle 1, validation of concepts within a theory has implications for the theoretical network as a whole. During concept validation, the location and linkages of a concept in a theory may change,

TABLE 13–1 General Principles Related to Testing of Theoretical Works

Principle	Implications of Principle		
	Concept Testing	Statement Testing	Theory Testing
1. Theoretical terms are usually interconnected within a network so that a sharp line between concept and theory testing is often not practical (see Hempel, 1966).	×	×	×
2. The logic of testing hypotheses in the form of statements or theoretical models, including use of auxiliary hypotheses, renders all test conclusions tentative (see Hempel, 1966; Smith, 2005).		×	×
3. The processes of theory testing and determining the construct validity of instruments used in theory testing are interrelated (see Cronbach & Meehl, 1967; Smith, 2005).	×	×	×
4. Theory testing is not locked to only one type of data or testing method, but may embrace qualitative and quantitative approaches depending on the purposes of the study.	×	×	×

which in turn alters the theory as a whole. An example of this occurs in Stuifbergen and Rogers' (1997) validation of concepts within a theory of health promotion for persons with chronic disabling conditions, which is discussed later in this chapter. The work of Stuifbergen and Rogers also demonstrates that qualitative methods, not just quantitative ones, may be involved in testing or validating aspects of theories (Principle 4). Still other principles addressed in Table 13–1 include the tentative nature of conclusions based on statement testing (Principle 2) and the iterative and reciprocal nature (Principle 3) of theory testing and construct validity of measures used in theory testing (Smith, 2005).

CONCEPT TESTING

Concepts have been a focal point of theoretic activity because they are critical in delineating problems or phenomena in clinical practice. Concepts such as insufficient milk supply (Gatti, 2008; Hill & Humenick, 1989), chronic fatigue (Bryant, Walton, & Phillips, 2015; Potempa, Lopez, Reid, & Lawson, 1986; Renner & Saligan, 2016), and chronic dyspnea (Bull, 2014; McCarley, 1999) are ones that have been of long-standing and continuing interest in nursing scholarship and practice. Whether concepts originate from synthesis of observations, derivation from other fields, analysis of existing ideas, or still other methods, it is often necessary to empirically validate the existence and clinical relevance of the concept and its purported properties. Even if a concept is embedded in a loose network of related concepts, it is sometimes useful to focus first on the empirical validation of that concept, especially if it is critical to developing a continuing program of research. Revising a concept embedded within a larger network, however, may necessitate modification of the network itself. For example, based on qualitative interviews, Stuifbergen and Rogers (1997) relocated the concept of demands of illness from a component of perceptual factors to barriers in their theoretical model of health promotion among persons with chronic disabling conditions.

Empirical validation of concepts is guided by three questions (see Box 13–1). Gathering the evidence to answer these questions and weighing that evidence as it supports or fails to support the credibility, relevance, and clarity of the concept is not a black-and-white or one-time matter. That is, new evidence may call into question earlier judgments. Further, by their very nature these three questions are directed at concepts in general and, thus, may not be well suited to every type of concept. User discretion is advised!

First, a working definition of a concept is required in order to determine whether there is evidence that the concept represents a phenomenon in reality. If possible, the definition should specify preliminary conceptual attributes of the concept as well as indicators so that instances of the concept can be identified. This definition can then be used to search the literature for supportive evidence as well as to design concept validation studies (see Waltz, Strickland, and Lenz [2010] for an example of how to operationalize concepts and Pedhazur and Schmelkin [1991] on construct validation).

BOX 13–1 Three Questions to Guide Concept Validation

Question 1. Is there evidence (and if so how strong and reliable is the evidence) that the concept represents a phenomenon in reality?

Question 2. What evidence is there that the concept is relevant to practice, in terms of client needs, clinical outcomes, or other meaningful clinical criteria?

Question 3. What evidence supports the purported attributes of the concept (Pedhazur and Schmelkin call these "reflective indicators" [1991, p. 54])?

A historical example with great influence for nursing care illustrates what is involved in validating if a concept truly represents a phenomenon in reality. Klaus and Kennell (1976) and Klaus et al. (1972) proposed that the concept of bonding—biologically based maternal behavior—applied to humans similar to its occurrence in animals. They noted that in animals, separating mother and offspring immediately after birth was associated with "deviant behavior" (Klaus et al., 1972, p. 460). What was unknown was whether the "bonding" concept represented a phenomenon that also occurred in human mothers. By providing an opportunity for extended contact shortly after birth (their operational definition of the conditions necessary for bonding to occur), Klaus et al. tested for the existence of attachment in human mothers. In noting later that mothers who had extra contact responded differently to their infants, they took that evidence to support a concept of human mother–infant bonding (Klaus & Kennell, 1976). As additional evidence accumulated and was evaluated critically by others, however, Klaus and Kennell (1982) modified their claims about the existence of bonding in humans to include broader origins than just the biological ones. Thus, the original Klaus and Kennell bonding concept was altered as additional evidence accrued.

Concept validation may also be part of a larger program of theory testing. For example, Lee and Winters (2004) included concept validation in their qualitative study testing rural nursing theory. They accomplished this by conducting a qualitative study "to explore the health perceptions and needs" of rural workers. The "concepts emerging from this study [were then compared] with those in a rural nursing theory base" (p. 51). Thus, concept validation may lead to some revision in concepts and the theories within which concepts are embedded (Principle 1 in Table 13–1).

Second, even if a concept appears to represent some phenomenon in reality, such existence in itself does not render the concept of high relevance to practice. That is, there must also be a good reason to believe that the introduction of the concept into scientific discourse can aid in meeting—at some level—the practice aims of the nursing discipline. One might ask:

1. What client needs does a concept address?
2. What guidance does the concept give to the content of nursing actions?
3. What clinical outcomes are clarified or enhanced by virtue of the insight provided by the concept?
4. How does the concept contribute to nursing knowledge development?

Evidence of relevance to practice may come from many sources. These include, but are not limited to, existing literature that identifies problems needing conceptual solutions, opinions of expert clinicians in the area the concept has relevance to, and perceptions of nursing clients. The long and continuing endurance of the concepts of insufficient milk supply, chronic fatigue, and chronic dyspnea cited earlier in this chapter attests to their continuing relevance to practice.

Third, evidence related to attributes of a concept clarifies the dimensions, components, or other features that are essential to that concept (see Chapter 10 regarding defining attributes of concepts). Procedures and methods for testing attributes of a concept have been extensively developed in relation to the areas of tests and measurement (see Pedhazur & Schmelkin, 1991; Waltz et al., 2010) and nursing diagnosis development and validation (see Appoloni, Herdman, Napoleao, de Carvalho, & Hortense, 2013; Avant, 1979; Fehring, 1986; Gordon & Sweeney, 1979). These respective literatures provide in-depth treatment of attribute validation. Our intent here is to give general guidelines for concept-attribute testing.

To facilitate concept testing, the theorist should specify in advance (1) whether the purported attributes are all equally central to the concept and (2) whether there is a hierarchical structure to attributes. By making a clear proposal about concept attributes, it is easier to interpret the results of testing. Further, testing and interpretation of results can be done with greater clarity if the theorist specifies the likely antecedents of the concept (called "formative indicators" by Pedhazur and Schmelkin [1991, p. 54]) in contrast to its defining attributes (Pedhazur and Schmelkin's "reflective indicators"). Stating in advance the boundaries of a concept and its attributes (see Chapter 10 on concept analysis) with a specific population is also helpful. Wide applicability makes a concept more useful. Initial careful testing with delimited populations, however, can aid in differentiating poorly identified attributes of a concept from later differences stemming from variations in its presentation in different populations. The work of Whitley (1997) illustrates the process of validating attributes of the nursing diagnoses of anxiety and fear in medical–surgical and psychiatric patients, as does Alfradique de Souza, Santana, and Cassiano's (2015) validation of the differences between the diagnoses impaired memory and chronic confusion. Subsequently, areas of difference in attributes can be tested in new groups (e.g., see Fry and Nguyen's [1996] test of the symptoms of depression in Australian and Vietnamese groups).

Attribute testing may take many forms. One of the most common is generating items that reflect discrete instances of the various attributes of a concept and subsequently analyzing these items through statistical procedures such as factor analysis. Such analysis aids in determining whether purported attributes indeed can be demonstrated empirically. In many respects, the processes of concept testing and instrument development overlap. For some practice-based concepts, such as confusion (Nagley & Byers, 1987), more clinically relevant methods of testing are needed. Nagley and Byers proposed the idea of clinical construct validity wherein "a test reflects the clinical correlates that comprise a phenomenon as viewed from the nursing perspective in nursing situations" (p. 619). For an example of testing defining attributes in the context of nursing diagnoses related to respiratory function, see Carlson-Catalano et al. (1998).

As noted in the introduction to this chapter, we consider concept, statement, and theory testing separately to distinguish among each type of testing, but frequently there is overlap among them. Often a concept is the focal point for theoretical work, but the concept itself may be seen by the theorist as occurring within a network of other concepts. The stage of evolution of a program of scholarship determines whether it is more useful to approach testing as concept-, statement-, or theory-focused.

STATEMENT TESTING

Testing the empirical validity of statements is probably the form of testing with which readers are most familiar. Research texts (see Polit & Beck, 2012) typically present hypotheses to be tested as statements of relationships between two or more variables. Depending on the nature of the concepts linked in statements, those statements usually are tested in descriptive–correlational or experimental designs. It is generally easier to demonstrate that evidence supports an association among concepts than it is to demonstrate that the association is causal in nature. This is because establishing a causal relationship requires use of methods that rule out other explanations for the findings. Application of such methods can be challenging, costly, or, in some cases, impossible for ethical reasons. Readers should refer to extant research texts for guidance in designing and conducting hypothesis-testing research.

In testing statements, the measures or indicators of concepts should be selected with great care. If a measure is not a good reflective indicator (Pedhazur & Schmelkin, 1991) of a concept, misleading conclusions can be made about the credibility of the statement being tested. On the other hand, when evidence from a study supports a statement being tested, it increases scientists' confidence about the credibility of the statement as well as the validity of measures used in the testing process (see Principle 3 in Table 13–1). Still, it is important to remember that judgments about the overall credibility of statements depend on the quantity and quality of accumulated evidence. As a result, not one study but the accumulated evidence across studies is usually considered in determining the credibility of a statement.

Drawing conclusions about the credibility of statements tested in various types of research is not a new aspect of inquiry in nursing or health sciences. For example, Susser (1991) weighed the thoroughness and quality of evidence about the causal relationship between maternal nutrition and infant birth weight, a long-standing outcome of interest to nurses and other health professionals. Among the conclusions of that review were the following: "Prenatal diet affects birth weight most, as it does maternal weight, in the third trimester in women starving and acutely hungry . . . Effects are otherwise more modest and conditional" (p. 1394). In a more recent study on air pollution reported in *Nursing Research*, Longo (2009) noted that, "Epidemiological results support the current . . . [hypothesis] that air pollution is associated with adverse cardiovascular functioning" (p. 29). Credibility of statements such as these may increase or decrease if new, high-quality evidence becomes available. What constitutes high-quality evidence may vary with the statement being tested. For example, randomized clinical trials may be appropriate for testing statements about the efficacy of clinical interventions but ill-suited for testing predictive statements about health disparities of groups.

Testing statements is an integral part of developing evidence-based practice. As repeated affirmative tests of a statement (usually framed as a research hypothesis in a study) accumulate, these tests lend increasing validity to the statement. For example, in a systematic review of studies related to weight management, an expert panel report from the National Heart, Lung, and Blood Institute (2013) rated the following statement to have high supporting evidence:

> With dietary intervention in overweight and obese adults, average weight loss is maximal at 6 months with smaller losses maintained for up to 2 years while treatment and follow-up tapers. Weight loss achieved by dietary techniques aimed at reducing daily energy intake ranges from 4 to 12 kg at a 6-month follow-up. Thereafter, slow weight regain is observed, with a total weight loss of 4 to 10 kg at 1 year and 3 to 4 kg at 2 years (p. 56).

By contrast, the following statement was rated as having low strength of evidence:

> In overweight and obese adults, when compared to typical protein diets (15 percent of total calories), high-protein diets (25 percent of total calories) do not result in more beneficial effects on CVD risk factors in the presence of weight loss and other macronutrient changes (p. 58).

Increasing supportive evidence leads to greater confidence in the credibility of a statement. Evidence statements in clinical guidelines are examples of statements about relationships related to health and health care and their associated level of evidence.

In another example salient to hospital-based nursing care, the Agency of Healthcare Research and Quality released an evidence report on staffing and patients' quality of care. After extracting relevant studies and weighing the evidence, the authors summarized one of their conclusions in the following statement: "Greater nurse staffing was associated with better outcomes in intensive care units and in surgical patients" (Kane, Shamliyan, Mueller, Duval, & Wilt, 2007, p. v). As shown by this example, an evidence report is based on patterns of evidence summarized across studies. Although an individual study usually is not sufficient to establish the credibility of an evidence statement, each study does contribute to the cumulative results needed for evidence-based conclusions to guide practice or policy.

Finally, keep in mind that there is not always a hard-and-fast line between concept, statement, and theory testing. For example, although a theory can be tested as a whole in some cases, it is often more feasible to test selected statements from a theory. Thus, statement testing may be part of a larger theory-testing enterprise. As a result, many of the concerns identified in the next section on theory testing also can apply to testing theoretically derived statements.

THEORY TESTING

Scope and Criteria for Theory Testing

Theory-testing research has been conducted in diverse nursing contexts: health promotion (Shin, Kang, Park, Cho, & Heitkemper, 2008); preventive care of women (Ehrenberger, Alligood, Thomas, Wallace, & Licavoli, 2002) and men (Nivens, Herman, Weinrich, & Weinrich, 2001); children's (Yeh, 2002), adolescents' (Verchota & Sawin, 2016), and older adults' health (Zauszniewski, Chung, & Krafcik, 2001); chronic illness care related to cancer (Berger & Walker, 2001), HIV (Bova, 2001), and heart disease (Beckie, Beckstead, & Webb, 2001); nursing performance (Doran, Sidani, Keatings, & Doidge, 2002); ethnically diverse populations (Jennings-Dozier, 1999; Villarruel & Denyes, 1997); and various countries (Demerouti, Bakker, Nachreiner, & Schaufeli, 2000; Kim, Reed, Hayward, Kang, & Koenig, 2011) and geographic communities (McCullagh, Lusk, & Ronis, 2002). Given its ubiquitous nature, it is important to understand this important dimension of nursing knowledge validation.

Theory testing is challenging because of the greater complexity of relationships inherent in theories compared to statements (e.g., see Figure 9–1 in the chapter on theory synthesis). Furthermore, assessing the empirical validity of a theory in nursing was hampered by lack of clarity about what constitutes sound theory-testing research. Consequently, Silva (1986) proposed seven evaluation criteria that studies aimed at testing conceptual models (grand theories) should ideally meet. Her work is particularly important because it has provided methodological reference points that have been missing from most previous literature on theory testing. Thus, our understanding of what constitutes adequate theory testing was sharpened by her work. Because the concern in this section is with testing a wide variety of middle-range theories that may inform us about nursing phenomena, we have adapted Silva's (1986) criteria to fit this more specific application:

1. The purpose of the study is to determine the empirical validity of a designated theory's assumptions or propositions (internal theoretical statements).
2. The theory is explicitly stated as the rationale for the theory-testing research.
3. The theory's internal structure (key propositions and their interrelationships) is explicitly stated so that its relationship to study hypotheses is clear.
4. The study hypotheses are clearly deduced from the theory's assumptions or propositions.
5. The study hypotheses are empirically tested in an appropriate research design using sound and relevant instruments and suitable study participants.
6. As a result of the empirical testing, evidence exists in support of the validity or invalidity of the designated assumptions or propositions of the theory.
7. This evidence is considered specifically as it supports, refutes, or explains relevant aspects of the theory.

Even these criteria are lacking in one regard, though. Consider that it is conceivable that hypotheses derived from a theory are compatible with it as well as other related theories and, additionally, that the hypotheses are consistently shown to be congruent with empirical observations. For example, the hypothesis that poor persons will experience more health problems than wealthy ones is compatible with several theoretical models. Similarly, predicting on theoretical grounds that patients receiving individualized nursing intervention will demonstrate more skill in self-care than those receiving routine care may be derivable from a number of theories. Further, testing hypotheses such as any of the above carries a low risk for any theories from which they are derived because they would be expected to be supported by the data. Indeed, both of the examples given are vague hypotheses that would be difficult to reject. Thus, theory testing is more complex than simply deriving hypotheses and testing them. Not only must researchers be able to derive hypotheses, but they should also do so in a way that puts a theory at high risk for falsification (Popper, 1965).

To be falsifiable, a theory must be able to predict with enough specificity that empirical results that are incompatible with the theory can be derived clearly (Fawcett, 1999, p. 95). In a classic example, Wallace (1971) illustrates this principle in operation.

> *For a simple example, the hypothesis that "all human groups are either stratified or not stratified" is untestable in principle because it does not rule out any logically possible empirical findings. The hypothesis that "all human groups are stratified," however, is testable because it asserts that the discovery of an unstratified human group, though logically possible, will not in fact occur. (p. 78)*

To repeat an old adage: A theory that predicts everything predicts nothing. Or, in the words of Popper (1965), "Every 'good' scientific theory is a prohibition: it forbids certain things to happen. The more a theory forbids, the better it is" (p. 36). Thus, we add still another criterion for theory testing:

8. The hypotheses used to test a specific theory are designed to put the theory at risk for falsification by virtue of their specificity and compatibility with only a limited set of outcomes.

Consistent with this last criterion, the more specific the predictions are that can be made from a theory, the more readily it can be falsified and the narrower the range of data that will support the theory.

In testing theories, the theorist must judge how well the results of testing fit with the theories. As theoretical predictions increase in precision, the judgment about "fit" becomes less ambiguous and less arbitrary (Blalock, 1979). Further, if the testing of highly specific hypotheses results in data that are very consistent with predictions, the theory is judged to be both falsifiable and empirically valid. Consider the following examples. The prediction that "*A* is associated with *B*" is less specific than the prediction that "in every case of *B*, it is preceded by the occurrence of *A*." As hypotheses formulated in nursing research move increasingly from the former type to the latter, the falsifiability of theories will increase.

Another dimension complicating theory testing (Principle 2 in Table 13–1) is assumptions made in designing testing conditions (Hempel, 1966, pp. 19–32). These assumptions are taken to be true and constitute what Hempel called *auxiliary assumptions*, or *auxiliary hypotheses* (p. 23). Assumptions include a wide range of explicit and implicit beliefs such as (1) adequate reliability and validity of measurement procedures used, (2) absence of contaminating circumstances during data collection, and

(3) accuracy of any scientific facts or theories assumed to be true in designing the research procedures. When results support a theory, the theorist erroneously may have discounted an alternate explanation of the results. Conversely, when results do not support a theoretical prediction, an error may lie not in the theory itself but in assumptions made related to the testing conditions. Thus, no one test will definitively refute or substantiate a theory. Theory testing is rather the weight of accumulated testing results in varied researches with greater weight given to more rigorous tests.

Replication of research that tests a promising theory is consequently a strategic aspect in building nursing science. Consequently, empirical validity is a conditional quality of theories; it is tied to the existing evidence pertinent to the theory. As further research is done, a theory that was judged empirically valid at one time may be considered less valid at a later time. Thus, as additional tests of a theory provide evidence that is compatible or incompatible with theoretical predictions, judgments about the empirical validity of the theory may change.

Examples of Theory Testing in Nursing

Tsai, Tak, Moore, and Palencia's (2003) theory-testing research illustrates many of the aspects of theory development and testing: linkages between grand theories and middle-range theories, specifying relationships in the theoretical model, applying appropriate testing procedures, and theory revision. These researchers used the Roy adaptation model as a framework to explicate a middle-range theory of chronic pain among older adults with arthritis. In their theory, the concepts of chronic pain (focal stimulus), disability and social support (contextual stimuli), and age and gender (residual stimuli) influence daily stress and subsequently depression among older adults with arthritis. Tests of the initial theory with path analysis showed that the theory had acceptable fit with the data and overall explained 35 percent of the variance in depression. Still, two individual paths were not statistically significant: those from age and gender to daily stress. Thus, the middle-range theory was subsequently revised by eliminating these two nonsignificant paths. Table 13–2 presents additional examples of theory-testing studies.

TABLE 13–2   Examples of Theory-Testing Research Articles

Author(s)	Article Title
Hoffman et al. (2009)	Testing a theoretical model of perceived self-efficacy for cancer-related fatigue self-management and optimal physical functional status
Ryan, Weiss, Traxel, and Brondino (2011)	Testing the integrated theory of health behavior change for postpartum weight management
Covell and Sidani (2013)	Nursing intellectual capital theory: testing selected propositions
Vellone et al. (2013)	Structural equation model testing the situation-specific theory of heart failure self-care
Verchota and Sawin (2016)	Testing components of a self-management theory in adolescents with type 1 diabetes mellitus

Johnson, Ratner, Bottorff, and Hayduk's (1993) classic study further illustrates the complexity of the theory-testing process. One of the purposes of the study was to test an early version of the Pender (1987) health promotion model (HPM). The HPM specified that two sets of factors (modifying factors and cognitive–perceptual factors) and cues to action influence the likelihood of health-promoting behaviors. The demographic characteristics indirectly influence health promotion behaviors by modifying cognitive–perceptual factors. Johnson et al. (1993) focused on three cognitive–perceptual factors hypothesized to directly influence health promotion behaviors: perceived control of health, perceived self-efficacy, and perceived health status. They focused on two modifying factors: demographic characteristics and biological characteristics.

Johnson et al. (1993) used structural equation modeling as the data analytic method because it was "the only means by which a simultaneous test of multiple variables can be accomplished" (p. 132). Although they used a delimited set of variables in their test, they argued that the components they selected "must fit the data if the overall model is to succeed" (p. 133). Tests of the HPM were carried out using a national health survey of over 1,000 adults. Johnson et al. reported that, "the model failed to explain observed relationships" (p. 136). The investigators noted that, contrary to the HPM, modifying factors exerted direct effects on health promotion behaviors. Finally, the investigators concluded that, "the causal structure of the HPM must be reconsidered with a view to fully specifying all of the key factors that affect health-promoting lifestyle and their interrelationships" (p. 138).

The discrepant findings reported by Johnson et al. (1993) point to the final problem faced by the theorist and researcher: How to best interpret the findings. Was the theory essentially "wrong," or were the testing conditions and related auxiliary assumptions in the testing situation in error? For example, in the theory test conducted by Johnson et al., most variables were measured by one-item indicators: Were these items valid and reliable indicators of the theory concepts? This question reflects one of the testing principles presented at the outset of this chapter: the interrelatedness of theory testing and instrument validity (Principle 3 in Table 13–1).

An additional challenge that may occur in theory-testing research is the need to create new measurement scales to test the theory. This may occur when a theory is new and suitable measures have yet to be developed, or when the theory is applied to a problem that requires context-specific measures. For example, self-efficacy is a concept that occurs in a number of theories, but self-efficacy measures need to fit the specific health situation, such as self-efficacy for carrying out needed dietary and exercise behaviors for weight loss.

Although it is customary to associate theory testing with quantitative methods, such a view is too restrictive. Qualitative methods may also be applied to theory testing and concept validation efforts. Examples of such applications include the previously mentioned research of Stuifbergen and Rogers (1997) related to a model of health promotion in chronic illness and Lee and Winters (2004) related to rural nursing theory.

One cautionary note must be made with regard to theory testing. Powerful statistical methods, such as structural equation modeling, now exist to test the fit of a model with available data (Tabachnick & Fidell, 2013). Through model modification, it is possible to achieve successively better fits of a model with the data. Data-derived

BOX 13–2   Applying Criteria for Theory Testing to an Article

Select an article that purports to test a theory, such as either of the following, which may be accessed at the links listed below:

- Hoffman AJ, von Eye A, Gift AG, Given BA, Given CW, Rothert M. Testing a theoretical model of perceived self-efficacy for cancer-related fatigue self-management and optimal physical functional status. *Nurs Res.* 2009;58(1):32–41. Available at https://www.ncbi.nlm.nih.gov/pmc/articles/PMC3108333/pdf/nihms100201.pdf
- Ryan P, Weiss M, Traxel N, Brondino M. Testing the integrated theory of health behavior change for postpartum weight management. *J Adv Nurs.* 2011;67(9):2047–2059. Available at https://www.ncbi.nlm.nih.gov/pmc/articles/PMC4547450/

Critically examine the article:

- First, did the authors test the overall theory, or just a part of it? Did the authors add concepts not already in the theory or change the theory before testing? If so, why was this done?
- Look at each of the eight criteria for theory testing presented in this chapter. Which ones were most clearly met, and which were least met?
- Were there difficulties the authors encountered in conducting the theory-testing research, such as lack of pre-existing validated measures, sample attrition, or small sample size?
- What limitations did the authors report that may have affected the validity of the theory testing?
- Did the authors recommend changes in the theory as a result of the testing?

model modifications, however, shift the context from justification to discovery. In other words, using the data to simultaneously test and then rebuild and retest a model undermines the credibility of theory testing. Such work should be considered developmental. Box 13–2 presents an exercise for interested readers to deepen understanding of theory testing and difficulties that may be encountered.

Finally, theories are more comprehensive in scope than individual statements of relationships. Consequently, theories provide a potentially broader impact on practice and research than an individual evidence statement or a specific clinical guideline. That is, theories that are well supported by evidence move the practice and research of a discipline by influencing how practitioners and researchers think about problems related to health and nursing care and the way solutions are sought. For example, in the science of human health behavior change there is now a wealth of behavioral theories to guide intervention studies (National Cancer Institute, 2005). Thus, interventions to change health behaviors are usually couched in terms of one or more of these guiding theories. Nursing as a somewhat younger science is still growing its theory base. The scope of nursing is also broader and not limited to just one facet of humans, such as behavior. Thus, nursing theories may be comparatively broader in their reach, covering biopsychosocial dimensions of persons. Developing and testing such theories and related theoretical models are challenging and complex (e.g., see the psychoneuroimmunological models related to living with HIV or breast cancer developed by

McCain, Gray, Walter, and Robins [2005]). Despite the challenges inherent in such work, it reflects the vision of nursing foreseen in the critical analysis of nursing by Bixler and Bixler in 1945 (see Chapter 1).

THE SCOPE OF NURSING KNOWLEDGE AND ITS CENTRAL CONCERNS

The launch of the journal *Nursing Research* in 1952 marked a point of origin from which to consider systematically developed nursing knowledge. As we end this 6th edition, that effort of knowledge development is into its 7th decade. If we step back further to Bixler and Bixler's articulation and vision of "nursing science" in 1945, that history of nursing knowledge development is reaching into its 8th decade. What have we learned over this time about the scope of and central concerns embraced in nursing knowledge? What challenges loom on the horizon?

Some, such as Thorne (2014), have articulated the idea of "core disciplinary knowledge," that is, "the intellectual structures within which the discipline delineates is unique [we might say, distinctive] focus of vision and social mandate" (p. 1). Ironically, despite decades of theorizing and research, Thorne notes that, "agreement as to what this constitutes can be maddeningly elusive" (p. 1). Yet clarity may be especially important at this juncture given the trends cited at the beginning of Chapter 1 (see the section titled "Theory Development in Nursing: A Beginner's Guide").

Are there areas of achievement in nursing science and practice that are defining of a distinct nursing perspective? A brief sampling of the scope and/or central concerns might include, but certainly not be limited to, the following achievements:

- The accumulated research associated with various conceptual models in nursing that has been studiously chronicled by Jacqueline Fawcett over several volumes of work (see Fawcett, 1993, 1995; Fawcett & DeSanto-Madeya, 2013).
- Theories and models developed by nurses related to symptoms and disease self-management and the associated research—both qualitative and quantitative (see Cashion, Gill, Hawes, Henderson, Saligan, 2016; Grady & Gough, 2014; Lenz, Pugh, Milligan, Gift, Suppe, 1997; Ryan & Sawin, 2009).
- Theories and research—both qualitative and quantitative—on transitions as a result of parenthood, life changes, or health events (see Meleis, Sawyer, Im, & Messias, 2000; Mercer, 1995; Mercer & Walker, 2006; Rubin, 1967).
- The growing body of validated nursing diagnoses (Herdman & Kamitsuru, 2014) and accumulated practice knowledge related to nursing interventions (Butcher, Bulechek, Dochterman, & Wagner, 2013) and nursing outcomes (Moorhead, Johnson, Maas, & Swanson, 2013).

Others might offer equally or even more compelling examples (see exercise in Box 13–3). Our intent is only to give a flavor of what nurse scholars have been about since the 1950s. Nurses and nursing as a practice discipline do not have exclusive interest in the examples cited above. Still, these areas reflect key components of the

BOX 13–3   Qualitative Review of Nursing Science Content

The aim of this exercise is to understand key foci of contemporary nursing science.

- We recommend that readers form a team of three to five people, with each person focusing on a key scholarly, nonspecialty journal in nursing, such as:
  - *International Journal of Nursing Studies*
  - *Journal of Nursing Scholarship*
  - *Journal of Advanced Nursing*
  - *Nursing Research*
  - *Worldviews of Evidence-Based Nursing*
  - *Research in Nursing & Health*
  - *Clinical Nursing Research*
- As a team, determine how many issues of each journal will be reviewed, what aspects of journal articles will be reviewed, and what information will be abstracted from articles, such as key variables, conceptual or theoretical frameworks, and key nursing care concerns addressed in articles.
- As a trial run, practice going over two to three articles together to develop a shared understanding of the project.
- Now forge out into the individual journals, meeting regularly to discuss findings, questions, and emerging insights. Focus more on the conceptual structure of findings than numerical frequency.
- Meet as a team to synthesize your findings. Share your findings! You may have found the elusive body of core nursing disciplinary knowledge.

person–health–environment–nursing metaparadigm (Fawcett, 1984), and as a result contribute to the distinctive perspective of nursing.

Nursing also shares cross-cutting concerns, such as concern for vulnerable populations and health disparities, with other health professions as well as the wider community. Often addressing these and related concerns entails collaborations with interdisciplinary teams and communities. In such research and practice environments, it is especially important to have a firm grasp on nursing core knowledge to ensure it is infused into collaborative efforts so that outcomes for patients and families benefit from nursing's broad vision of health.

As we look to the future, Grace, Willis, Roy, and Jones (2016) remind us that "philosophical, conceptual/theoretical, and empirical inquiry on behalf of professional practice" (p. 61) comprises the central onus of scholars in the practice discipline of nursing. Thus, for nursing scholars to fully reflect this vision, they must have "an in-depth historic understanding of the goals and perspectives of the [nursing] discipline" (Grace et al., p. 68). Despite the importance of scientific inquiry in this disciplinary mix, theoretical inquiry is essential in deepening understanding and envisioning new possibilities. Similarly, philosophical studies are needed in nursing, not only to critique, but also to clarify and enlighten across the spectrum of ethical and epistemological issues of nursing and human caring.

Closing Commentary

As we pointed out in the first chapter of this book, nursing has generated theory at many levels. But only when a theory is sufficiently refined and enables users to specify measurable models of reality does it become amenable to rigorous testing. Well-articulated theories decrease the arbitrariness of judgments about their merits. This is especially important if a theory is used in defining directions for policy and practice. Testability of a theory and its empirical validity are of equal or greater importance in nursing as a practice discipline than basic sciences. The public trust in a profession warrants using the very best procedures in making scientific judgments that have human import.

In a practice discipline such as nursing, interdependence of theory development and testing is essential to build a sound body of knowledge for practice. Sustained and diversified development of the theoretic base of nursing practice requires that nurses manifest not only energy and thought in their work, but also long-term commitment. Such commitment is clear when scholarly projects of nurses can be organized into programs of scholarship. For graduate students, it is useful to begin defining that program early and framing its evolution into the future with a passion for the substance of nursing (Meleis, 1987).

References

Alfradique de Souza P, Santana RF, Cassiano KM. Differential validation of nursing diagnoses of impaired memory and chronic confusion. *J Nurs UFPE Online*. 2015;9(7):9078–9085. Retrieved June 8, 2017, at http://www.revista.ufpe.br/revistaenfermagem/index.php/revista/article/view/7915/pdf_8465

Appoloni AH, Herdman H, Napoleao AA, de Carvalho EC, Hortense P. Concept analysis and validation of the nursing diagnosis, delayed survival recovery. *Int J Nurs Knowl*. 2013;24(3):115–121.

Avant K. Nursing diagnosis: Maternal attachment. *Adv Nurs Sci*. 1979;2(1):45–55.

Beckie TM, Beckstead JW, Webb MS. Modeling women's quality of life after cardiac events. *West J Nurs Res*. 2001;23:179–194.

Berger AM, Walker SN. An explanatory model of fatigue in women receiving adjuvant breast cancer chemotherapy. *Nurs Res*. 2001;50:42–52.

Bixler G, Bixler RW. The professional status of nursing. *Am J Nurs*. 1945;45:730–735.

Blalock HM. Dilemmas and strategies of theory construction. In: Snizek WE, Fuhrman ER, Miller MK, eds. *Contemporary Issues in Theory and Research: A Metasociological Perspective*. Westport, CT: Greenwood Press; 1979.

Bova C. Adjustment to chronic illness among HIV-infected women. *J Nurs Scholarsh*. 2001;33:217–223.

Bryant AL, Walton AL, Phillips B. Cancer-related fatigue: Scientific progress has been made in 40 years. *Clin J Oncol Nurs*. 2015;19(2):137–139.

Bull A. Primary care of chronic dyspnea in adults. *Nurse Pract*. 2014;39(8):34–40.

Butcher HK, Bulechek GM, Dochterman JMMC, Wagner C, eds. *Nursing Interventions Classification*. 6th ed. St. Louis, MO: Elsevier/Mosby; 2013.

Carlson-Catalano J, Lunney M, Paradiso C, Bruno J, Luise BK, Martin T, et al. Clinical validation of ineffective breathing pattern, ineffective airway clearance, and impaired gas exchange. *Image*. 1998;30(3):243–248.

Cashion AK, Gill J, Hawes R, Henderson WA, Saligan L. National Institutes of Health Symptom Science Model sheds light on patient symptoms. *Nurs Outlook.* 2016;64(5):499–506.

Covell CL, Sidani S. Nursing intellectual capital theory: Testing selected propositions. *J Adv Nurs.* 2013;69(11):2432–2445.

Coward DD. Critical multiplism: A research strategy for nursing science. *Image.* 1990;22:163–167.

Cronbach LJ, Meehl PE. Construct validity in psychological tests. In: Jackson DN, Messick S, eds. *Problems in Human Assessment.* New York, NY: McGraw-Hill; 1967, pp. 57–77.

Demerouti E, Bakker AB, Nachreiner F, Schaufeli WB. A model of burnout and life satisfaction amongst nurses. *J Adv Nurs.* 2000;32:454–464.

Doran DI, Sidani S, Keatings M, Doidge D. An empirical test of the Nursing Role Effectiveness Model. *J Adv Nurs.* 2002;38:29–39.

Ehrenberger HE, Alligood MR, Thomas SP, Wallace DC, Licavoli CM. Testing a theory of decision-making derived from King's systems framework in women eligible for a cancer clinical trial. *Nurs Sci Q.* 2002;15:156–163.

Fawcett J. *Analysis and Evaluation of Nursing Theories.* Philadelphia, PA: Davis; 1993.

Fawcett J. *Analysis and Evaluation of Conceptual Models of Nursing.* 3rd ed. Philadelphia, PA: Davis; 1995.

Fawcett J. The metaparadigm of nursing: Present status and future refinements. *Image.* 1984;16:84–87.

Fawcett J. *The Relationship of Theory and Research.* 3rd ed. Philadelphia, PA: Davis; 1999.

Fawcett J, DeSanto-Madeya S. *Contemporary Nursing Knowledge: Analysis and Evaluation of Nursing Models and Theories.* 3rd ed. Philadelphia, PA: Davis; 2013.

Fehring R. Validating diagnostic labels: Standardized methodology. In: Hurley ME, ed. *Classification of Nursing Diagnoses: Proceedings of the Sixth Conference.* St. Louis, MO: Mosby; 1986.

Fry A, Nguyen T. Culture and the self: Implications for the perception of depression by Australian and Vietnamese nursing students. *J Adv Nurs.* 1996;23:1147–1154.

Gatti L. Maternal perceptions of insufficient milk supply in breastfeeding. *J Nurs Scholarsh.* 2008;49(4):355–363.

Gordon M, Sweeney MA. Methodological problems and issues in identifying and standardizing nursing diagnoses. *Adv Nurs Sci.* 1979;2(1):1–15.

Grace PJ, Willis DG, Roy C, Jones DA. Profession at the crossroads: A dialog concerning the preparation of nursing scholars and leaders. *Nurs Outlook.* 2016;64:61–70.

Grady PA, Gough LL. Self-management: A comprehensive approach to management of chronic conditions. *Am J Public Health.* 2014;104(8):e25–e31.

Hempel CG. *Philosophy of Natural Science.* Englewood Cliffs, NJ: Prentice Hall; 1966.

Herdman TH, Kamitsuru S. *Nursing Diagnoses 2015–17: Definitions and Classification.* 10th ed. Oxford, UK: Wiley Blackwell; 2014.

Hill PD, Humenick SS. Insufficient milk supply. *Image.* 1989;21:145–148.

Hoffman AJ, von Eye A, Gift AG, Given BA, Given CW, Rothert M. Testing a theoretical model of perceived self-efficacy for cancer-related fatigue self-management and optimal physical functional status. *Nurs Res.* 2009;58(1):32–41.

Jennings-Dozier K. Predicting intentions to obtain a Pap smear among African American and Latina women: Testing the theory of planned behavior. *Nurs Res.* 1999;48:198–205.

Johnson JL, Ratner PA, Bottorff JL, Hayduk LA. An exploration of Pender's health promotion model using LISREL. *Nurs Res.* 1993;42:132–138.

Kane RL, Shamliyan T, Mueller C, Duval S, Wilt T. *Nursing Staffing and Quality of Patient Care.* Evidence Report/Technology Assessment No. 151. Prepared by the Minnesota Evidence-based Practice Center under Contract No. 290-02-0009. AHRQ Publication No. 07-E005. Rockville, MD: Agency for Healthcare Research and Quality; March 2007.

Kim S-S, Reed PG, Hayward RD, Kang Y, Koenig HG. Spirituality and psychological well-being: Testing a theory of family interdependence among family caregivers and their elders. *Res Nurs Health.* 2011;34:103–115.

Klaus MH, Jerauld R, Kreger MC, McAlpine W, Steffa M, Kennell JH. Maternal attachment: Importance of the first postpartum days. *N Engl J Med.* 1972;286:460–463.

Klaus MH, Kennell JH. *Maternal–Infant Bonding.* St. Louis, MO: Mosby; 1976.

Klaus MH, Kennell JH. *Parent–Infant Bonding.* 2nd ed. St. Louis, MO: Mosby; 1982.

Lee HJ, Winters CA. Testing rural nursing theory: Perceptions and needs of service providers. *Online J Rural Nurs Health Care.* 2004;4:51–63.

Lenz ER, Pugh LC, Milligan RA, Gift A, Suppe F. The middle-range theory of unpleasant symptoms: An update. *Adv Nurs Sci.* 1997;19(3):14–27.

Longo BM. The Kilauea Volcano adult health study. *Nurs Res.* 2009;58:23–31.

Marx MH. The general nature of theory construction. In: Marx MH, ed. *Theories in Contemporary Psychology.* New York, NY: Macmillan; 1963.

McCain NL, Gray DP, Walter JM, Robins J. Implementing a comprehensive approach to the study of health dynamics using the psychoneuroimmunology paradigm. *Adv Nurs Sci.* 2005;28:320–332.

McCarley C. A model of chronic dyspnea. *Image.* 1999;31:231–236.

McCullagh M, Lusk SL, Ronis DL. Factors influencing use of hearing protection among farmers: A test of the Pender Health Promotion Model. *Nurs Res.* 2002;51:33–39.

Meleis AI. ReVisions in knowledge development: A passion for substance. *Sch Inq Nurs Pract.* 1987;1(1):5–19.

Meleis AI, Sawyer LM, Im EO, Messias DK, Schumacher K. Experiencing transitions: An emerging middle-range theory. *Adv Nurs Sci.* 2000;23(1):12–28.

Mercer RT. *Becoming a Mother: Research on Maternal Role Identity from Rubin to the present.* New York, NY: Springer; 1995.

Mercer RT, Walker LO. A review of nursing interventions to foster becoming a mother. *J Obstet Gynecol Neonatal Nurs.* 2006;35(5):568–582.

Moorhead S, Johnson M, Maas M, Swanson E, eds. *Nursing Outcomes Classification.* 5th ed. St. Louis, MO: Elsevier/Mosby; 2013.

Nagley SJ, Byers PH. Clinical construct validity. *J Adv Nurs.* 1987;12:617–619.

National Cancer Institute. *Theory-at-a-Glance: A Guide for Health Promotion Practice.* 2nd ed. Washington, DC: U. S. Department of Health and Human Services; 2005. Available at https://cancercontrol.cancer.gov/brp/research/theories_project/theory.pdf

National Heart, Lung, and Blood Institute. *Managing Overweight and Obesity in Adults: Systematic Evidence Review from the Obesity Expert Panel.* 2013. Available at https://www.nhlbi.nih.gov/health-topics/managing-overweight-obesity-in-adults

Nivens AS, Herman J, Weinrich SP, Weinrich MC. Cues to participation in prostate cancer screening: A theory for practice. *Oncol Nurs Forum.* 2001;28:1449–1156.

Pedhazur EJ, Schmelkin LP. *Measurement, Design, and Analysis: An Integrated Approach.* Hillsdale, NJ: Erlbaum; 1991.

Pender NJ. *Health Promotion in Nursing Practice.* 2nd ed. Norwalk, CT: Appleton & Lange; 1987.

Polit DF, Beck CT. *Nursing Research: Generating and Assessing Evidence for Nursing Practice.* 9th ed. Philadelphia, PA: Lippincott Williams & Wilkins; 2012.

Popper KR. *Conjectures and Refutations.* New York, NY: Basic Books; 1965.

Potempa K, Lopez M, Reid C, Lawson L. Chronic fatigue. *Image.* 1986;18:165–169.

Renner M, Saligan LN. Understanding cancer-related fatigue: Advancing the science. *Fatigue.* 2016;4(4):189–192.

Rubin R. Attainment of the maternal role: Part I. Processes. *Nurs Res.* 1967;16:237–245.

Ryan P, Sawin KJ. The individual and family self-management theory: Background and perspectives on context, process, and outcomes. *Nurs Outlook.* 2009;57(4):217–225.

Ryan P, Weiss M, Traxel N, Brondino M. Testing the integrated theory of health behavior change for postpartum weight management. *J Adv Nurs.* 2011;67(9):2047–2059.

Schumacher KL, Gortner SR. (Mis)conceptions and reconceptions about traditional science. *Adv Nurs Sci.* 1992;14(4):1–11.

Shin KR, Kang Y, Park HJ, Cho MO, Heitkemper M. Testing and developing the health promotion model in low-income, Korean elderly women. *Nurs Sci Q.* 2008;21:173–178.

Silva MC. Research testing nursing theory: State of the art. *Adv Nurs Sci.* 1986;9(1):1–11.

Silva MC, Sorrell JM. Testing of nursing theory: Critique and philosophical expansion. *Adv Nurs Sci.* 1992;14(4):12–23.

Smith GT. On construct validity: Issues of method and measurement. *Psychol Assess.* 2005;17:396–408.

Stuifbergen AK, Rogers S. Health promotion: An essential component of rehabilitation for persons with chronic disabling conditions. *Adv Nurs Sci.* 1997;19(4):1–20.

Susser M. Maternal weight gain, infant birth weight, and diet: Causal sequences. *Am J Clin Nutr.* 1991;53:1384–1396.

Tabachnick BG, Fidell LS. *Using Multivariate Statistics.* 6th ed. Boston, MA: Pearson; 2013.

Thorne S. What constitutes core disciplinary knowledge? *Nurs Inq.* 2014;21(1):1–2.

Tsai P, Tak S, Moore C, Palencia I. Testing a theory of chronic pain. *J Adv Nurs.* 2003;43:158–169.

Vellone E, Riegel B, D'Agostino F, Fida R, Rocco G, Cocchieri A, et al. Structural equation model testing the situation-specific theory of heart failure self-care. *J Adv Nurs.* 2013;69(11):2481–2492.

Verchota G, Sawin K. Testing components of a self-management theory in adolescents with type 1 diabetes mellitus. *Nurs Res.* 2016;65(6):487–495.

Villarruel AM, Denyes MJ. Testing Orem's theory with Mexican Americans. *Image.* 1997;29:283–288.

Wallace WL. *The Logic of Science in Sociology.* New York, NY: Aldine; 1971.

Waltz CF, Strickland OL, Lenz ER. *Measurement in Nursing and Health Research.* 4th ed. New York, NY: Springer/Davis; 2010.

Weaver K, Olson JK. Understanding paradigms used for nursing research. *J Adv Nurs.* 2006;53:459–469.

Whitley GG. Three phases of research in validating nursing diagnoses. *West J Nurs Res.* 1997;19:379–399.

Yeh C. Health-related quality of life in pediatric patients with cancer: A structural equation approach with the Roy Adaptation Model. *Cancer Nurs.* 2002;25:74–80.

Zauszniewski JA, Chung C, Krafcik K. Social cognitive factors predicting the health of elders. *West J Nurs Res.* 2001;23:490–503.

Additional Readings

Acton GJ, Irvin BL, Hopkins BA. Theory-testing research: Building the science. *Adv Nurs Sci.* 1991;14(1):52–61.

Behi R, Nolan M. Deduction: Moving from the general to the specific. *Br J Nurs.* 1995;4:341–344.

Coates VE. Measuring constructs accurately: A prerequisite to theory testing. *J Psychiatr Ment Health Nurs.* 1995;2:287–293.

Dulock HL, Holzemer WL. Substruction: Improving the linkage from theory to research. *Nurs Sci Q*. 1991;4:83–87.

Fawcett J. Testing nursing theory. In: *Analysis and Evaluation of Nursing Theories*. Philadelphia, PA: Lippincott; 1993.

Field M. Causal inference in behavioral research. *Adv Nurs Sci*. 1979;2(1):81–93.

Gibbs JP. Part 3: Test of theories. In: *Sociological Theory Construction*. Hinsdale, IL: Dryden Press; 1972.

Hall JM, Stevens PE. Rigor in feminist research. *Adv Nurs Sci*. 1991;13(3):16–29.

Hinshaw AS. Theoretical model testing: Full utilization of data. *West J Nurs Res*. 1984;6:5–9.

Jacobs MK. Can nursing theory be tested? In: Chinn PL, ed. *Nursing Research Methodology*. Rockville, MD: Aspen; 1986.

McQuiston CM, Campbell JC. Theoretical substruction: A guide for theory testing research. *Nurs Sci Q*. 1997;10:117–123.

Mullins NC. Empirical testing. In: *The Art of Theory: Construction and Use*. New York, NY: Harper & Row; 1971.

Platt JR. Strong inference. *Science*. 1964;146:347–352.

Reynolds PD. Testing theories. In: *A Primer in Theory Construction*. Indianapolis, IN: Bobbs-Merrill; 1971.

Sandelowski M. The problem of rigor in qualitative research. *Adv Nurs Sci*. 1986;8(3):27–37.

Wallace WL. Tests of hypotheses; decisions to accept or reject hypotheses; logical inference; theories. In: *The Logic of Science of Sociology*. New York, NY: Aldine; 1971.

Zetterberg HL. *On Theory and Verification in Sociology*. Totowa, NJ: Bedminster Press; 1965.

INDEX

Note: Page numbers in *italics* denote figures; those followed by "t" denote tables.